Clinical Care for Older Adults with Cardiovascular Disease: Current Challenges and Perspectives Ahead

Clinical Care for Older Adults with Cardiovascular Disease: Current Challenges and Perspectives Ahead

Editors

Claudio Montalto
Nuccia Morici
Aung Myat

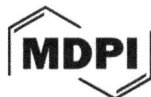

Basel • Beijing • Wuhan • Barcelona • Belgrade • Novi Sad • Cluj • Manchester

Editors
Claudio Montalto
De Gasperis Cardio Center,
Niguarda Hospital
Milan
Italy

Nuccia Morici
IRCCS Santa Maria Nascente,
Fondazione Don Gnocchi
Milan
Italy

Aung Myat
Sussex Cardiac Centre
Brighton
UK

Editorial Office
MDPI
St. Alban-Anlage 66
4052 Basel, Switzerland

This is a reprint of articles from the Special Issue published online in the open access journal *Journal of Clinical Medicine* (ISSN 2077-0383) (available at: https://www.mdpi.com/journal/jcm/special_issues/Care_Elderly).

For citation purposes, cite each article independently as indicated on the article page online and as indicated below:

Lastname, A.A.; Lastname, B.B. Article Title. *Journal Name* **Year**, *Volume Number*, Page Range.

ISBN 978-3-7258-0101-5 (Hbk)
ISBN 978-3-7258-0102-2 (PDF)
doi.org/10.3390/books978-3-7258-0102-2

© 2024 by the authors. Articles in this book are Open Access and distributed under the Creative Commons Attribution (CC BY) license. The book as a whole is distributed by MDPI under the terms and conditions of the Creative Commons Attribution-NonCommercial-NoDerivs (CC BY-NC-ND) license.

Contents

About the Editors . . . . **vii**

Preface . . . . **ix**

Tzu-Ping Yu and Ju-Yi Chen
Unexplained Left Ventricular Hypertrophy with Symptomatic High-Grade Atrioventricular Block in Elderly Patients: A Case Report
Reprinted from: *J. Clin. Med.* **2022**, *11*, 3522, doi:10.3390/jcm11123522 . . . . **1**

Alessandro Caracciolo, Renato Francesco Maria Scalise, Fabrizio Ceresa, Gianluca Bagnato, Antonio Giovanni Versace, Roberto Licordari, et al.
Optimizing the Outcomes of Percutaneous Coronary Intervention in Patients with Chronic Kidney Disease
Reprinted from: *J. Clin. Med.* **2022**, *11*, 2380, doi:10.3390/jcm11092380 . . . . **12**

Tomoyuki Morisawa, Masakazu Saitoh, Shota Otsuka, Go Takamura, Masayuki Tahara, Yusuke Ochi, et al.
Hospital-Acquired Functional Decline and Clinical Outcomes in Older Cardiac Surgical Patients: A Multicenter Prospective Cohort Study
Reprinted from: *J. Clin. Med.* **2022**, *11*, 640, doi:10.3390/jcm11030640 . . . . **29**

Vincenzo Livio Malavasi, Anna Chiara Valenti, Sara Ruggerini, Marcella Manicardi, Carlotta Orlandi, Daria Sgreccia, et al.
Kidney Function According to Different Equations in Patients Admitted to a Cardiology Unit and Impact on Outcome
Reprinted from: *J. Clin. Med.* **2022**, *11*, 891, doi:10.3390/jcm11030891 . . . . **39**

Moritz Benjamin Immohr, Hug Aubin, Ralf Westenfeld, Sophiko Erbel-Khurtsidze, Igor Tudorache, Payam Akhyari, et al.
Heart Transplantation of the Elderly—Old Donors for Old Recipients: Can We Still Achieve Acceptable Results?
Reprinted from: *J. Clin. Med.* **2022**, *11*, 929, doi:10.3390/jcm11040929 . . . . **53**

Nastasia Marinus, Carlo Vigorito, Francesco Giallauria, Paul Dendale, Raf Meesen, Kevin Bokken, et al.
Frailty Test Battery Development including Physical, Socio-Psychological and Cognitive Domains for Cardiovascular Disease Patients: A Preliminary Study
Reprinted from: *J. Clin. Med.* **2022**, *11*, 1926, doi:10.3390/jcm11071926 . . . . **63**

Lorenzo Falsetti, Vincenzo Zaccone, Emanuele Guerrieri, Giulio Perrotta, Ilaria Diblasi, Luca Giuliani, et al.
Implementation of EHMRG Risk Model in an Italian Population of Elderly Patients with Acute Heart Failure
Reprinted from: *J. Clin. Med.* **2022**, *11*, 2982, doi:10.3390/jcm11112982 . . . . **85**

Daniele Luiso, Marta Herrero-Torrus, Neus Badosa, Cristina Roqueta, Sonia Ruiz-Bustillo, Laia C. Belarte-Tornero, et al.
Quality of Life in Older Patients after a Heart Failure Hospitalization: Results from the SENECOR Study
Reprinted from: *J. Clin. Med.* **2022**, *11*, 3035, doi:10.3390/jcm11113035 . . . . **94**

Manuel Méndez-Bailon, Noel Lorenzo-Villalba, Jorge Rubio-Garcia, María Carmen Moreno-García, Guillermo Ropero-Luis, Eduardo Martínez-Litago, et al.
Clinical Characteristics and Prognostic Relevance of Different Types of Caregivers for Elderly Patients with Acute Heart Failure—Analysis from the RICA Registry
Reprinted from: *J. Clin. Med.* **2022**, *11*, 3516, doi:10.3390/jcm11123516 . . . . **106**

Yong Hoon Kim, Ae-Young Her, Seung-Woon Rha, Cheol Ung Choi, Byoung Geol Choi, Ji Bak Kim, et al.
Comparison of 3-Year Outcomes between Early and Delayed Invasive Strategies in Older and Younger Adults with Non-ST-Segment Elevation Myocardial Infarction Undergoing New-Generation Drug-Eluting Stent Implantation
Reprinted from: *J. Clin. Med.* **2022**, *11*, 4780, doi:10.3390/jcm11164780 . . . . **115**

Francesca Mantovani, Gianluca Campo, Elisa Guerri, Francesco Manca, Massimo Calzolari, Giovanni Tortorella, et al.
Management and Outcomes in the Elderly with Non-ST-Elevation Acute Coronary Syndromes Admitted to Spoke Hospitals with No Catheterization Laboratory Facility
Reprinted from: *J. Clin. Med.* **2022**, *11*, 6179, doi:10.3390/jcm11206179 . . . . **131**

About the Editors

Marc Maresca

Marc Maresca was born on 25 October 1974. He is an assistant professor at the Institute of Molecular Sciences of Marseille (ISM2, UMR-CNRS 7313). Research performed at this multidisciplinary institute aims at combining different techniques (cell biology, microbiology, toxicology, nuclear magnetic resonance, mass spectrometry, chromatography, chemometrics, peptide synthesis) in order to understand biological mechanisms (eukaryotic and prokaryotic systems). Dr Marc MARESCA is specialized in using and characterizing in vitro cell models for toxicity studies, including human intestine epithelium and brain cell models as demonstrated by his publications in both subjects. Part of his research is on food-contaminants and their toxicity, including pesticides and mycotoxins (particularly deoxynivalenol but also ochratoxin, patulin and fumonisin). He has published major articles on the effects of deoxynivalenol and its derivatives on the human gut. He also has expertise in antibiotic development (particularly antimicrobial peptides) and works to understand their mechanisms of action (pore-forming activity, safety of antibiotics to human and animal cells).

Preface

Life is a battle and thus living organisms have developed strategies to win this war. Among the different strategies employed by micro-organisms to dominate their habitat is the production of toxins including bacteria and fungi and their use as bioweapons. Mycotoxins are secondary metabolites produced by molds that play such a role.

For many years, one of these mycotoxins, the food-associated trichothecene Deoxynivalenol (DON or vomitoxin) has attracted the attention of scientists. This is due, in part, to its high prevalence in animal/human food and feed products, as demonstrated through the successful use of urinary biomarkers confirming the exposure of humans to substantial doses of this toxin. DON is also one of the most hazardous mycotoxins; it affects the functions of nerve, endocrine, immune and intestinal cells. In addition to its toxicity to animal cells (this could be considered as collateral damage), DON is also known to affect plant cell functions; such effects certainly play a role during the colonization of wheat and cereals by DON-producing fungi such as Fusarium species. The toxicity of DON seems to depend on the presence of an epoxide function which allows its binding to ribosomes, causing the so-called "ribotoxic stress" effect, and the activation of specific kinases (including PKR and MAP kinases), eventually leading to the inhibition of the protein synthesis and to cell death. Due to its ability to activate PKR and MAP kinases, DON also acts as a proinflammatory signal at low doses whereas higher doses are immunosuppressive due to cellular toxicity. In animals, as well as affecting systemic and intestinal immunity, DON also impacts the functions of the brain and endocrine cells, causing anorexia and vomiting. Food not only contains native toxin, but also large amounts of plant and fungal derivatives of DON (including the fungal metabolites 3 and 15 acetyl-DON (3 and 15ADON) and the plant derivative 3-O-glucoside-DON (D3G)) and possibly, although no study has yet confirmed it, of animal derivatives (i.e., 3 and 15-glucuronide DON) potentially present in meat and animal-derived products. New DON derivatives were also recently found in plants and food products, including DON-oligoglycosides, DON-glutathione, DON-S-Cysteine, DON-S-Cysteinyl-glycine, and DON-sulfonate. Although previous research has shed light on the mechanisms of action of DON, important questions remain. For example, little is known about the ability of the fungi to transmit from the soil to the cereals, and about the levels of DON and DON metabolites in different plant tissues during natural and experimental contamination.

Data on the effects of DON and its metabolites on plant cells are also scarce. Similarly, how DON enters the cells (animal or plant cells) and how it binds/acts on ribosomes is not perfectly characterized. Finally, if ribosomes are the only target of DON, how the toxin could activate different kinases, depending on the toxin dose, remains a mystery. We hope that some of these questions will be answered in this Special Issue that focuses on one of the most studied and relevant food-associated mycotoxins.

Claudio Montalto, Nuccia Morici, and Aung Myat
Editors

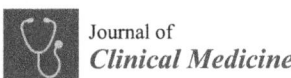

Case Report

Unexplained Left Ventricular Hypertrophy with Symptomatic High-Grade Atrioventricular Block in Elderly Patients: A Case Report

Tzu-Ping Yu and Ju-Yi Chen *

Department of Internal Medicine, National Cheng Kung University Hospital, College of Medicine, National Cheng Kung University, Tainan 704, Taiwan; g860920@gmail.com
* Correspondence: juyi@mail.ncku.edu.tw

Abstract: Left ventricular hypertrophy (LVH) is common among older adults. Amidst all causes, Fabry disease (FD) should be considered when LVH occurs with family history, specific clinical manifestations, or cardiac alert signs. Here, we report a case of a 76-year-old male who presented late onset concentric LVH with symptomatic high-grade atrioventricular (AV) block. After dual-chamber pacemaker implantation, interrogation revealed frequent right ventricular (RV) pacing with a wide QRS duration. The patient developed heart failure symptoms with rapid deterioration of LV systolic function. Pacing-induced cardiomyopathy (PICM) was suspected, and the pacemaker was upgraded to biventricular pacing. Further FD surveys were performed, including biochemical examinations, cardiac biopsies, and genetic sequencing, and the patient was ultimately diagnosed with a cardiac variant of FD. Particularly, we strongly suggest that physiologic pacing should be initially considered for patients with FD who have symptomatic high-grade AV block, rather than traditional RV pacing to prevent PICM.

Keywords: unexplained hypertrophy; elderly; Fabry disease; high-grade atrioventricular block

Citation: Yu, T.-P.; Chen, J.-Y. Unexplained Left Ventricular Hypertrophy with Symptomatic High-Grade Atrioventricular Block in Elderly Patients: A Case Report. *J. Clin. Med.* 2022, 11, 3522. https://doi.org/10.3390/jcm11123522

Academic Editor: Juan F. Delgado Jiménez

Received: 31 May 2022
Accepted: 14 June 2022
Published: 19 June 2022

Publisher's Note: MDPI stays neutral with regard to jurisdictional claims in published maps and institutional affiliations.

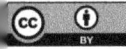

Copyright: © 2022 by the authors. Licensee MDPI, Basel, Switzerland. This article is an open access article distributed under the terms and conditions of the Creative Commons Attribution (CC BY) license (https:// creativecommons.org/licenses/by/ 4.0/).

1. Introduction

Left ventricular hypertrophy (LVH) is a common, but ominous, discovery in older adults that is associated with an increased risk of cardiovascular morbidity and mortality. Although hypertension, valvulopathies, and obesity elucidate most causes of LVH, it is crucial to consider other rare causes if unexplained LVH persists. Less common causes of LVH include numerous myocardial disorders, such as hypertrophic cardiomyopathy (HCM), infiltrative diseases, metabolic disorders, mitochondrial diseases, and some syndromic conditions [1–3]. Amidst all possible causes, Fabry disease (FD) should be considered when LVH is accompanied by a family history of FD, specific clinical manifestations of FD, or certain cardiac alert signs [4–6]. Clinicians have discussed specific cardiac alert signs of FD intensely, which may possibly reveal more clues and increase cardiologists' vigilance in investigating FD. FD is an inherited lysosomal storage disorder that results in multisystem diseases. The reported prevalence of FD varies widely, ranging from 1:17,000 to 1:117,000 [4,6]. Cardiovascular complications are the leading cause of impaired quality of life and death in all FD patients [4–6]. Early detection of FD before irreversible organ damage occurs, as well as the prompt initiation of effective treatment, are considered extremely important. Nonetheless, the diagnosis of FD is burdensome because the full picture of the disease is not yet recognized, and caution is lacking regarding the FD-related symptoms or signs. The final diagnosis of FD is usually made years after the onset of primary symptoms or signs, and many cases have been greatly underdiagnosed.

Herein we report a case of a 76-year-old male who was diagnosed as FD with symptomatic high-grade atrioventricular (AV) block. Furthermore, we have proposed an algorithm by which to evaluate patients with unexplained LVH, in order to support the diagnostic and therapeutic management of FD with high-grade AV block.

2. Case Presentation

In 2008, a 63-year-old male with no known underlying diseases was referred due to recurrent palpitation. A 12-lead electrocardiogram (ECG) showed sinus rhythm with ventricular pre-excitation (Figure 1A). Seeking a link between palpitations and abnormal rhythm, the 24-h Holter monitor described no tachyarrhythmia. Transthoracic echocardiogram (TTE) showed concentric left ventricular hypertrophy (LVH) with adequate systolic function (Figure 1D,E).

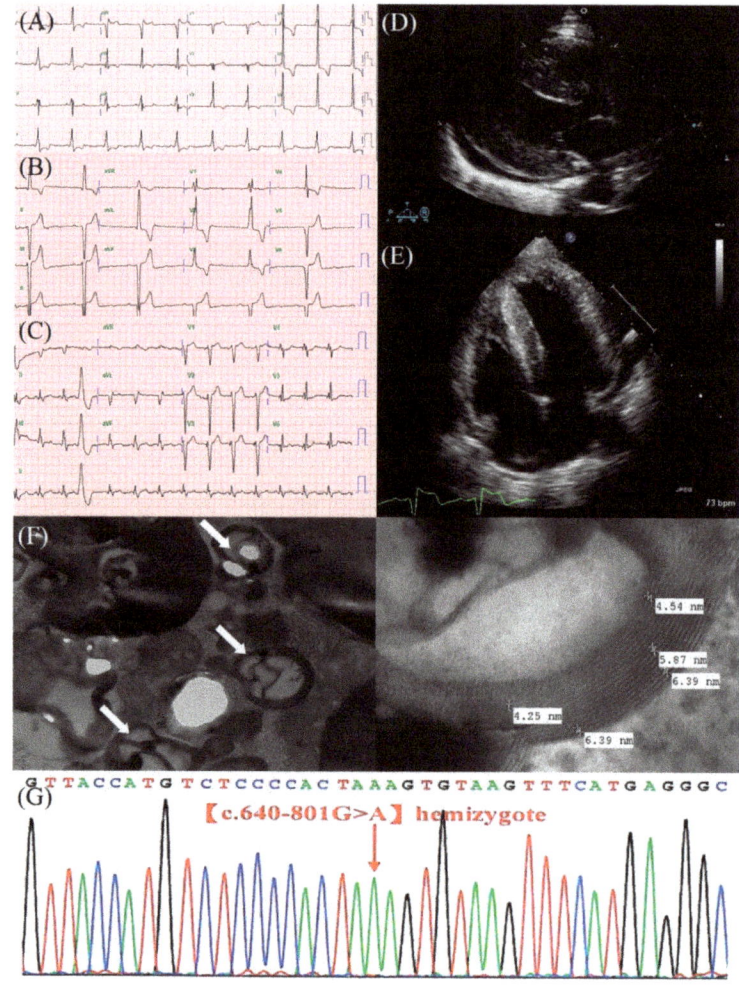

Figure 1. (**A**) The initial 12-lead ECG showed short PR-interval and LVH pattern. (**B**) The 12-lead ECG showed sinus rhythm with 3:1 AV block. (**C**) The 12-lead ECG showed biventricular pacing rhythm. (**D,E**) The initial TTE for the patient showed the generalized LVH pattern ((**D**): parasternal long axis view and (**E**): apical four chamber view). (**F**) The pathology showed the typical features of FD on electron microscopy (arrows indicate zebra bodies, with a periodicity of 5–6 nm in the cardiomyocytes). (**G**) The genetic study shows c.640-801G>A polymorphism (cardiac variants of FD).

From 2008 to 2015, the patient was repeatedly referred due to recurring unexplained palpitations and occasional retrosternal oppression. Holter monitor and TTE continued to have similar findings from his primary reports in 2008 (Table 1). In 2016, he visited the emergency department once, owing to episodic dizziness with near syncope. A 12-lead ECG showed bradycardia (37 bpm) and 3:1 atrioventricular (AV) block (Figure 1B). Emergent temporary transvenous pacing was performed, and then he was admitted for permanent pacemaker implantation (Medtronic, DDDR mode). Following discharge, he was followed regularly by his private cardiologist. Since 2017, his pacemaker interrogation reports have recorded right ventricular (RV) pacing, dependent as predominant rhythm without prominent symptoms. From 2019 to 2021, he began to feel dyspnea on exertion and increasingly aggravated, which met the criteria for New York Heart Association (NYHA) functional class III. TTE revealed impaired left ventricular (LV) systolic function (LV ejection fraction [EF] 20%). Under the impression of heart failure with reduced ejection fraction, standard treatments were prescribed and titrated to the optimized dosage (drugs: carvedilol, furosemide, ramipril, and spironolactone). However, he was still symptomatic, and rapid deterioration of LV systolic function was noted by TTE, with widening of pacing QRS on ECG (Table 1). Hence, pacing-induced cardiomyopathy (PICM) was assumed, so that the upgrading of his permanent pacemaker to cardiac resynchronization therapy (CRT: biventricular pacemaker) was executed. After upgradation, both TTE and ECG (Table 1) displayed markedly improved heart function, and his symptoms subsided, thus supporting the diagnosis of PICM.

Table 1. Clinical history.

Year	Age	Symptoms	Evaluation	Management
2008	63	Palpitation	**ECG**: Sinus rhythm, ventricular preexcitation, LVH (Figure 1A) **Holter**: Normal **TTE**: Concentric LVH, impaired LV relaxation (Figure 1D,E)	OPD follow-up
2011	66	Palpitation and chest tightness	**ECG**: Sinus rhythm, ventricular preexcitation, LVH **Holter**: Normal	OPD follow-up
2015	70	Palpitation and chest tightness	**Holter**: Normal **TTE**: Concentric LVH, LV diastolic dysfunction, adequate LV systolic function, LVEF = 76%, E/e′: 20.2, LV mass index: 273.0 g/m^2 **Treadmill test**: Positive for ischemia	PCI, OPD follow-up
2016	71	Dizziness	**ECG**: 3:1 AV block (Figure 1B)	PPM (DDDR), OPD follow-up
2017	72	X	**ECG**: Ventricular pacing rhythm, QRS = 180 ms	OPD follow-up
2019	74	DOE	**ECG**: Ventricular pacing rhythm, QRS = 180 ms **TTE**: Concentric LVH, apical LV hypokinesis, borderline LV systolic function, LVEF = 53%, E/e′: 17.0, LV mass index: 292.9 g/m^2	HF drugs, OPD follow-up

Table 1. Cont.

Year	Age	Symptoms	Evaluation	Management
2021	76	Aggravated DOE	**ECG**: Ventricular pacing rhythm, QRS = 200 ms **ECG (s/p CRT)**: Biventricular pacing rhythm, QRS = 160 ms (Figure 1C) **TTE**: Concentric LVH, large apical LV akinesis, impaired LV systolic function, LVEF = 20%, E/e': 21.4, LV mass index: 160.0 g/m^2 **TTE (s/p CRT)**: Concentric LVH, apical LV hypokinesis, LVEF = 35%, E/e': 11.9, LV mass index: 214.5 g/m^2	CRT, HF drugs, ERT, OPD follow-up

ECG: electrocardiogram, TTE: transthoracic echocardiogram, LVH: left ventricular hypertrophy, LV: left ventricular, OPD: outpatient department, g/m^2: grams per square meter, LVEF: left ventricular ejection fraction, PCI: percutaneous coronary intervention, HF: heart failure, DOE: dyspnea on exertion, PPM: permanent pacemaker, DDDR: dual-chamber with rate modulation, s/p: status post, CRT: cardiac resynchronization therapy, ERT: enzyme replacement therapy.

On the other hand, because of his constantly unexplained concentric LVH with intensified symptoms, extra investigations were launched. After excluding the common secondary causes of LVH, such as valvular heart diseases, systemic hypertension, and obesity, other rare diseases, including familial HCM, infiltrative diseases, and metabolic storage disorders, were under-differentiated. According to his clinical manifestations, ECG and TTE interpretations, FD was initially suspected. Accordingly, we began comprehensive FD survey (Table 2). However, the patient denied family history of FD, and no extracardiac presentations had been revealed. In accordance with the entire results of his FD survey, this patient was consequently diagnosed with cardiac variants of FD, and further received enzyme replacement therapy (agalsidase beta 1 mg/kg every other week).

Table 2. Fabry disease survey.

Examination	Results	Reference Value
α-Gal A activity	1.17 μmol/h (borderline)	N > 1.5 Borderline: 0.6~1.5 (μmol/h)
Plasma Lyso-Gb3	11.95 ng/mL (elevated)	N < 0.8 (ng/mL)
Endomyocardial biopsy	Cardiomyocytes are focally vacuolated with a lace-like appearance. The electron microscope showed laminated lysosomal inclusions (zebra bodies) (Figure 1F).	Compatible with FD
Genetic sequencing	Genotype: c.640-801G>A (Figure 1G)	Also known as IVS4+919G>A and c.936+919G>A, Cardiac variant of FD [7]

α-Gal A: α-galactosidase A, Lyso-Gb3: globotriaosylsphingosine, N: normal value, FD: Fabry disease.

3. Discussion

3.1. Differential Diagnosis of Elderly LVH

In older adult patients, LVH can develop from primary cardiomyopathy or secondary to extrinsic stimuli (pressure or volume overload). Extrinsic stimuli are the most common causes, including systemic hypertension, valvular diseases (e.g., aortic stenosis), and obesity, which all need to be carefully excluded first. For unexplained LVH, rare myocardial disorders, including HCM, infiltrative diseases (e.g., amyloidosis and sarcoidosis), metabolic disorders (e.g., FD, Pompe disease, and *PRKAG2* syndrome), and mitochondrial diseases, should be thoroughly investigated. In the present case, the patient presented with late onset LVH, with symptomatic high-grade AV block and without extracardiac comorbidities, suggesting that HCM, cardiac amyloidosis, and FD were the most probable causes. Other rare diseases (e.g., sarcoidosis and mitochondrial diseases) usually develop at earlier ages and tend to present broad extracardiac features [3]. Pompe disease can sometimes be late onset but is often characterized by progressive skeletal muscle weakness or loss of respiratory function [8]. PRKAG2 syndrome usually displays LVH with conduction abnormalities (e.g., ventricular pre-excitation), yet onset is mostly in childhood. As mentioned above, we prioritized HCM, cardiac amyloidosis, and FD when considering the patient's differential diagnosis.

Hypertrophic cardiomyopathy (HCM). HCM is the most common inherited cardiomyopathy and relates to imperative cause of sudden cardiac death (SCD), especially the obstructive type. As such, it should be placed at high hierarchy in the scheme of elderly LVH. HCM typically manifests as the early onset of asymmetric septal hypertrophy but could be late onset and highly variable (e.g., apical, concentric, and right ventricular hypertrophy). Favorable determinants of HCM are family history of HCM or SCD, as well as dynamic LV outflow tract obstruction or systolic anterior motion of mitral valve presenting on echocardiogram [1]. Advanced diagnostic methods include cardiac biopsy (myofibrillar disarray and fibrosis) and genetic sequencing (genetic mutations in sarcomere or sarcomere-associated proteins). Diagnosis of HCM is challenging, given phenotypic heterogeneity, numerous unknown genetic mutations, and often a clinical diagnosis of exclusion [1].

Cardiac amyloidosis. As for cardiac amyloidosis, the more likely cause of elderly LVH is wild-type transthyretin amyloidosis (ATTRwt), previously called age-related amyloidosis. ATTRwt gives rise to amyloidotic cardiomyopathy, resulting from the deposition of misfolded or misassembled transthyretins that are prone to form amyloid fibrils aggregates within the myocardium. The majority of patients typically present with diastolic heart failure or atrial fibrillation in old age. ECG findings, such as low voltage, pseudoinfarct pattern, or AV block, may possibly be seen. Echocardiogram has demonstrated a generalized concentric hypertrophy, biatrial dilation, and mainly diastolic dysfunction [9]. Establishing a diagnosis of ATTRwt is difficult, due to the lack of definitive biomarkers, and the clinical characteristics frequently mimic the diseases coexisting in advanced age, although cardiac scintigraphy with 99 m Tc-diphosphonates may play a useful role in the diagnosis of ATTRwt [10]. Final diagnosis is usually made by cardiac biopsy, which directly identifies the amyloid fibrils using Congo red staining and specifies the type by immunohistochemistry or mass spectrometry.

Fabry disease (FD). FD is an X-linked recessive genetic disease, resulting in insufficient activity of lysosomal enzyme, α-galactosidase A (α-Gal A), which causes accumulation of glycosphingolipids, especially globotriaosylceramide (Gb3) and its deacylated derivative globotriaosylsphingosine (lyso-Gb3). These cumulative sediments within cells may eventually cause organ destruction (Figure 2) [5]. Typical FD clinical manifestations contain extracardiac involvements, comprising hypo- or anhidrosis, angiokeratomas, cornea verticillata, gastrointestinal manifestations, renal insufficiency, premature stroke, neuropathic pain, tinnitus or hearing impairment, and cardiac involvements (i.e., Fabry cardiomyopathy), including LVH, heart failure and conduction abnormalities. Classic FD symptoms normally present during early childhood but can be delayed in heterozygous cases. A late onset phenotype (i.e., cardiac variants) presents chiefly cardiac involvements, especially LVH, as a primary sign after the fourth decade of life [3,5,11,12]. The disease course of this phenotype is still largely unknown but tends to develop severe cardiac diseases in elderly individuals [11]. According to numerous studies, FD should be considered when unexplained LVH is found in combination with specific cardiac alert signs recorded by ECG, echocardiography, or cardiac magnetic resonance imaging (CMR) (Table 3) [3–5]. Both family history of FD and extracardiac presentations should be carefully scrutinized. Nevertheless, the lack of extracardiac manifestations and late onset phenotype may account for the absence of family history of FD. The earliest cardiac signs are subtle ECG changes, as well as LVH patterns with repolarization abnormalities or short PR interval. In advanced cases, sinus bradycardia, high voltage QRS, conduction disturbances, T wave inversion, or ST-segment deviation may be observed. FD patients are at relatively high risk of developing conduction diseases (e.g., any degree of AV block and arrhythmia). Consequently, regular 24-h Holter monitoring is recommended. Echocardiography is the most crucial instrument for initial diagnosis and monitoring of Fabry cardiomyopathy. The early stage is characterized by concentric ventricular hypertrophy without LV outflow tract (OT) obstruction, for which the LV systolic function is generally normal. Other particular findings may be noted, including prominent papillary muscles, early diastolic dysfunction, and right ventricular hypertrophy. As Fabry cardiomyopathy progresses, a regional wall (esp. basal inferolateral wall) hypo- or akinesis may develop. The non-invasive gold standard for detecting FD is CMR with gadolinium contrast agents. It provides accurate assessment of LV size, mass, and myocardial fibrosis involvement. Representative CMR features include late gadolinium enhancement (LGE) distinctively starting from the basal inferolateral wall and reduced T1 values in the affected area [4,5,13].

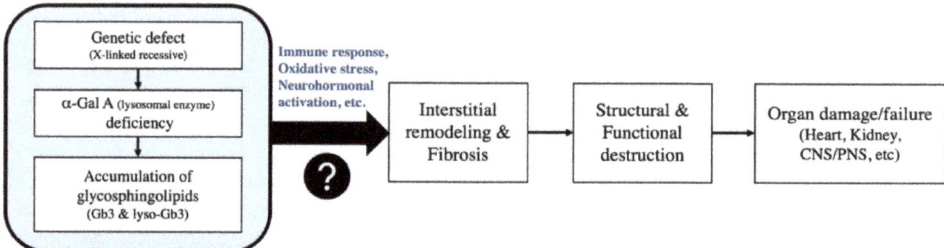

Figure 2. Brief concepts of the pathophysiology of FD [14,15]. α-Gal A: α-galactosidase A, Gb3: globotriaosylceramide, lyso-Gb3: globotriaosylsphingosine, CNS: central nervous system, PNS: peripheral nervous system.

Table 3. Diagnosis and management of FD.

Cardiac Imaging	Cardiac Alert Signs [4,13]
ECG	Short PR interval, AV block, chronotropic incompetence
2D-Echocardiography	Concentric LVH, prominent papillary muscles, diastolic dysfunction
CMR	LGE in the basal inferolateral wall, reduced T1 values
Diagnostic examinations	**Diagnostic criteria [3,4,7,12]**
α-Gal A activity	N > 1.5, borderline: 0.6~1.5 (μmol/h)
Plasma Lyso-Gb3	N < 0.8 (ng/mL)
Endomyocardial biopsy	General: diffuse vacuolization with lace-like appearance. The electron microscope: laminated lysosomal inclusions (zebra bodies), focal loss of myofilaments.
Genetic sequencing (Pathogenic variants)	Classical phenotype: more than 840 private mutations, e.g., p.R227X, p.R220X, p.R342X Late-onset phenotype: p.R301Q, p.R363H, p.F113L, p.N215S, IVS4+919G>A

Table 3. Cont.

Disease-specific therapies	Detailed information [4,14,15]
ERT	IV agalsidase alpha and beta (approved), pegunigalsidase alfa (ongoing trials)
Pharmacological chaperone	Oral Miglastat (approved)
SRT	Oral lucerastat, venglustat (ongoing trials)
Gene-based therapy	Gene transfer, mRNA (ongoing trials)

FD: Fabry disease, ECG: electrocardiogram, AV: atrioventricular, 2D: 2 dimensional, LVH: left ventricular hypertrophy, CMR: cardiac magnetic resonance imaging, LGE: late gadolinium enhancement, α-Gal A: α-galactosidase A, Lyso-Gb3: globotriaosylsphingosine, N: normal value, ERT: enzyme replacement therapy, IV: intravenous administration, SRT: substrate reduction therapy, mRNA: messenger ribonucleic acid.

Relative to the present case, HCM, cardiac amyloidosis (ATTRwt), and FD (cardiac variants) may likely be causes, in line with the patient's clinical presentations. Therefore, we differentiated between HCM, ATTRwt, and cardiac variants of FD, in terms of image interpretations (ECG and TTE). According to his initial ECG showing, as well as LVH with pre-excitation pattern and without low voltage QRS or pseudoinfarct pattern (Figure 1A), cardiac variants of FD was the most suspicious culprit. According to his echocardiography, which revealed generalized ventricular hypertrophy without LVOT obstruction (Figure 1D,E), this feature seemed to comply with cardiac amyloidosis or FD but was atypical for HCM. In brief, both cardiac variants of FD and ATTRwt were the likely suspects and held for further investigation. To distinguish these two diseases, biochemical blood tests for FD were first arranged due to currently available non-invasive examinations. Finally, cardiac biopsy and genetic sequencing were performed to confirm diagnosis. After thoroughly tracing the patient's clinical history (Table 1) and clarifying the clinical findings, this patient clearly could have been diagnosed with a cardiac variant of FD since 2008.

3.2. Diagnosis of FD

Patients with suspicion of FD should undergo certain biochemical and genetic examinations (Table 3) [4–6]. In general, male patients with FD typically have reduced or absent α-Gal A activity and elevated lyso-Gb3 level, as measured in dried blood spot or blood leukocytes, which are adequate to confirm FD diagnosis. However, in females, X-chromosome inactivation results in widely variable clinical phenotypes and α-Gal A activity may be normal or slightly defective. Hence, the diagnosis of FD in females requires genetic sequencing. On the whole, all FD diagnoses should eventually be verified by genetic sequencing, which is helpful for establishing the relationship between the disease phenotype and genotype, and further permits cascade screening for high-risk family members [4,5,7]. Endomyocardial biopsy may be performed in patients with genetic variants of unknown significance, or under unusual phenotypic manifestations, which offer definitive evidence of FD by demonstrating lace-like appearance, vacuolization, and representative lysosomal inclusions (zebra bodies) on electron microscopy [4].

3.3. Management of FD

To date, the management of FD includes disease-specific therapy, as well as therapies to manage multiorgan diseases. Approved FD-specific treatments include enzyme replacement therapy (ERT) and pharmacological chaperone therapy, while other novel therapeutic approaches, such as substrate reduction therapy, gene therapy, and mRNA-based therapy, are still in development (Table 3) [14,15]. To begin with, ERT is indicated in all symptomatic patients with an established FD diagnosis, which can delay FD advancement and reduce the burden of cardiac events when started at earlier stage [5]. Specifically, in patients with late-onset FD, studies have revealed that ERT decreases LV mass and wall thickness but does not significantly improve heart function (neither systolic nor diastolic), although evidence is limited [5,16]. Most studies further illustrate the poor response of ERT in the heart when applied in the advanced stage, particularly in patients with extensive fibrosis [4,5]. Importantly, cardiac fibrosis stands as a negative cardiac beneficial factor for ERT. Hence, it should be administered as early as possible, before substantial fibrosis development, and the assessment of fibrosis progression by CMR should be considered before and during ERT, in order to evaluate the patient's prognosis and treatment effectiveness [4,11]. Next, chaperone therapy is only prescribed for patients with amenable *GLA* pathogenic variants, but the effectiveness of this therapy is still debatable. Lastly, other novel treatments, including substrate reduction therapy, result in decreased Gb3 synthesis, which directly lower the cellular load. All gene therapy or mRNA-based therapy aims to restore the defective α-Gal A activity [15,17]. These new therapies will expand in the foreseeable future and hold promise for FD patients. Although FD-specific treatments have changed the natural history of FD, cardiac involvements remain the main prognostic determinant. Updated recommendations on the management of cardiovascular diseases of FD have been published in recent documents [4–6].

3.4. Management of FD with Symptomatic High-Grade AV Block

Symptomatic high-grade AV block should be treated following the current guidelines [18]. After receiving dual-chamber pacemaker implantation, this patient revealed that he had been in a setting of high-burden RV pacing for years with aggravating heart failure symptoms. A recent study proposed that chronic RV pacing dependence can cause electromechanical dyssynchrony between the ventricles and sequential maladaptive cardiac remodeling. Ultimately, LV systolic dysfunction, as a decrement in LVEF, will be displayed (i.e., pacing-induced cardiomyopathy, PICM) [19]. The most effective treatment for PICM is to upgrade to a physiologic pacing system (e.g., biventricular pacing, His bundle pacing, and left bundle area pacing) [19,20]. After upgradation, a significant improvement of LV systolic function was observed [20].

In FD patients receiving pacemakers, great concern exists about the adverse effect of non-physiological RV pacing with higher risk of developing PICM. From a pathophysiologic perspective, RV pacing contributes to fundamentally altered electrical pattern of ventricular activation. Disturbed electrical activation leads to impaired contraction and redistribution of myocardial strain [19]. These effects cause an abnormal cardiomyocyte metabolism and revised regional perfusion. Besides, in FD patients, deposits (Gb3 and lyzo-Gb3) accumulation and fibrosis replacement within the heart may increase the chance of ventricular dyssynchrony and catalyze the process of cardiac remodeling. For these reasons, physiologic pacing should be initially considered in FD patients who require pacing. However, routine insertion of physiologic pacing systems in patients with low burden of RV pacing (<40%) or preserved systolic function (LVEF > 50%) has not emerged as the standard of care in recent guidelines [18,21]. We strongly suggest that physiologic pacing, rather than traditional RV pacing, be considered for FD patients with symptomatic high-grade AV block, in order to prevent PICM. This novel recommendation still lacks adequate clinical trials to validate the effectiveness in FD patients.

All in all, this article focuses on two key concepts. First, physicians should keep FD in mind when noticing unexplained LVH in combination with specific cardiac alert signs. Earlier detection of the disease and initiation of FD-specific treatments leads to a superior prognosis. Secondly, we have raised a novel and important issue that physiologic pacing systems might play a crucial role in FD patients with AV block requiring pacing, especially in patients who already have impaired LV systolic function. Further, we have provided a comprehensive algorithm (Figure 3), based on elderly patients with unexplained LVH, to guide the diagnostic and therapeutic approaches of FD with symptomatic high-grade AV block, which may be useful to support clinical judgement. Future research should focus on validating the pros and cons of the physiologic pacing system in FD patients and investigate the beneficial effects of FD-specific treatments of the cardiac variants of FD patients specifically.

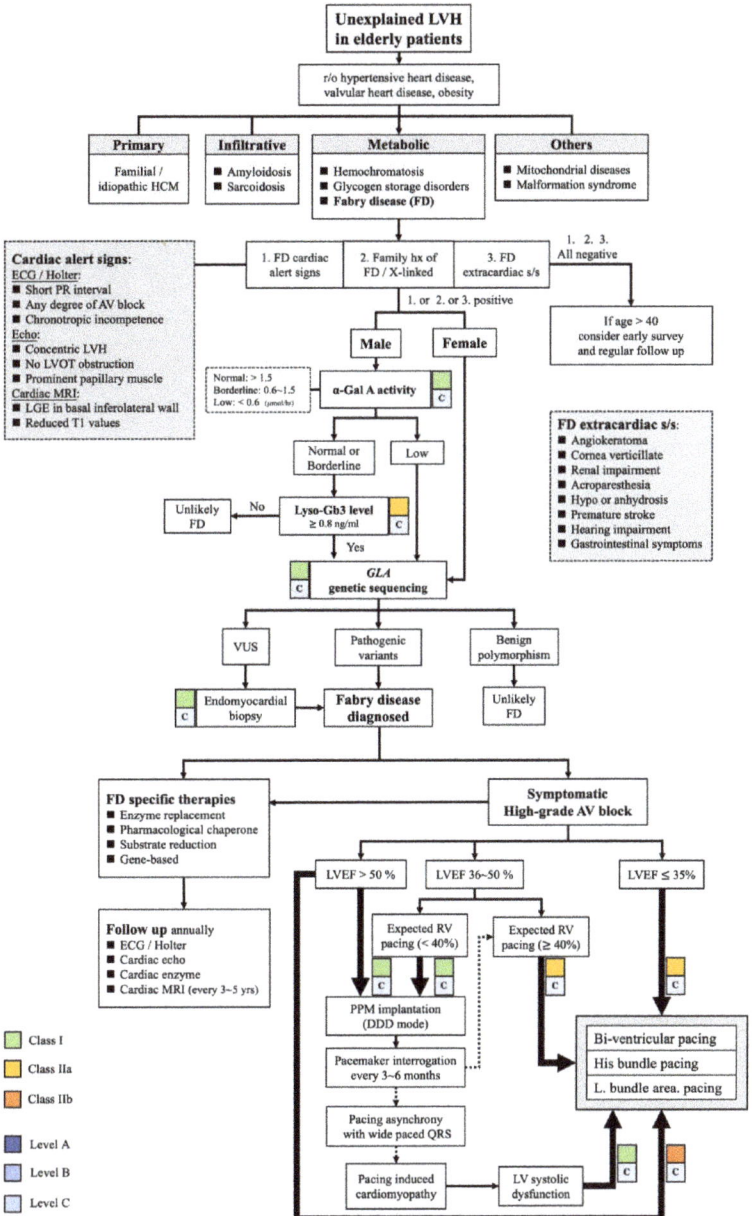

Figure 3. A hypothetical algorithm to evaluate elderly patients who have unexplained LVH to the diagnostic and therapeutic management of FD with high-grade AV block. LVH: left ventricular hypertrophy, r/o: rule out, HCM: hypertrophic cardiomyopathy, FD: Fabry disease, hx: history, LVOT: left ventricular outflow tract, MRI: magnetic resonance imaging, LGE: late gadolinium enhancement, s/s: symptoms/signs, α-Gal A: α-galactosidase A, Lyso-Gb3: globotriaosylsphingosine, *GLA*: α-galactosidase A gene, VUS: variants of unknown significance, RV: right ventricular, LVEF: left ventricular ejection fraction, PPM: permanent pacemaker, DDD: dual-chamber pacing. Classes I, IIa, IIb: the classes of recommendation based on existing studies or guidelines. Levels A, B, C: the levels of evidence based of existing studies [4,18,20,21].

4. Conclusions

Overall, this article focuses on two key concepts. First, physicians should keep FD in mind when noticing unexplained LVH in combination with specific cardiac alert signs. Earlier detection of the disease and initiation of FD-specific treatments leads to a superior prognosis. Second, we have raised a novel issue that physiologic pacing systems play a crucial role in patients with FD who have AV block requiring pacing, especially in patients who already have impaired LV systolic function. Furthermore, we provided a comprehensive algorithm (Figure 2), based on elderly patients with unexplained LVH, to guide the diagnostic and therapeutic approaches of FD with symptomatic high-grade AV block. Future research should focus on validating the pros and cons of the physiologic pacing system in patients with FD and investigating the beneficial effects of FD-specific treatments of the cardiac variants of patients with FD specifically.

Author Contributions: Conception and design: T.-P.Y. and J.-Y.C.; data acquisition: T.-P.Y. and J.-Y.C.; literature review, as well as drafting and finalizing the article: T.-P.Y.; critical revision of the article for important intellectual content: T.-P.Y. and J.-Y.C.; supervised the literature search and revision and approved the final version: J.-Y.C. All authors have read and agreed to the published version of the manuscript.

Funding: The authors would like to thank the Ministry of Science and Technology of the Republic of China, Taiwan, for financially supporting this research under contracts MOST 109-2218-E-006-024, MOST 110-2218-E-006-017, and MOST 110-2218-E-006-015.

Institutional Review Board Statement: Ethics approval was obtained from National Cheng Kung University's Institutional Review Board, case A-EC-111-005.

Data Availability Statement: The datasets used during the current study are available from the corresponding author on reasonable request.

Conflicts of Interest: The authors declare that they have no competing interests.

Abbreviations

FD	Fabry disease
LVH	Left ventricular hypertrophy
HCM	Hypertrophic cardiomyopathy
AV	Atrioventricular
ECG	Electrocardiogram
TTE	Transthoracic echocardiography
RV	Right ventricular
LV	Left ventricular
EF	Ejection fraction
PICMOPD	Pacing-induced cardiomyopathyOutpatient department
SCD	Sudden cardiac death
ATTRwt	Wild-type transthyretin amyloidosis
α-Gal A	α-galactosidase A
Gb3	Globotriaosylceramide
Lyso-Gb3	Globotriaosylsphingosine
CMR	Cardiac magnetic resonance imaging
OT	Outflow tract
ERT	Enzyme replacement therapy

References

1. Geske, J.B.; Ommen, S.R.; Gersh, B.J. Hypertrophic Cardiomyopathy: Clinical Update. *JACC Heart Fail.* **2018**, *6*, 364–375. [CrossRef]
2. Arad, M.; Maron, B.J.; Gorham, J.M.; Johnson, W.H.; Saul, J.P.; Perez-Atayde, A.R.; Spirito, P.; Wright, G.B.; Kanter, R.J.; Seidman, C.E.; et al. Glycogen Storage Diseases Presenting as Hypertrophic Cardiomyopathy. *N. Engl. J. Med.* **2005**, *352*, 362–372. [CrossRef] [PubMed]

3. Yousef, Z.; Elliott, P.; Cecchi, F.; Escoubet, B.; Linhart, A.; Monserrat, L.; Namdar, M.; Weidemann, F. Left ventricular hypertrophy in Fabry disease: A practical approach to diagnosis. *Eur. Heart J.* **2012**, *34*, 802–808. [CrossRef] [PubMed]
4. Linhart, A.; Germain, D.P.; Olivotto, I.; Akhtar, M.M.; Anastasakis, A.; Hughes, D.; Namdar, M.; Pieroni, M.; Hagège, A.; Cecchi, F.; et al. An expert consensus document on the management of cardiovascular manifestations of Fabry disease. *Eur. J. Heart Fail.* **2020**, *22*, 1076–1096. [CrossRef] [PubMed]
5. Pieroni, M.; Moon, J.C.; Arbustini, E.; Barriales-Villa, R.; Camporeale, A.; Vujkovac, A.C.; Elliott, P.M.; Hagege, A.; Kuusisto, J.; Linhart, A.; et al. Cardiac Involvement in Fabry Disease: Jacc Review Topic of the Week. *J. Am. Coll. Cardiol.* **2021**, *77*, 922–936. [CrossRef]
6. Hagège, A.; Réant, P.; Habib, G.; Damy, T.; Barone-Rochette, G.; Soulat, G.; Donal, E.; Germain, D.P. Fabry disease in cardiology practice: Literature review and expert point of view. *Arch. Cardiovasc. Dis.* **2019**, *112*, 278–287. [CrossRef]
7. Hwu, W.L.; Chien, Y.H.; Lee, N.C.; Chiang, S.C.; Dobrovolny, R.; Huang, A.C.; Yeh, H.Y.; Chao, M.C.; Lin, S.J.; Kitagawa, T.; et al. Newborn Screening for Fabry Disease in Taiwan Reveals a High Incidence of the Later-Onset Gla Mutation C.936+919g>a (Ivs4+919g>a). *Hum. Mutat.* **2009**, *30*, 1397–1405. [CrossRef]
8. Tarnopolsky, M.; Katzberg, H.; Petrof, B.J.; Sirrs, S.; Sarnat, H.B.; Myers, K.; Dupré, N.; Dodig, D.; Genge, A.; Venance, S.L.; et al. Pompe Disease: Diagnosis and Management. Evidence-Based Guidelines from a Canadian Expert Panel. *Can. J. Neurol. Sci.* **2016**, *43*, 472–485. [CrossRef]
9. Adam, R.D.; Coriu, D.; Jercan, A.; Bădeliță, S.; Popescu, B.A.; Damy, T.; Jurcuț, R. Progress and challenges in the treatment of cardiac amyloidosis: A review of the literature. *ESC Heart Fail.* **2021**, *8*, 2380–2396. [CrossRef]
10. Perugini, E.; Guidalotti, P.L.; Salvi, F.; Cooke, R.M.; Pettinato, C.; Riva, L.; Leone, O.; Farsad, M.; Ciliberti, P.; Bacchi-Reggiani, L.; et al. Noninvasive Etiologic Diagnosis of Cardiac Amyloidosis Using 99mtc-3,3-Diphosphono-1,2-Propanodicarboxylic Acid Scintigraphy. *J. Am. Coll. Cardiol.* **2005**, *46*, 1076–1084. [CrossRef]
11. Hsu, T.R.; Hung, S.C.; Chang, F.P.; Yu, W.C.; Sung, S.H.; Hsu, C.L.; Dzhagalov, I.; Yang, C.F.; Chu, T.H.; Lee, H.J.; et al. Later Onset Fabry Disease, Cardiac Damage Progress in Silence: Experience with a Highly Prevalent Mutation. *J. Am. Coll. Cardiol.* **2016**, *68*, 2554–2563. [CrossRef] [PubMed]
12. Fan, Y.; Chan, T.-N.; Chow, J.; Kam, K.; Chi, W.-K.; Chan, J.; Fung, E.; Tong, M.; Wong, J.; Choi, P.; et al. High Prevalence of Late-Onset Fabry Cardiomyopathy in a Cohort of 499 Non-Selective Patients with Left Ventricular Hypertrophy: The Asian Fabry Cardiomyopathy High-Risk Screening Study (Asian-Fame). *J. Clin. Med.* **2021**, *10*, 2160. [CrossRef] [PubMed]
13. Esposito, R.; Santoro, C.; Mandoli, G.E.; Cuomo, V.; Sorrentino, R.; La Mura, L.; Pastore, M.C.; Bandera, F.; D'Ascenzi, F.; Malagoli, A.; et al. Cardiac Imaging in Anderson-Fabry Disease: Past, Present and Future. *J. Clin. Med.* **2021**, *10*, 1994. [CrossRef] [PubMed]
14. Vardarli, I.; Weber, M.; Rischpler, C.; Führer, D.; Herrmann, K.; Weidemann, F. Fabry Cardiomyopathy: Current Treatment and Future Options. *J. Clin. Med.* **2021**, *10*, 3026. [CrossRef] [PubMed]
15. Yim, J.; Yau, O.; Yeung, D.; Tsang, T. Fabry Cardiomyopathy: Current Practice and Future Directions. *Cells* **2021**, *10*, 1532. [CrossRef] [PubMed]
16. Germain, D.P.; Elliott, P.; Falissard, B.; Fomin, V.V.; Hilz, M.J.; Jovanovic, A.; Kantola, I.; Linhart, A.; Mignani, R.; Namdar, M.; et al. The effect of enzyme replacement therapy on clinical outcomes in male patients with Fabry disease: A systematic literature review by a European panel of experts. *Mol. Genet. Metab. Rep.* **2019**, *19*, 100454. [CrossRef]
17. Miller, J.J.; Kanack, A.J.; Dahms, N.M. Progress in the understanding and treatment of Fabry disease. *Biochim. Biophys. Acta (BBA) Gen. Subj.* **2020**, *1864*, 129437. [CrossRef]
18. Kusumoto, F.M.; Schoenfeld, M.H.; Barrett, C.; Edgerton, J.R.; Ellenbogen, K.A.; Gold, M.R.; Goldschlager, N.F.; Hamilton, R.M.; Joglar, J.A.; Kim, R.J.; et al. 2018 Acc/Aha/Hrs Guideline on the Evaluation and Management of Patients with Bradycardia and Cardiac Conduction Delay: A Report of the American College of Cardiology/American Heart Association Task Force on Clinical Practice Guidelines and the Heart Rhythm Society. *Circulation* **2019**, *140*, e382–e482.
19. Merchant, F.M.; Mittal, S. Pacing Induced Cardiomyopathy. *J. Cardiovasc. Electrophysiol.* **2020**, *31*, 286–292. [CrossRef]
20. Khurshid, S.; Obeng-Gyimah, E.; Supple, G.E.; Schaller, R.; Lin, D.; Owens, A.T.; Epstein, A.E.; Dixit, S.; Marchlinski, F.E.; Frankel, D.S. Reversal of Pacing-Induced Cardiomyopathy Following Cardiac Resynchronization Therapy. *JACC Clin. Electrophysiol.* **2017**, *4*, 168–177. [CrossRef]
21. Slotwiner, D.J.; Raitt, M.H.; Munoz, F.D.-C.; Mulpuru, S.K.; Nasser, N.; Peterson, P.N. Impact of Physiologic Pacing Versus Right Ventricular Pacing Among Patients With Left Ventricular Ejection Fraction Greater Than 35%: A Systematic Review for the 2018 ACC/AHA/HRS Guideline on the Evaluation and Management of Patients With Bradycardia and Cardiac Conduction Delay: A Report of the American College of Cardiology/American Heart Association Task Force on Clinical Practice Guidelines and the Heart Rhythm Society. *J. Am. Coll. Cardiol.* **2019**, *74*, 988–1008.

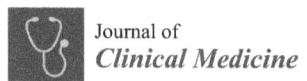

Review

Optimizing the Outcomes of Percutaneous Coronary Intervention in Patients with Chronic Kidney Disease

Alessandro Caracciolo [1], Renato Francesco Maria Scalise [1], Fabrizio Ceresa [2], Gianluca Bagnato [1], Antonio Giovanni Versace [1], Roberto Licordari [1], Silvia Perfetti [1], Francesca Lofrumento [1], Natasha Irrera [1], Domenico Santoro [1], Francesco Patanè [2], Gianluca Di Bella [1], Francesco Costa [1,*] and Antonio Micari [3,*]

[1] Department of Clinical and Experimental Medicine, Policlinic "Gaetano Martino", University of Messina, 98100 Messina, Italy; caracciolo.alessandro.ac@gmail.com (A.C.); rfm.scalise@gmail.com (R.F.M.S.); gianbagnato@gmail.com (G.B.); antonio.versace@polime.it (A.G.V.); robertolicordari@gmail.com (R.L.); silvia.perfetti@hotmail.it (S.P.); francesca.lofrumetno@studenti.unime.it (F.L.); natasha.irrera@unime.it (N.I.); domenico.santoro@unime.it (D.S.); gianluca.dibella@unime.it (G.D.B.)
[2] Department of Cardio-Thoraco-Vascular Surgery, Division of Cardiac Surgery, Papardo Hospital, 98158 Messina, Italy; ceresa77@hotmail.com (F.C.); f_patane@hotmail.it (F.P.)
[3] Department of Biomedical and Dental Sciences and Morphological and Functional Imaging, University of Messina, 98100 Messina, Italy
* Correspondence: dottfrancescocosta@gmail.com (F.C.); antonio.micari@unime.it (A.M.)

Abstract: Percutaneous coronary intervention (PCI) is one of the most common procedures performed in medicine. However, its net benefit among patients with chronic kidney disease (CKD) is less well established than in the general population. The prevalence of patients suffering from both CAD and CKD is high, and is likely to increase in the coming years. Planning the adequate management of this group of patients is crucial to improve their outcome after PCI. This starts with proper preparation before the procedure, the use of all available means to reduce contrast during the procedure, and the implementation of modern strategies such as radial access and drug-eluting stents. At the end of the procedure, personalized antithrombotic therapy for the patient's specific characteristics is advisable to account for the elevated ischemic and bleeding risk of these patients.

Keywords: chronic kidney disease; percutaneous coronary intervention; contrast-induced nephropathy

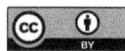

1. Introduction

Percutaneous coronary intervention (PCI) is one of the most common procedures performed in medicine [1]. PCI improves survival in acute coronary syndrome and helps to control anginal symptoms in chronic coronary disease [2,3]; however, its net benefit among patients with chronic kidney disease (CKD) is less well established. The use of contrast dye, arterial wall instrumentation, and the potential for microembolization are associated with potential renal harm which is amplified in patients with pre-existing CKD, potentially reducing the clinical benefit of PCI, especially in an elective setting.

The clinical impact of PCI in patients with stable CAD has been widely studied in recent years: in the ISCHEMIA trial [4], 5179 patients with stable coronary disease and moderate to severe inducible ischemia by imaging test were randomized to an immediate invasive strategy with coronary angiography or an initial approach with medical therapy alone. Over a median of 3.2 years, the primary outcome of cardiovascular death, myocardial infarction, resuscitated cardiac arrest, or hospitalization for unstable angina or heart failure was similar in the two treatment groups, confirming the modest impact of an initial invasive strategy in patients with stable angina and the potential for early related complications. This concept is even more important for patients with CKD, especially in its more severe forms. CKD and coronary artery disease (CAD) are strictly related, and are associated with a higher risk of thrombotic and bleeding complications [5]. In fact, lower values of glomerular filtration rate (GFR) below

60–75 mL/min/1.73 m² are associated with a linear increase in CAD risk and a tripled risk of cardiovascular mortality when reaching GFR drops below 15 mL/min/1.73 m² [6]. In addition, the impaired renal elimination of antithrombotic drugs exposes patients with CAD and PCI to a higher risk of bleeding complications.

There is a paucity of data regarding the impact of PCI on patients with CKD, especially those in advanced stages or those treated with dialysis, who are often excluded from clinical trials. Recently, the ISCHEMIA CKD trial included 777 patients with advanced renal insufficiency (eGFR < 30 mL/min) in the context of the larger ISCHEMIA trial population. As observed in the main population, an early routine invasive strategy failed to reduce the incidence of death or myocardial infarction, and an excess of stroke, death or the initiation of dialysis was observed compared to the initial approach with medical therapy alone [7]. In addition, for CKD, no benefits of an early invasive strategy were evident with regard to angina-related health status [2].

Hence, the PCI benefit window for CKD patients is narrow. After careful patient selection, careful technological and organizational strategies should be implemented in order to allow a positive trade-off, balancing the risk of the procedure with the potential benefits. In this review, we will discuss strategies to minimize PCI's potential for harm in CKD patients, in addition to the current evidence for pharmacological and device therapies in this domain.

2. Contrast-Induced Nephropathy Prophylaxis Strategies

Contrast-induced nephropathy (CIN) is defined as the impairment of renal function, with either a relative 25% increase or an absolute 0.5 mg/dL increase within 48–72 h of intravenous contrast administration. CIN is associated with an increased risk of all-cause death and ischemic events, and should be thoroughly prevented [8]. Several pathophysiological mechanisms of CIN have been proposed. Contrast dye might exert direct renal toxicity mediated by free radicals and oxidative stress, or indirect toxicity through medullary hypoxia due to a vasodilation/vasoconstriction imbalance.

The risk of CIN depends on patient's characteristics and procedural variables. Patients with pre-existing renal impairment are exposed to the highest risk of CIN, in direct relation to serum creatinine level [9]. Diabetes mellitus is a mild risk factor, but in the presence of renal dysfunction it has a synergistic effect that exposes patients to a four-fold higher risk of CIN [10–13]. Advanced age, heart failure, haemodynamic instability, anaemia, dehydration, female sex, procedural bleeding, nephrotoxic drugs, and type and dose of contrast are additional risk factors that increase the risk of CIN, especially when renal impairment coexists [14–20]. There are no effective treatments for CIN, so prevention represents the most important strategy. The risk of CIN should be estimated in every patient considering clinical history and renal function. An estimated glomerular filtration rate (eGFR) lower than 60 mL/min is suggestive of a high risk for CIN [21]. In this setting, reducing the total volume of contrast administered is key to preventing CIN. A ratio of total contrast volume administered (in mL) to eGFR (in mL/min) higher than 3.7 exposes patients to a higher risk of CIN [17,18]. Several methods [15,17,22–25] have been proposed to identify high-risk patients, but there is no evidence that suggest their systematic use. Nevertheless, it is recommended that particular attention should be paid to the pre- and post-procedural clinical management of patients that present clinical characteristics associated with an increased risk of CIN [26]. Nephrotoxic drugs should be suspended before the procedure, and drugs that have an impact on renal function should be carefully evaluated for their benefit/risk ratio [21]. Studies on CIN prophylaxis have focused on three main strategies: fluid administration, pharmacological prevention, and renal replacement therapies.

2.1. Fluid Administration

Hydration represents the most important strategy for CIN prevention before and after PCI in patients with CKD. Fluids administration expands plasma volume, determines a downregulation of the renin–angiotensin–aldosterone system, reduces renal cortical vasoconstriction, dilutes contrast agents, and prevents tubular obstruction [27]. The European Society of Cardiology recommends (class I, level of evidence C) to administer isotonic saline to all patients with moderate to severe CKD (1 mL/kg/h or 0.5 mL/kg/h in patients with LVEF $\leq$ 35% or NYHA > 2) 12 h before and 24 h after the procedure [28]. Intravenous hydration has been found to be more effective in reducing CIN than oral hydration, although intravenous administration appears to be less manageable in acute patients and in day-hospital settings [29,30]. A meta-analysis of six trials showed no differences between intravenous and oral hydration in CIN reduction, suggesting that further adequately powered trials are needed [31]. Intravenous hydration with 0.9% isotonic saline was found to be more effective in CIN reduction when compared to other solutions [32]. Fluid administration in patients with renal impairment is often performed at a flow significantly lower than that assumed to give protection because of the concern of volume overload, especially in patients with left ventricle dysfunction [33]. Different combined strategies of hydration and diuretics have been tested under the assumption that a higher urine output relates to a greater contrast dilution and lower contrast toxicity. Loop diuretics showed a negative effect probably related to volume depletion and consequent vasoconstriction [34]. Interestingly, it has been demonstrated that increased diuresis, concurrently obtained with diuretics from fluid administration matched with urine output, not only prevents dehydration but also reduces CIN occurrence [35]. On the basis of this evidence, an automated hydration system was developed (Renal Guard System™, Renal Guard Solutions, Inc., Milford, MA, USA). The Renal Guard consists of a collection bag for the urine with a computed monitoring system and an intravenous infusion system. After an initial bolus of 250 mL isotonic saline and furosemide (0.25–0.5 mg/kg) that stimulates the diuresis, the saline solution is constantly infused at a volume corresponding to the volume of urine that flows into the collection bag, minimizing the risk of fluid depletion or overload. The Renal Guard System™ was tested for efficacy and safety in a clinical trial, and it was associated with a statistically significant reduction in CIN and the need for renal replacement therapy [36–38]. Interestingly, the comparison of the mean volume of fluids administered with the Renal Guard System™ and the typical hydration protocol (4000 mL vs. 1750 mL) in relation to timing (6 h vs. 24 h) emphasized the beneficial effect of hydration [37].

2.2. Pharmacological Prevention

Several pharmacological therapies have been evaluated for CIN prevention [39] in patients with CKD, producing mainly contrasting results. Among those tested, N-acetylcysteine, bicarbonate and statins represent the most promising molecules.

N-Acetylcysteine has been tested for CIN prevention on the basis of its antioxidant and vasodilator effects. A protective role of N-acetylcysteine was demonstrated in an initial study [40], but this was not confirmed in the subsequent clinical trials [41–43] that showed conflicting results, nor in the pooled data from the meta-analysis [44–52]. A multitude of elements may have contributed to the heterogeneity of these results, e.g., differences in patient selection, the definition of CIN, contrasting agent types, concomitant fluid administration, or different administration route [53]. Interesting, it was observed that the greater protective effect of N-acetylcysteine was in patients that received small amounts of contrast (<140 mL) [43]. Additional studies that tested higher cumulative doses of N-acetylcysteine compared with the most used protocol demonstrated a protective effect [54], suggesting a dose-dependent mechanism. A subsequent meta-analysis regarding the protective effect of high doses of N-acetylcysteine suggested that the most beneficial effect might be obtained in patients at high risk of CIN [55]. The beneficial effect of high doses of N-acetylcysteine on CIN prevention was confirmed in patients with STEMI [56], and it was also associated with a reduction in hospital deaths. Furthermore, in patients with myocardial infarction treated with intravenous N-acetylcysteine, a smaller size of infarcted area and protection of the left ventricular function were observed [57,58]. In acute ischemic settings, N-acetylcysteine antioxidant properties are potentially able to lessen oxidative stress related to reperfusion, and it has been demonstrated that this compound reduces platelet inhibition with a potential reduction in thrombotic burden [59]. A combination of hydration with sodium bicarbonate and N-acetylcysteine immediately before and up to 12 h after PCI reduced CIN occurrence compared to hydration with isotonic saline [60]. Conversely, in a trial of patients undergoing coronary angiography who were randomized to hydration with isotonic saline associated with oral N-acetylcysteine or hydration with bicarbonate, no differences emerged in terms of CIN prevention [48].

Alkalization therapy has been tested for CIN prevention in patients with CKD on the basis of a potential protective effect of renal tubular epithelial cells related to the reduction in renal tubules acidification with potential antioxidant effects [61], but conflicting results emerged. It was initially observed that hydration with bicarbonate was more effective in CIN reduction as compared to hydration with saline [62], but a subsequent study [63] and a meta-analysis did not confirm this data [64]. More recently, a randomized controlled trial showed no difference between intravenous sodium bicarbonate over intravenous isotonic saline or oral acetylcysteine over placebo for the prevention of CIN, need for dialysis, or death in patients with CKD undergoing coronary or non-coronary angiography [65].

Statins have been tested for CIN prevention in patients with CKD on the basis of their pleiotropic effect that includes anti-inflammatory activity and the improvement of endothelial function [66]. It was initially demonstrated that, in statin-naïve patients with acute coronary syndrome undergoing coronary angiography, a pre-treatment with rosuvastatin reduced CIN occurrence [67]. A meta-analysis of 124 trials and 28,240 patients comparing different strategies of CIN prevention in patients undergoing PCI demonstrated an important protective effect of premedication with statins [68] that, in accordance with another meta-analysis, was found to be independent of the hydration protocol. On the basis of these results, the European Society of Cardiology recommends (class IIa, level of evidence C) high-dose statins in statin-naïve patients.

Proton pump inhibitors (PPIs) have been demonstrated to reduce the rate of recurrent gastrointestinal bleeding in high-risk patients receiving aspirin [69]. Prior observational studies suggested a possible increased risk of cardiovascular ischemic events when PPI therapy was administered concomitantly with clopidogrel [70]. However, randomized trials did not support such concerns [71,72]. ESC guidelines endorse the routine association of PPI during DAPT treatment with class IB recommendations [73].

2.3. Renal Replacement Therapies

Haemodialysis and hemofiltration have been proposed for CIN prevention in patients with CKD because of their effectiveness in removing contrast agents from circulation. Several studies evaluating haemodialysis immediately after an angiographic procedure [74–77] failed to demonstrate a beneficial effect. It has been proposed that the lack of clinical benefit of haemodialysis could be related to the nephrotoxicity of the procedure that determines a pro-inflammatory, pro-coagulative, hypotensive and hypovolemic effect [78]. Hemofiltration, as compared to haemodialysis, is often found to be more manageable because fluid and solute removal are performed with better volume control and more haemodynamic stability. Indeed, a randomised study demonstrated that hemofiltration reduces CIN occurrence and 1-year mortality in patients with severe CKD. A subsequent study [79] compared two different protocols of hemofiltration in patients with severe CKD; one group was treated with hemofiltration for 6 h before and for 18/24 h after the procedure, while the other group was treated for 18/24 h after the procedure. An important reduction in CIN occurrence was observed in the group treated with hemofiltration before and after the procedure. On the basis of these results, the European Society of Cardiology recommends (class IIb, level of evidence B) hemofiltration for 6 h before and for 24 h after a given procedure for patients with severe CKD undergoing complex PCI, while prophylactic haemodialysis is not recommended (class III, level of evidence B) [28].

3. Transradial Artery Access

Transradial access (TRA) for percutaneous coronary angiography and intervention has become the default route over the transfemoral approach (TFA) on the basis of several advantages [80]. Among these advantages is an important reduction in renal complications [81–84]. Different mechanisms have been implicated to explain the nephroprotective effect of TRA over TFA, including a lower incidence of major bleeding [20,85], embolization [86,87] and hypotension, but also a lower use of contrast agents. Several studies have evaluated the benefit of TRA on renal outcome with heterogeneous results [88–90]. In the pivotal MATRIX-Access randomized trial, TRA was demonstrated to reduce major bleeding and all-cause mortality compared to TFA [91]. A prespecified sub-analysis of this study revealed a reduction in acute kidney injury occurrence in the TRA cohort compared to the TFA cohort [92]. Interestingly, a subsequent multistate and competing risk model analysis suggested that the reduction in mortality was mainly mediated by the reduction in acute kidney injury [93]. Finally, a large meta-analysis of 14 studies and 46,816 patients confirmed that TRA was associated with a lower occurrence of acute kidney injury after coronary angiography or PCI [94], compared to TFA.

4. Contrast Dye Reduction for Coronary Angiography and PCI

In recent years, new procedural approaches have been introduced to reduce contrast administration with the aim of performing ultra-low contrast angiography and virtually zero-contrast PCI. The implementation of these techniques could reduce the need for contrast during the procedure to a minimum. For example, catheter engagement in the coronary ostia could be performed without contrast by focusing on calcium distribution using a high frame rate [95]. Moreover, correct cannulation could be confirmed without contrast by injecting 10–20 mL of isotonic saline and observing temporal changes in the electrocardiogram (i.e., T wave or ST segment modification) [96] or, alternatively, by cautiously advancing a coronary guidewire [97]. A total of 15 mL of contrast is usually sufficient to perform a reliable coronary angiography [98] by injecting 2–3 mL of contrast to visualize the left coronary artery and 2 mL for the right coronary artery. Contrast medium should be removed from the catheter prior to every drug administration or catheter exchange, and contrast must be refilled before subsequent angiography. When clear angiographic images are available, PCI without contrast may be attempted (during the same session or in a staged procedure) using different techniques, intravascular imaging, and functional tests. Large guiding catheters (usually 7 Fr) are preferable as they give stable support and accommodate multiple guidewires, stents and IVUS probes. Multiple guidewires should trace the course of the vessels shown on the reference angiography, and represent a map used to track major reference points during the procedure (e.g., ostia, bifurcations etc.). Once the correct position of the guide wire has been verified, an IVUS evaluation can be performed. IVUS is able to accurately define plaque burden and reference vessel dimensions, allowing the selection of the optimal stent size [97,98]. Several landmarks such as calcification, ribs, surgical clips, the catheter, or guidewires are useful to gain the correct position for stent placement. After stent implantation, correct stent expansion and possible dissections can be assessed by IVUS. IVUS co-registration to merge angiography and intravascular probe position could further increase PCI accuracy. The physiological evaluation of coronary plaque can be used to guide the procedure and confirm the effectiveness of the intervention [99]. In non-complex anatomy, rotational atherectomy can be performed without contrast, because calcifications of the wall vessel usually mark the location and the extent of the lesion [100]. If vessel perforation, distal embolization, or other complications that cannot be ruled out by IVUS or functional tests are suspected, a small contrast injection can elucidate the problem.

5. Revascularization Strategy

Coronary atherosclerosis in patients with CKD is typically associated with a higher burden of calcification, and more frequently involves the left, main, or three vessels resulting in high lesion complexity [101–103]. A correlation between the severity of renal impairment and coronary lesion complexity expressed by an inverse relationship between the eGFR and the SYNTAX (SYNergy between PCI with TAXUS™ and Cardiac Surgery) Score has been demonstrated [104]. In the clinical setting of ACS, CKD affects nearly 30–40% of patients and it has been demonstrated to be an independent predictor of death and MACCE with a correlation between the severity of CKD and the event rate [105–107]. Despite this, patients with ACS and CKD less frequently receive optimal medical treatment and early invasive strategies [107,108]. ACS diagnosis in patients with CKD may be delayed due to atypical presentation without chest pain, ECG abnormalities, or mild elevations in cardiac necrosis markers. Furthermore, CKD (particularly end-stage renal disease) has been adopted as an exclusion criteria for large ACS clinical trials, so the efficacy/safety profile of different treatments remain uninvestigated against the disease [109]. Interestingly, CKD patients with ACS undergoing PCI have been evaluated with three-vessel grayscale and virtual histology intravascular ultrasound (IVUS) imaging [110]. Longer atherosclerotic lesions with augmented necrotic core-to-fibrous cap ratios, higher plaque burdens, greater luminal inclusions, and the coexistence of these elements of complexity have been proposed as evidence for the increased risk of periprocedural complications [111,112].

The choice of the best strategy of revascularization is critical to improve the patient's prognosis. Several studies have shown that drug-eluting stents (DES) are superior to bare-metal stents (BMS) in reducing MACE at a distance [113], irrespective of clinical and procedural characteristics [114]. Similar results have been obtained in the CKD population. Crimi et al. compared the impact of BMS vs. DES (paclitaxel-PES; zotarolimus-ZES-S; everolimus-EES-eluting stent) implantation in patients with CKD (GFR < 60 mL/min/1.73 m^2) in a post hoc analysis of the PRODIGY trial. A total of 2003 patients with stable or unstable CAD were randomized 1:1:1:1:1 to BMS-EES-PES-ZES. The study showed that CKD at baseline was associated with a two-fold higher risk of stent thrombosis (ST) and MACE, and EES halved ST risk at 2 years after PCI in CKD patients compared with BMS and PES [115]. Bangalore et al. evaluated, in an observational study, the impact of different revascularization strategies in CKD patients with multivessel disease, comparing outcomes for CABG and PCI with everolimus-eluting stents. This study showed that, in patients with CKD, CABG was associated with a higher short-term risk of death, stroke, and repeat revascularization, while PCI was associated with a higher long-term risk of repeat revascularization and myocardial infarction. In the subgroup of patients on dialysis, the results favored CABG over PCI [116].

6. Secondary Prevention Antithrombotic Drug

To improve the prognosis of patients with CKD, the correct management of antithrombotic therapy as a secondary prevention factor is of great importance. Despite huge improvements in antithrombotic therapy for secondary prevention, the prevalence of CKD patients within the randomized populations of pivotal clinical studies has been low. In the PLATO trial, comparing ticagrelor vs. clopidogrel in patients with ACS, the proportion of CKD patients was only 21.3%, while dialysis was a study exclusion criteria. Similarly, in the TRITON TIMI 38 trial testing prasugrel vs. clopidogrel in ACS patients, the proportion of CKD patients was only 15.1%, and patients with CKD stage >4 were rare [117,118].

CKD patients carry both a higher ischemic and bleeding risk [119]. The coagulation cascade is imbalanced towards more thrombotic activity: the concentration of prothrombotic factors including fibrinogen, tissue factor and higher inflammatory milieu increase the risk of thrombotic complications [120]. The endothelial injuries associated with CKD also favor the loss of antithrombotic properties [121]. On the other hand, CKD might impair α-granule release and prostaglandin metabolism, impairing platelet aggregation [122]. Circulating fibrinogen fragments interfere by competitive binding to the glycoprotein IIb/IIIa receptor, resulting in decreased adhesion and aggregation and increased bleeding liability [123]. In addition, altered drug metabolism increases plasma concentration and the risk of antithrombotic overdosing in CKD patients.

Multiple studies have shown a high platelet reactivity in patients with CKD [124,125]. In the ADAPT-DES registry, authors compared platelet function in patients with and without CKD, demonstrating that those with CKD had higher platelet reactivity with a linear relationship to the renal function of platelet function testing [126]. Similarly, Angiolillo et al. observed that diabetic patients with CKD had markedly elevated platelet reactivity with a reduced response to the active metabolite of clopidogrel, suggesting altered $P2Y_{12}$-mediated signaling [127]. High platelet reactivity with reduced responsiveness to clopidogrel (the best-studied P2Y12I) resulted in an increase in MACE and ACS in patients treated with PCI [128,129]. In the CREDO (Clopidogrel for the Reduction of Events During Observation) trial, the CKD group patients did not show the same benefit in terms of reduction in death, myocardial infarction, or stroke, with respect to the placebo of the non-CKD group [130]. The evidence for potent P2Y12i is limited in CKD patients. A small single-center study enrolling non ST-elevation myocardial infarction patients with CKD demonstrated significantly lower P2Y12 reaction unit (PRU) values in the group treated with ticagrelor versus the clopidogrel group [131]. In another small study, prasugrel demonstrated no difference in the pharmacokinetics and pharmacodynamics of subjects with CKD in terms of platelet inhibition contrary to clopidogrel [132,133]. A comparison of three P2Y12Is (ticagrelor, prasugrel and clopidogrel) in CKD patients with ACS undergoing PCI were available in the subgroup analysis of the two RCTs (TRITON TIMI 38 and PLATO studies). The TRITON TIMI 38 subgroup analysis included 1490 patients with a creatinine clearance < 60 mL/min. In this group, the benefit of prasugrel treatment compared with clopidogrel was similar to that of the overall population without significant interaction between the treatment groups and the CKD group [117]. The CKD sub-group of the PLATO trial was composed of 3237 patients who were followed over a mean of 9 months. No interaction was noted between the CKD and treatment groups; this data suggests a similar net benefit ratio in patients with CKD compared to the normal population ($p = 0.13$). On the other hand, all-cause mortality was lower in the ticagrelor group, with a 36% reduction (3.9 versus 5%; $p = 0.01$). The results were not significant for non-CKD patients [134]. The SWEDEHEART registry compared two P2Y12Is (ticagrelor and clopidogrel) in patients undergoing PCI for ACS and suffering with CKD. The registry defined two groups: moderate CKD (30–60 mL/min) and severe CKD (<30 mL/min). In the moderate CKD group, lower rates of death, myocardial infarction, and stroke at the 1-year follow-up were registered in the ticagrelor group compared with the clopidogrel group (adjusted HR, 0.82; 95% CI, 0.7–0.97). No benefit was observed for the patients with severe CKD (adjusted HR, 0.95; 95% CI, 0.69–1.29). Bleeding with the need for hospitalization was similar between the two groups in the moderate CKD setting (OR, 1.13; 95% CI, 0.84–1.51), while a trend towards higher bleeding rates was recorded in patients in the severe CKD group treated with ticagrelor (adjusted HR, 1.79; 95% CI, 1.00–3.21) [135]. The TRILOGY ACS trial (Targeted Platelet Inhibition to Clarify the Optimal Strategy to Medically Manage Acute Coronary Syndromes) was a randomized study comparing prasugrel and clopidogrel over 30 months in combination with aspirin in an ACS medically managed setting. A prespecified subgroup analysis showed that patients with moderate or severe CKD had an excessive risk of ischemic and bleeding events, and there were no differences between prasugrel and clopidogrel in terms of outcome in these subgroups [136].

Dual antiplatelet therapy duration should be selected on a single-patient basis, taking into consideration clinical characteristics [137,138] and CKD [139]. In a post hoc analysis of the PRODIGY trial, CKD did not appear as a treatment modifier for DAPT duration with respect to ischemic events, and longer DAPT was associated with excessive bleeding in moderate and severe CKD [140]. On the other hand, CKD is included in several risk scores as a criterium for high ischemic and bleeding risk. In a sub-analysis of the PRECISE-DAPT population, shorter-term DAPT was associated with improved outcomes for patients that were considered at higher ischemic and bleeding risk, supporting the concept that when both ischemic and bleeding risk are high, bleeding risk prevention with shorter-term DAPT is preferred [141]. Concomitant treatment with proton pump inhibitors while patients are on DAPT magnifies the benefit of antithrombotic therapy by limiting gastrointestinal bleeding [72,142], and should be maintained throughout.

7. VKA/NOAC for Atrial Fibrillation (AF) in Patients with CKD

Atrial fibrillation and CKD have a high prevalence in the adult population, and frequently co-exist in the same patient. Patients with AF and CKD have both thromboembolic and hemorrhagic risk factors that significantly contribute to elevated mortality and morbidity in this population [143]. This framework particularly concerns the metabolism of the four currently available NOAC compounds that are all partially excreted by the kidneys: 80% of dabigatran is eliminated thorough renal clearance, while 50%, 35%, and 27% of edoxaban, rivaroxaban, and apixaban are eliminated this way, respectively. To date, no RCT has investigated the clinical role of VKA for thromboprophylaxis in AF patients with severe or end-stage kidney disease and, unfortunately, the main trials with NOACs excluded patients with an eGFR lower than 30 mL/min. Beyond that, on the basis of pharmacokinetic analysis, rivaroxaban, apixaban, and edoxaban (but not dabigatran) are approved in Europe for patients with severe CKD eGFR: 15–29 mL/min) with a reduced dose regimen.

Patients with AF undergoing PCI are an increasingly large group [144] and, in this specific clinical setting, CKD is a crucial variable to consider to properly tailor antithrombotic treatment, as this a major criterion for higher bleeding risk [145]. The AGUSTUS trial, with a 2 × 2 design, evaluated the safety of apixaban AVK, aspirin, and placebo in patients with ACS and/or undergoing PCI. Within the study population, eGFR was >80 mL/min in 30% of patients, >50–80mL/min in 52% of patients, and 30–50 mL/min for 19% of patients. Patients treated with apixaban—compared with VKA—had a lower rate of death, hospitalization and bleeding, independent of renal function [146]. Data from the REDUAL-PCI study are aligned with these results. Patients with AF who had undergone PCI were assigned to triple therapy (VKA, aspirin, and clopidogrel or ticagrelor) or dual therapy with dabigatran (110 mg or 150 mg) and clopidogrel or ticagrelor. Dual therapy with dabigatran 110 mg, compared with VKA, reduced the risk of major bleeding events or clinically relevant non-major bleeding events irrespective of eGFR class (p for interaction = 0.19). Likewise, dual therapy with dabigatran 150 mg reduced the risk of major bleeding events or clinically relevant non-major bleeding events irrespective of eGFR class, compared with VKA. No significant differences in the prevention of thromboembolic events or unplanned revascularization emerged between dual therapy with dabigatran 110 mg or triple therapy, irrespective of eGFR class. Dual therapy with dabigatran 150 mg, compared with triple therapy, had a similar risk for thromboembolic events or unplanned revascularization in patients with eGFR from 30 to <80 mL/min, and a lower risk with eGFR $\geq$ 80 mL/min (p for interaction = 0.02) [147].

8. Optimal Medical Therapy for CKD

8.1. Hypertension Treatment

Hypertension is the second most important cause of CKD and an independent risk factor for cardiovascular events [148]. The evidence suggests that blood pressure (BP) targets should be lowered to <140/90 mmHg with the aim of moving towards 130/80 mmHg [149,150]. The SPRINT trial demonstrated that a more ambitious systolic BP target < 120 mmHg reduces CV events and all-cause mortality compared to a target of <140 mmHg [151]. CKD guidelines suggest a combination of renin angiotensin system (RAS) blockers with calcium channel blockers (CCBs) as a first-choice therapy [152]. Other therapeutic agents, such as beta-blockers, spironolactone, diuretics (amiloride, thiazide, thiazide-like diuretics or loop diuretics), and alpha-blockers could be added as second-line therapy options [153]. Many therapeutic agents should be considered and monitored carefully for their impact on renal function and potassium levels, especially in patients with eGFR < 45 mL/min/1.73 m^2 and serum potassium levels > 5.0 mmol/L.

8.2. Lipid Control

According to ESC guidelines, patients with advanced CKD are considered to be at high or very high risk of cardiovascular disease, with LDL targets of 70 mg/dL and 55 mg/dL, respectively [154]. The KDIGO organization developed practice guidelines for the management of dyslipidemia in CKD patients in which the use of statins or a statin/ezetimibe combination was recommended in non-dialysis patients with end-stage CKD. For dialysis patients who are already on lipid-lowering agents at the time of dialysis initiation, the continuation of these drugs is recommended, especially in cases where there is evidence of atherosclerotic cardiovascular disease [155].

The metabolisms of statins are mainly explained by the liver (and minimally by the kidneys), so dose adjustment with CKD and hemodialysis is not necessary, with the exception of hydrophilic statins such as pravastatin and rosuvastatin. This particular kind of statin has a higher risk of myopathy and rhabdomyolysis in CKD patients [156]. For rosuvastatin, a dose adjustment in non-dialysis severe renal impairment with a starting dose of 5 mg, once daily, and a maximal recommended dose of 10 mg, once daily, is suggested.

9. Conclusions

The prevalence of patients suffering from both CAD and CKD is high and is likely to increase in the coming years. Planning adequate management of this group of patients is crucial to improve their outcome after PCI. This starts with proper preparation before the procedure, the use of all available means to reduce contrast use during the procedure, and the implementation of modern strategies such as radial access and drug-eluting stents. At the end of the procedure, a personalized antithrombotic therapy plan based on patient's characteristics is advisable in light of their elevated ischemic and bleeding risk (Figure 1).

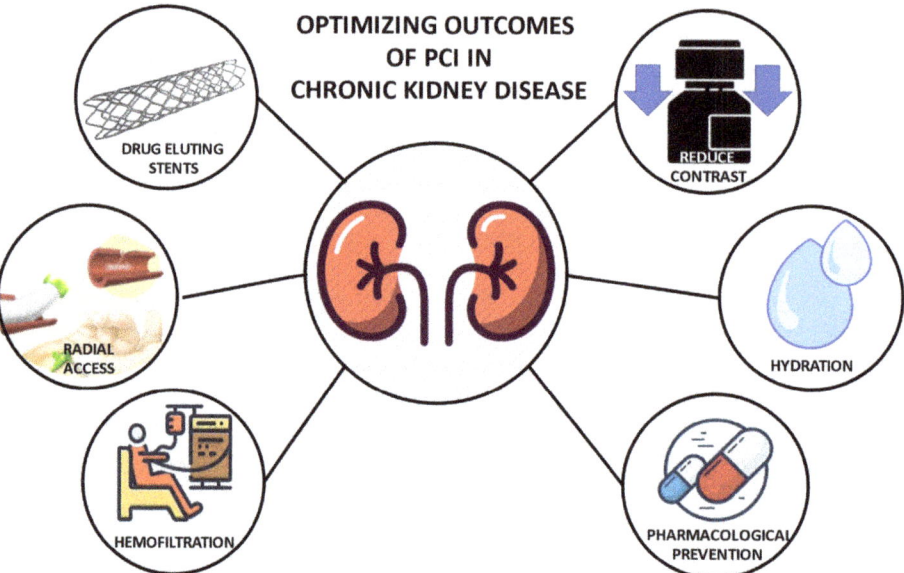

Figure 1. Strategies to optimize PCI outcomes in patients with chronic kidney disease.

Author Contributions: A.C. drafted, and revised critically the manuscript; R.F.M.S. wrote original draft; G.B. drafted and critically revised the manuscript; A.G.V. drafted and critically revised the manuscript; R.L. drafted and critically revised the manuscript; F.C. (Fabrizio Ceresa) drafted and critically revised the manuscript; S.P. drafted and critically revised the manuscript; F.L. drafted and critically revised the manuscript; N.I. drafted and critically revised the manuscript; D.S. drafted and critically revised the manuscript; F.P. drafted and critically revised the manuscript; G.D.B. drafted and critically revised the manuscript; F.C. (Francesco Costa) conceptualized, drafted, and critically revised the manuscript. A.M. drafted and critically revised the manuscript. All authors have read and agreed to the published version of the manuscript.

Funding: This research received no external funding.

Institutional Review Board Statement: Not applicable.

Informed Consent Statement: Not applicable.

Data Availability Statement: The data presented in this study are available in manuscript.

Conflicts of Interest: The authors declare no conflict of interest.

References

1. Caracciolo, A.; Mazzone, P.; Laterra, G.; Garcia-Ruiz, V.; Polimeni, A.; Galasso, S.; Saporito, F.; Carerj, S.; D'Ascenzo, F.; Marquis-Gravel, G.; et al. Antithrombotic Therapy for Percutaneous Cardiovascular Interventions: From Coronary Artery Disease to Structural Heart Interventions. *J. Clin. Med.* **2019**, *8*, 2016. [CrossRef] [PubMed]
2. Spertus, J.A.; Jones, P.G.; Maron, D.J.; O'Brien, S.M.; Reynolds, H.; Rosenberg, Y.; Stone, G.W.; Harrell, F.E.; Boden, W.E.; Weintraub, W.S.; et al. Health-Status Outcomes with Invasive or Conservative Care in Coronary Disease. *N. Engl. J. Med.* **2020**, *382*, 1408–1419. [CrossRef] [PubMed]
3. Zijlstra, F.; Hoorntje, J.C.; De Boer, M.-J.; Reiffers, S.; Miedema, K.; Ottervanger, J.P.; Hof, A.W.V.T. Long-Term Benefit of Primary Angioplasty as Compared with Thrombolytic Therapy for Acute Myocardial Infarction. *N. Engl. J. Med.* **2008**, *341*, 1413–1419. [CrossRef] [PubMed]
4. Maron, D.J.; Hochman, J.S.; Reynolds, H.R.; Bangalore, S.; O'Brien, S.M.; Boden, W.E.; Chaitman, B.R.; Senior, R.; López-Sendón, J.; Alexander, K.P.; et al. Initial Invasive or Conservative Strategy for Stable Coronary Disease. *N. Engl. J. Med.* **2020**, *382*, 1395–1407. [CrossRef]
5. Visseren, F.L.J.; Mach, F.; Smulders, Y.M.; Carballo, D.; Koskinas, K.C.; Bäck, M.; Benetos, A.; Biffi, A.; Boavida, J.-M.; Capodanno, D.; et al. 2021 ESC Guidelines on cardiovascular disease prevention in clinical practiceDeveloped by the Task Force for cardiovascular disease prevention in clinical practice with representatives of the European Society of Cardiology and 12 medical societies With the special contribution of the European Association of Preventive Cardiology (EAPC). *Eur. Heart J.* **2021**, *42*, 3227–3337. [CrossRef] [PubMed]
6. Manjunath, G.; Tighiouart, H.; Ibrahim, H.; MacLeod, B.; Salem, D.N.; Griffith, J.L.; Coresh, J.; Levey, A.S.; Sarnak, M.J. Level of kidney function as a risk factor for atherosclerotic cardiovascular outcomes in the community. *J. Am. Coll. Cardiol.* **2003**, *41*, 47–55. [CrossRef]
7. Bangalore, S.; Maron, D.J.; O'Brien, S.M.; Fleg, J.L.; Kretov, E.I.; Briguori, C.; Kaul, U.; Reynolds, H.; Mazurek, T.; Sidhu, M.S.; et al. Management of Coronary Disease in Patients with Advanced Kidney Disease. *N. Engl. J. Med.* **2020**, *382*, 1608–1618. [CrossRef]
8. Crimi, G.; Leonardi, S.; Costa, F.; Ariotti, S.; Tebaldi, M.; Biscaglia, S.; Valgimigli, M. Incidence, prognostic impact, and optimal definition of contrast-induced acute kidney injury in consecutive patients with stable or unstable coronary artery disease undergoing percutaneous coronary intervention. insights from the all-comer PRODIGY trial. *Catheter. Cardiovasc. Interv.* **2015**, *86*, E19–E27. [CrossRef]
9. McCullough, P.A.; Wolyn, R.; Rocher, L.L.; Levin, R.N.; O'Neill, W.W. Acute renal failure after coronary intervention: Incidence, risk factors, and relationship to mortality. *Am. J. Med.* **1997**, *103*, 368–375. [CrossRef]
10. Gruberg, L.; Mintz, G.S.; Mehran, R.; Dangas, G.; Lansky, A.J.; Kent, K.M.; Pichard, A.D.; Satler, L.F.; Leon, M.B. The prognostic implications of further renal function deterioration within 48 h of interventional coronary procedures in patients with pre-existent chronic renal insufficiency. *J. Am. Coll. Cardiol.* **2000**, *36*, 1542–1548. [CrossRef]
11. Rudnick, M.R.; Goldfarb, S.; Wexler, L.; Ludbrook, P.A.; Murphy, M.J.; Halpern, E.F.; Hill, J.A.; Winniford, M.; Cohen, M.B.; VanFossen, D.B.; et al. Nephrotoxicity of ionic and nonionic contrast media in 1196 patients: A randomized trial. *Kidney Int.* **1995**, *47*, 254–261. [CrossRef] [PubMed]
12. Thomsen, H.S.; Morcos, S.K. Contrast media and the kidney: European Society of Urogenital Radiology (ESUR) Guidelines. *Br. J. Radiol.* **2003**, *76*, 513–518. [CrossRef] [PubMed]
13. Aspelin, P.; Aubry, P.; Fransson, S.-G.; Strasser, R.; Willenbrock, R.; Berg, K.J. Nephrotoxic Effects in High-Risk Patients Undergoing Angiography. *N. Engl. J. Med.* **2003**, *348*, 491–499. [CrossRef] [PubMed]

14. Koreny, M.; Karth, G.D.; Geppert, A.; Neunteufl, T.; Priglinger, U.; Heinz, G.; Siostrzonek, P. Prognosis of patients who develop acute renal failure during the first 24 hours of cardiogenic shock after myocardial infarction. *Am. J. Med.* **2002**, *112*, 115–119. [CrossRef]
15. Mehran, R.; Aymong, E.D.; Nikolsky, E.; Lasic, Z.; Iakovou, I.; Fahy, M.; Mintz, G.S.; Lansky, A.J.; Moses, J.W.; Stone, G.W.; et al. A simple risk score for prediction of contrast-induced nephropathy after percutaneous coronary intervention: Development and initial validation. *J. Am. Coll. Cardiol.* **2004**, *44*, 1393–1399. [CrossRef] [PubMed]
16. Jo, S.-H.; Youn, T.-J.; Koo, B.-K.; Park, J.-S.; Kang, H.-J.; Cho, Y.-S.; Chung, W.-Y.; Joo, G.-W.; Chae, I.-H.; Choi, D.-J.; et al. Renal Toxicity Evaluation and Comparison Between Visipaque (Iodixanol) and Hexabrix (Ioxaglate) in Patients with Renal Insufficiency Undergoing Coronary Angiography: The RECOVER Study: A Randomized Controlled Trial. *J. Am. Coll. Cardiol.* **2006**, *48*, 924–930. [CrossRef]
17. Laskey, W.K.; Jenkins, C.; Selzer, F.; Marroquin, O.C.; Wilensky, R.L.; Glaser, R.; Holmes, D.R., Jr.; Cohen, H.A. Volume-to-creatinine clearance ratio: A pharmacokinetically based risk factor for prediction of early creatinine increase after percutaneous coronary intervention. *J. Am. Coll. Cardiol.* **2007**, *50*, 584–590. [CrossRef]
18. Marenzi, G.; Assanelli, E.; Campodonico, J.; Lauri, G.; Marana, I.; De Metrio, M.; Moltrasio, M.; Grazi, M.; Rubino, M.; Veglia, F.; et al. Contrast volume during primary percutaneous coronary intervention and subsequent contrast-induced nephropathy and mortality. *Ann. Intern. Med.* **2009**, *150*, 170–177. [CrossRef]
19. Solomon, R.J.; Natarajan, M.K.; Doucet, S.; Sharma, S.K.; Staniloae, C.S.; Katholi, R.; Gelormini, J.L.; Labinaz, M.; Moreyra, A.E. Cardiac Angiography in Renally Impaired Patients (CARE) Study. *Circulation* **2007**, *115*, 3189–3196. [CrossRef]
20. Ohno, Y.; Maekawa, Y.; Miyata, H.; Inoue, S.; Ishikawa, S.; Sueyoshi, K.; Noma, S.; Kawamura, A.; Kohsaka, S.; Fukuda, K. Impact of periprocedural bleeding on incidence of contrast-induced acute kidney injury in patients treated with percutaneous coronary intervention. *J. Am. Coll. Cardiol.* **2013**, *62*, 1260–1266. [CrossRef]
21. Solomon, R.; Deray, G. How to prevent contrast-induced nephropathy and manage risk patients: Practical recommendations. *Kidney Int.* **2006**, *69*, S51–S53. [CrossRef] [PubMed]
22. Capodanno, D.; Ministeri, M.; Dipasqua, F.; Dalessandro, V.; Cumbo, S.; Gargiulo, G.; Tamburino, C. Risk prediction of contrast-induced nephropathy by ACEF score in patients undergoing coronary catheterization. *J. Cardiovasc. Med.* **2016**, *17*, 524–529. [CrossRef] [PubMed]
23. Gurm, H.S.; Seth, M.; Kooiman, J.; Share, D. A Novel Tool for Reliable and Accurate Prediction of Renal Complications in Patients Undergoing Percutaneous Coronary Intervention. *J. Am. Coll. Cardiol.* **2013**, *61*, 2242–2248. [CrossRef] [PubMed]
24. Brown, J.R.; DeVries, J.T.; Piper, W.D.; Robb, J.F.; Hearne, M.J.; Lee, P.M.V.; Kellet, M.A.; Watkins, M.W.; Ryan, T.J.; Silver, M.T.; et al. Serious renal dysfunction after percutaneous coronary interventions can be predicted. *Am. Heart J.* **2008**, *155*, 260–266. [CrossRef] [PubMed]
25. McCullough, P.A.; Adam, A.; Becker, C.R.; Davidson, C.; Lameire, N.; Stacul, F.; Tumlin, J. Risk Prediction of Contrast-Induced Nephropathy. *Am. J. Cardiol.* **2006**, *98*, 27–36. [CrossRef] [PubMed]
26. Ronco, F.; Azzalini, L.; Briguori, C.; Cosmai, L.; D'Amico, M.; Di Luca, M.; Esposito, G.; Granatelli, A.; Maddestra, N.; De Marco, F.; et al. Documento di consenso SICI-GISE/SIN: Danno renale acuto da mezzo di contrasto in cardiologia interventistica. *G Ital. Cardiol.* **2019**, *20*, 29–43.
27. Does Hydration Prevent Radiocontrast-Induced Acute Renal Failure? *Nephrol. Dial. Transplant.* **1999**, *14*, 1064–1066. Available online: https://academic.oup.com/ndt/article/14/5/1064/1816200 (accessed on 28 February 2022). [CrossRef]
28. Members, T.F.; Windecker, S.; Kolh, P.; Alfonso, F.; Collet, J.-P.; Cremer, J.; Falk, V.; Filippatos, G.; Hamm, C.W.; Head, S.J.; et al. 2014 ESC/EACTS Guidelines on myocardial revascularization: The Task Force on Myocardial Revascularization of the European Society of Cardiology (ESC) and the European Association for Cardio-Thoracic Surgery (EACTS)Developed with the special contribution of the European Association of Percutaneous Cardiovascular Interventions (EAPCI). *Eur. Heart J.* **2014**, *35*, 2541–2619. [CrossRef]
29. Bader, B.; Berger, E.; Heede, M.; Silberbaur, I.; Duda, S.; Risler, T.; Erley, C. What is the best hydration regimen to prevent contrast media-induced nephrotoxicity? *Clin. Nephrol.* **2004**, *62*, 1–7. [CrossRef]
30. Trivedi, H.S.; Moore, H.; Nasr, S.; Aggarwal, K.; Agrawal, A.; Goel, P.; Hewett, J. A Randomized Prospective Trial to Assess the Role of Saline Hydration on the Development of Contrast Nephrotoxicity. *Nephron Clin. Pract.* **2003**, *93*, c29–c34. [CrossRef]
31. Hiremath, S.; Akbari, A.; Shabana, W.; Fergusson, D.; Knoll, G.A. Prevention of Contrast-Induced Acute Kidney Injury: Is Simple Oral Hydration Similar To Intravenous? A Systematic Review of the Evidence. *PLoS ONE* **2013**, *8*, e60009. [CrossRef] [PubMed]
32. Mueller, C.; Buerkle, G.; Buettner, H.J.; Petersen, J.; Perruchoud, A.P.; Eriksson, U.; Marsch, S.; Roskamm, H. Prevention of Contrast Media–Associated Nephropathy: Randomized Comparison of 2 Hydration Regimens in 1620 Patients Undergoing Coronary Angioplasty. *Arch. Intern. Med.* **2002**, *162*, 329–336. [CrossRef] [PubMed]
33. Liu, Y.; Li, H.; Chen, S.; Chen, J.; Tan, N.; Zhou, Y.; Liu, Y.; Ye, P.; Ran, P.; Duan, C.; et al. Excessively High Hydration Volume May Not Be Associated With Decreased Risk of Contrast-Induced Acute Kidney Injury After Percutaneous Coronary Intervention in Patients With Renal Insufficiency. *J. Am. Heart Assoc.* **2016**, *5*, e003171. [CrossRef] [PubMed]
34. Solomon, R.; Werner, C.; Mann, D.; D'Elia, J.; Silva, P. Effects of Saline, Mannitol, and Furosemide on Acute Decreases in Renal Function Induced by Radiocontrast Agents. *N. Engl. J. Med.* **1994**, *331*, 1416–1420. [CrossRef] [PubMed]

35. Stevens, M.A.; McCullough, P.A.; Tobin, K.J.; Speck, J.P.; Westveer, D.C.; Guido-Allen, D.A.; Timmis, G.C.; O'Neill, W.W. A prospective randomized trial of prevention measures in patients at high risk for contrast nephropathy: Results of the P.R.I.N.C.E. Study. Prevention of Radiocontrast Induced Nephropathy Clinical Evaluation. *J. Am. Coll. Cardiol.* **1999**, *33*, 403–411. [CrossRef]
36. Renal Insufficiency After Contrast Media Administration Trial II (REMEDIAL II). *Circulation* **2011**, *124*, 1260–1269. Available online: https://www.ahajournals.org/doi/10.1161/CIRCULATIONAHA.111.030759?url_ver=Z39.88-2003&rfr_id=ori:rid:crossref.org&rfr_dat=cr_pub%20%200pubmed (accessed on 1 March 2022). [CrossRef] [PubMed]
37. Prevention of Contrast Nephropathy by Furosemide With Matched Hydration: The MYTHOS (Induced Diuresis With Matched Hydration Compared to Standard Hydration for Contrast Induced Nephropathy Prevention) Trial. *JACC Cardiovasc. Interv.* **2012**, *5*, 92–97. Available online: https://www.sciencedirect.com/science/article/pii/S1936879811007874?via%3Dihub (accessed on 1 March 2022).
38. Prevention of Contrast-Induced Acute Kidney Injury by Furosemide With Matched Hydration in Patients Undergoing Interventional Procedures: A Systematic Review and Meta-Analysis of Randomized Trials. *JACC Cardiovasc. Interv.* **2017**, *10*, 355–363. Available online: https://www.sciencedirect.com/science/article/pii/S1936879816319823?via%3Dihub (accessed on 1 March 2022). [CrossRef]
39. Briguori, C.; Marenzi, G. Contrast-induced nephropathy: Pharmacological prophylaxis. *Kidney Int.* **2006**, *69*, S30–S38. [CrossRef]
40. Tepel, M.; van der Giet, M.; Schwarzfeld, C.; Laufer, U.; Liermann, D.; Zidek, W. Prevention of Radiographic-Contrast-Agent–Induced Reductions in Renal Function by Acetylcysteine. *N. Engl. J. Med.* **2000**, *343*, 180–184. [CrossRef]
41. Acetylcysteine Protects against Acute Renal Damage in Patients with Abnormal Renal Function Undergoing a Coronary Procedure. *J. Am. Coll. Cardiol.* **2002**, *40*, 1383–1388. Available online: https://www.sciencedirect.com/science/article/pii/S0735109702023082?via%3Dihub (accessed on 1 March 2022). [CrossRef]
42. Acetylcysteine for Prevention of Acute Deterioration of Renal Function Following Elective Coronary Angiography and Intervention: A Randomized Controlled Trial. Clinical Pharmacy and Pharmacology. *JAMA* **2003**, *289*, 553–558. Available online: https://jamanetwork.com/journals/jama/fullarticle/195894 (accessed on 1 March 2022).
43. Briguori, C.; Manganelli, F.; Scarpato, P.; Elia, P.P.; Golia, B.; Riviezzo, G.; Lepore, S.; Librera, M.; Villari, B.; Colombo, A.; et al. Acetylcysteine and contrast agent-associated nephrotoxicity. *J. Am. Coll. Cardiol.* **2002**, *40*, 298–303. [CrossRef]
44. Kshirsagar, A.V.; Poole, C.; Mottl, A.; Shoham, D.; Franceschini, N.; Tudor, G.; Agrawal, M.; Denu-Ciocca, C.; Ohman, E.M.; Finn, W.F. N-acetylcysteine for the prevention of radiocontrast induced nephropathy: A meta-analysis of prospective controlled trials. *J. Am. Soc. Nephrol.* **2004**, *15*, 761–769. [CrossRef] [PubMed]
45. Isenbarger, D.W.; Kent, S.M.; O'Malley, P.G. Meta-analysis of randomized clinical trials on the usefulness of acetylcysteine for prevention of contrast nephropathy. *Am. J. Cardiol.* **2003**, *92*, 1454–1458. [CrossRef]
46. Alonso, A.; Lau, J.; Jaber, B.L.; Weintraub, A.; Sarnak, M.J. Prevention of radiocontrast nephropathy with N-acetylcysteine in patients with chronic kidney disease: A meta-analysis of randomized, controlled trials. *Am. J. Kidney Dis.* **2004**, *43*, 1–9. [CrossRef]
47. Pannu, N.; Manns, B.; Lee, H.; Tonelli, M. Systematic review of the impact of N-acetylcysteine on contrast nephropathy. *Kidney Int.* **2004**, *65*, 1366–1374. [CrossRef]
48. Guru, V.; Fremes, S.E. The role of N-acetylcysteine in preventing radiographic contrast-induced nephropathy. *Clin. Nephrol.* **2004**, *62*, 77–83. [CrossRef]
49. Bagshaw, S.M.; Ghali, W.A. Acetylcysteine for prevention of contrast-induced nephropathy after intravascular angiography: A systematic review and meta-analysis. *BMC Med.* **2004**, *2*, 38. [CrossRef]
50. Misra, D.; Leibowitz, K.; Gowda, R.M.; Shapiro, M.; Khan, I.A. Role of N-acetylcysteine in prevention of contrast-induced nephropathy after cardiovascular procedures: A meta-analysis. *Clin. Cardiol.* **2004**, *27*, 607–610. [CrossRef]
51. Nallamothu, B.K.; Shojania, K.G.; Saint, S.; Hofer, T.; Humes, H.D.; Moscucci, M.; Bates, E.R. Is acetylcysteine effective in preventing contrast-related nephropathy? A meta-analysis. *Am. J. Med.* **2004**, *117*, 938–947. [CrossRef]
52. Duong, M.H.; MacKenzie, T.A.; Malenka, D.J. N-acetylcysteine prophylaxis significantly reduces the risk of radiocontrast-induced nephropathy: Comprehensive meta-analysis. *Catheter. Cardiovasc. Interv.* **2005**, *64*, 471–479. [CrossRef] [PubMed]
53. Kelly, A.M.; Dwamena, B.; Cronin, P.; Bernstein, S.J.; Carlos, R.C. Meta-analysis: Effectiveness of Drugs for Preventing Contrast-Induced Nephropathy. *Ann. Intern. Med.* **2008**, *148*, 284–294. [CrossRef] [PubMed]
54. Baker, C.S.R.; Wragg, A.; Kumar, S.; De Palma, R.; Baker, L.R.I.; Knight, C.J. A rapid protocol for the prevention of contrast-induced renal dysfunction: The RAPPID study. *J. Am. Coll. Cardiol.* **2003**, *41*, 2114–2118. [CrossRef]
55. Trivedi, H.; Daram, S.; Szabo, A.; Bartorelli, A.L.; Marenzi, G. High-dose N-acetylcysteine for the Prevention of Contrast-induced Nephropathy. *Am. J. Med.* **2009**, *122*, 874.e9–874.e15. [CrossRef] [PubMed]
56. Marenzi, G.; Assanelli, E.; Marana, I.; Lauri, G.; Campodonico, J.; Grazi, M.; de Metrio, M.; Galli, S.; Fabbiocchi, F.; Montorsi, P.; et al. N-Acetylcysteine and Contrast-Induced Nephropathy in Primary Angioplasty. *N. Engl. J. Med.* **2006**, *354*, 2773–2782. [CrossRef] [PubMed]
57. Arstall, M.A.; Yang, J.; Stafford, I.; Betts, W.H.; Horowitz, J.D. N-Acetylcysteine in Combination With Nitroglycerin and Streptokinase for the Treatment of Evolving Acute Myocardial Infarction. *Circulation* **1995**, *92*, 2855–2862. [CrossRef] [PubMed]
58. Šochman, J.; Kolc, J.; Vrána, M.; Fabián, J. Cardioprotective effects of N-acetylcysteine: The reduction in the extent of infarction and occurrence of reperfusion arrhythmias in the dog. *Int. J. Cardiol.* **1990**, *28*, 191–196. [CrossRef]

59. Anfossi, G.; Russo, I.; Massucco, P.; Mattiello, L.; Cavalot, F.; Trovati, M. N-Acetyl-L-Cysteine Exerts Direct Anti-Aggregating Effect on Human Platelets—Anfossi. *Eur. J. Clin. Investig.* **2001**, *314*, 452–461. Available online: https://onlinelibrary.wiley.com/doi/abs/10.1046/j.1365-2362.2001.00815.x (accessed on 3 March 2022). [CrossRef]
60. Recio-Mayoral, A.; Chaparro, M.; Prado, B.; Cózar, R.; Méndez, I.; Banerjee, D.; Kaski, J.C.; Cubero, J.; Cruz, J.M. The renoprotective effect of hydration with sodium bicarbonate plus N-acetylcysteine in patients undergoing emergency percutaneous coronary intervention: The RENO Study. *J. Am. Coll. Cardiol.* **2007**, *49*, 1283–1288. [CrossRef]
61. Stacul, F.; Contrast Media Safety Committee of European Society of Urogenital Radiology (ESUR); van der Molen, A.J.; Reimer, P.; Webb, J.A.W.; Thomsen, H.S.; Morcos, S.K.; Almén, T.; Aspelin, P.; Bellin, M.-F.; et al. Contrast induced nephropathy: Updated ESUR Contrast Media Safety Committee guidelines. *Eur. Radiol.* **2011**, *21*, 2527–2541. [CrossRef]
62. Huber, W.; Huber, T.; Baum, S.; Franzen, M.; Schmidt, C.; Stadlbauer, T.; Beitz, A.; Schmid, R.M.; Schmid, S. Sodium Bicarbonate Prevents Contrast-Induced Nephropathy in Addition to Theophylline: A Randomized Controlled Trial. *Medicine* **2016**, *95*, e3720. [CrossRef] [PubMed]
63. Kooiman, J.; Sijpkens, Y.W.J.; Van Buren, M.; Groeneveld, J.H.M.; Ramai, S.R.S.; Van Der Molen, A.J.; Aarts, N.J.M.; Van Rooden, C.J.; Cannegieter, S.C.; Putter, H.; et al. Randomised trial of no hydration vs. sodium bicarbonate hydration in patients with chronic kidney disease undergoing acute computed tomography-pulmonary angiography. *J. Thromb. Haemost.* **2014**, *12*, 1658–1666. [CrossRef] [PubMed]
64. Sodium Bicarbonate for the Prevention of Contrast Induced-Acute Kidney Injury: A Systematic Review and Meta-Analysis. *Am. Soc. Nephrol.* **2009**, *10*, 1584–1592. Available online: https://cjasn.asnjournals.org/content/4/10/1584 (accessed on 3 March 2022).
65. Weisbord, S.D.; Gallagher, M.; Jneid, H.; Garcia, S.; Cass, A.; Thwin, S.-S.; Conner, T.A.; Chertow, G.M.; Bhatt, D.L.; Shunk, K.; et al. Outcomes after Angiography with Sodium Bicarbonate and Acetylcysteine. *N. Engl. J. Med.* **2018**, *378*, 603–614. [CrossRef] [PubMed]
66. Antonopoulos, A.S.; Margaritis, M.; Lee, R.; Channon, K.; Antoniades, C. Statins as anti-inflammatory agents in atherogenesis: Molecular mechanisms and lessons from the recent clinical trials. *Curr. Pharm. Des.* **2012**, *18*, 1519–1530. [CrossRef]
67. Leoncini, M.; Toso, A.; Maioli, M.; Tropeano, F.; Villani, S.; Bellandi, F. Early high-dose rosuvastatin for contrast-induced nephropathy prevention in acute coronary syndrome: Results from the PRATO-ACS Study (Protective Effect of Rosuvastatin and Antiplatelet Therapy On contrast-induced acute kidney injury and myocardial damage in patients with Acute Coronary Syndrome). *J. Am. Coll. Cardiol.* **2014**, *63*, 71–79. [CrossRef]
68. Giacoppo, D.; Gargiulo, G.; Buccheri, S.; Aruta, P.; Byrne, R.A.; Cassese, S.; Dangas, G.; Kastrati, A.; Mehran, R.; Tamburino, C.; et al. Preventive Strategies for Contrast-Induced Acute Kidney Injury in Patients Undergoing Percutaneous Coronary Procedures: Evidence From a Hierarchical Bayesian Network Meta-Analysis of 124 Trials and 28,240 Patients. *Circ. Cardiovasc. Interv.* **2017**, *10*, e004383. [CrossRef]
69. Lai, K.C.; Lam, S.K.; Chu, K.M.; Wong, B.C.Y.; Hui, W.M.; Hu, W.H.C.; Lau, G.K.K.; Wong, W.M.; Yuen, M.F.; Chan, A.O.O.; et al. Lansoprazole for the prevention of recurrences of ulcer complications from long-term low-dose aspirin use. *N. Engl. J. Med.* **2002**, *346*, 2033–2038. [CrossRef]
70. Shah, N.H.; LePendu, P.; Bauer-Mehren, A.; Ghebremariam, Y.T.; Iyer, S.V.; Marcus, J.; Nead, K.T.; Cooke, J.; Leeper, N.J. Proton Pump Inhibitor Usage and the Risk of Myocardial Infarction in the General Population. *PLoS ONE* **2015**, *10*, e0124653. [CrossRef]
71. O'Donoghue, M.L.; Braunwald, E.; Antman, E.M.; A Murphy, S.; Bates, E.R.; Rozenman, Y.; Michelson, A.D.; Hautvast, R.W.; Lee, P.N.V.; Close, S.L.; et al. Pharmacodynamic effect and clinical efficacy of clopidogrel and prasugrel with or without a proton-pump inhibitor: An analysis of two randomised trials. *Lancet Lond. Engl.* **2009**, *374*, 989–997. [CrossRef]
72. Bhatt, D.L.; Cryer, B.L.; Contant, C.F.; Cohen, M.; Lanas, A.; Schnitzer, T.J.; Shook, T.L.; Lapuerta, P.; Goldsmith, M.A.; Laine, L.; et al. Clopidogrel with or without Omeprazole in Coronary Artery Disease. *N. Engl. J. Med.* **2010**, *363*, 1909–1917. [CrossRef] [PubMed]
73. Valgimigli, M.; Bueno, H.; Byrne, R.A.; Collet, J.P.; Costa, F.; Jeppsson, A.; Jüni, P.; Kastrati, A.; Kolh, P.; Mauri, L.; et al. 2017 ESC Focused Update on Dual Antiplatelet Therapy in Coronary Artery Disease Developed in Collaboration with EACTS. *Eur. Heart J.* **2018**, *53*, 34–78. Available online: https://academic.oup.com/eurheartj/article/39/3/213/4095043?login=false (accessed on 12 April 2022).
74. Moon, S.S.; Bäck, S.E.; Kurkus, J.; Nilsson-Ehle, P. Hemodialysis for elimination of the nonionic contrast medium iohexol after angiography in patients with impaired renal function. *Nephron* **1995**, *70*, 430–437. [CrossRef] [PubMed]
75. Lehnert, T.; Keller, E.; Gondolf, K.; Ffner, T.S.; Dt, H.P.; Schollmeyer, P. Effect of haemodialysis after contrast medium administration in patients with renal insufficiency. *Nephrol. Dial. Transplant.* **1998**, *13*, 358–362. [CrossRef] [PubMed]
76. Sterner, G.; Frennby, B.; Kurkus, J.; Nyman, U. Does Post-angiographic Hemodialysis Reduce the Risk of Contrast-medium Nephropathy? *Scand. J. Urol. Nephrol.* **2000**, *34*, 323–326. [CrossRef] [PubMed]
77. Vogt, B.; Ferrari, P.; Schönholzer, C.; Marti, H.-P.; Mohaupt, M.; Wiederkehr, M.; Cereghetti, C.; Serra, A.; Huynh-Do, U.; Uehlinger, D.; et al. Prophylactic hemodialysis after radiocontrast media in patients with renal insufficiency is potentially harmful. *Am. J. Med.* **2001**, *111*, 692–698. [CrossRef]
78. Marenzi, G.; Bartorelli, A.L. Recent advances in the prevention of radiocontrast-induced nephropathy. *Curr. Opin. Crit. Care* **2004**, *10*, 505–509. [CrossRef]

79. Marenzi, G.; Lauri, G.; Campodonico, J.; Marana, I.; Assanelli, E.; De Metrio, M.; Grazi, M.; Veglia, F.; Fabbiocchi, F.; Montorsi, P.; et al. Comparison of Two Hemofiltration Protocols for Prevention of Contrast-induced Nephropathy in High-risk Patients. *Am. J. Med.* **2006**, *119*, 155–162. [CrossRef]
80. Scalise, R.F.M.; Salito, A.M.; Polimeni, A.; Garcia-Ruiz, V.; Virga, V.; Frigione, P.; Andò, G.; Tumscitz, C.; Costa, F. Radial Artery Access for Percutaneous Cardiovascular Interventions: Contemporary Insights and Novel Approaches. *J. Clin. Med.* **2019**, *8*, 1727. [CrossRef]
81. Acute kidney Injury after Percutaneous Coronary Intervention: Rationale of the AKI-MATRIX (Acute Kidney Injury-Minimizing Adverse Hemorrhagic Events by TRansradial Access Site and Systemic Implementation of angioX) Sub-Study. *Catheter. Cardiovasc. Interv.* **2015**, *86*, 950–987. Available online: https://onlinelibrary.wiley.com/doi/10.1002/ccd.25932 (accessed on 3 March 2022). [CrossRef]
82. Steinvil, A.; Garcia-Garcia, H.M.; Rogers, T.; Koifman, E.; Buchanan, K.; Alraies, M.C.; Torguson, R.; Pichard, A.D.; Satler, L.F.; Ben-Dor, I.; et al. Comparison of Propensity Score–Matched Analysis of Acute Kidney Injury After Percutaneous Coronary Intervention With Transradial Versus Transfemoral Approaches. *Am. J. Cardiol.* **2017**, *119*, 1507–1511. [CrossRef] [PubMed]
83. Andò, G.; Costa, F.; Boretti, I.; Trio, O.; Valgimigli, M. Benefit of radial approach in reducing the incidence of acute kidney injury after percutaneous coronary intervention: A meta-analysis of 22,108 patients. *Int. J. Cardiol.* **2015**, *179*, 309–311. [CrossRef] [PubMed]
84. Andò, G.; Costa, F.; Trio, O.; Oreto, G.; Valgimigli, M. Impact of vascular access on acute kidney injury after percutaneous coronary intervention. *Cardiovasc. Revascularization Med. Mol. Interv.* **2016**, *17*, 333–338. [CrossRef] [PubMed]
85. Valgimigli, M.; Gagnor, A.; Calabrò, P.; Frigoli, E.; Leonardi, S.; Mazzarotto, P.; Rubartelli, P.; Briguori, C.; Andò, G.; Repetto, A.; et al. Radial versus femoral access in patients with acute coronary syndromes undergoing invasive management: A randomised multicentre trial. *Lancet* **2015**, *385*, 2465–2476. [CrossRef]
86. Vuurmans, T.; Byrne, J.; Fretz, E.; Janssen, C.; Hilton, J.D.; Klinke, W.P.; Djurdjev, O.; Levin, A. Chronic kidney injury in patients after cardiac catheterisation or percutaneous coronary intervention: A comparison of radial and femoral approaches (from the British Columbia Cardiac and Renal Registries). *Heart Br. Card Soc.* **2010**, *96*, 1538–1542. [CrossRef]
87. Scolari, F.; Ravani, P.; Gaggi, R.; Santostefano, M.; Rollino, C.; Stabellini, N.; Colla, L.; Viola, B.F.; Maiorca, P.; Venturelli, C.; et al. The challenge of diagnosing atheroembolic renal disease: Clinical features and prognostic factors. *Circulation* **2007**, *116*, 298–304. [CrossRef]
88. Azzalini, L.; Jolicoeur, E.M. The use of radial access decreases the risk of vascular access-site-related complications at a patient level but is associated with an increased risk at a population level: The radial paradox. *EuroIntervention* **2014**, *10*, 531–532. [CrossRef]
89. Damluji, A.; Cohen, M.G.; Smairat, R.; Steckbeck, R.; Moscucci, M.; Gilchrist, I.C. The incidence of acute kidney injury after cardiac catheterization or PCI: A comparison of radial vs. femoral approach. *Int. J. Cardiol.* **2014**, *173*, 595–597. [CrossRef]
90. Gili, S.; D'Ascenzo, F.; Di Summa, R.; Conrotto, F.; Cerrato, E.; Chieffo, A.; Boccuzzi, G.; Montefusco, A.; Ugo, F.; Omedé, P.; et al. Radial Versus Femoral Access for the Treatment of Left Main Lesion in the Era of Second-Generation Drug-Eluting Stents. *Am. J. Cardiol.* **2017**, *120*, 33–39. [CrossRef]
91. Valgimigli, M.; Frigoli, E.; Leonardi, S.; Vranckx, P.; Rothenbühler, M.; Tebaldi, M.; Varbella, F.; Calabrò, P.; Garducci, S.; Rubartelli, P.; et al. Radial versus femoral access and bivalirudin versus unfractionated heparin in invasively managed patients with acute coronary syndrome (MATRIX): Final 1-year results of a multicentre, randomised controlled trial. *Lancet* **2018**, *392*, 835–848. [CrossRef]
92. Andò, G.; Cortese, B.; Russo, F.; Rothenbühler, M.; Frigoli, E.; Gargiulo, G.; Briguori, C.; Vranckx, P.; Leonardi, S.; Guiducci, V.; et al. Acute Kidney Injury After Radial or Femoral Access for Invasive Acute Coronary Syndrome Management: AKI-MATRIX. *J. Am. Coll. Cardiol.* **2017**, *69*, 2592–2603. [CrossRef] [PubMed]
93. Rothenbühler, M.; Valgimigli, M.; Odutayo, A.; Frigoli, E.; Leonardi, S.; Vranckx, P.; Turturo, M.; Moretti, L.; Amico, F.; Uguccioni, L.; et al. Association of acute kidney injury and bleeding events with mortality after radial or femoral access in patients with acute coronary syndrome undergoing invasive management: Secondary analysis of a randomized clinical trial. *Eur. Heart J.* **2019**, *40*, 1226–1232. [CrossRef] [PubMed]
94. Wang, C.; Chen, W.; Yu, M.; Yang, P. Comparison of acute kidney injury with radial vs. femoral access for patients undergoing coronary catheterization: An updated meta-analysis of 46,816 patients. *Exp. Ther. Med.* **2020**, *20*, 1. [CrossRef] [PubMed]
95. Lai, J.; Akindavyi, G.; Fu, Q.; Li, Z.L.; Wang, H.M.; Wen, L.H. Research Progress on the Relationship between Coronary Artery Calcification and Chronic Renal Failure. *Chin. Med. J. Engl.* **2018**, *131*, 608–614. [CrossRef] [PubMed]
96. Kim, J.K.; Kim, N.-H.; Shin, I.S.; Noh, D.H.; Kim, Y.C.; Kim, S.H.; Choi, J.H.; Park, E.M.; Lee, S.J.; Yun, K.H.; et al. Alteration of Ventricular Repolarization by Intracoronary Infusion of Normal Saline in Patients With Variant Angina. *Korean Circ. J.* **2009**, *39*, 223–227. [CrossRef] [PubMed]
97. Sacha, J.; Gierlotka, M.; Feusette, P.; Dudek, D. Ultra-low contrast coronary angiography and zero-contrast percutaneous coronary intervention for prevention of contrast-induced nephropathy: Step-by-step approach and review. *Adv. Interv. Cardiol.* **2019**, *15*, 127–136. [CrossRef] [PubMed]
98. Nayak, K.R.; Mehta, H.S.; Price, M.J.; Russo, R.J.; Stinis, C.T.; Moses, J.W.; Mehran, R.; Leon, M.B.; Kandzari, D.E.; Teirstein, P.S. A novel technique for ultra-low contrast administration during angiography or intervention. *Catheter. Cardiovasc. Interv.* **2010**, *75*, 1076–1083. [CrossRef]

99. Imaging—And Physiology-Guided Percutaneous Coronary Intervention without Contrast Administration in Advanced Renal Failure: A Feasibility, Safety, and Outcome Study. *Eur. Heart J.* **2016**, *37*, 3090–3095. Available online: https://academic.oup.com/eurheartj/article/37/40/3090/2420804?login=false (accessed on 3 March 2022). [CrossRef]
100. Karimi Galougahi, K.; Mintz, G.S.; Karmpaliotis, D.; Ali, Z.A. Zero-contrast percutaneous coronary intervention on calcified lesions facilitated by rotational atherectomy. *Catheter. Cardiovasc. Interv.* **2017**, *90*, E85–E89. [CrossRef]
101. Hruska, K.; Mathew, S.; Lund, R.; Fang, Y.; Sugatani, T. Cardiovascular risk factors in chronic kidney disease: Does phosphate qualify? *Kidney Int. Suppl.* **2011**, *79*, S9–S13. [CrossRef]
102. Madhavan, M.V.; Tarigopula, M.; Mintz, G.S.; Maehara, A.; Stone, G.W.; Généreux, P. Coronary artery calcification: Pathogenesis and prognostic implications. *J. Am. Coll. Cardiol.* **2014**, *63*, 1703–1714. [CrossRef] [PubMed]
103. Chonchol, M.; Whittle, J.; Desbien, A.; Orner, M.B.; Petersen, L.A.; Kressin, N.R. Chronic kidney disease is associated with angiographic coronary artery disease. *Am. J. Nephrol.* **2008**, *28*, 354–360. [CrossRef] [PubMed]
104. Coskun, U.; Kilickesmez, K.O.; Abaci, O.; Kocas, C.; Bostan, C.; Yildiz, A.; Baskurt, M.; Arat, A.; Ersanli, M.K.; Gurmen, T. The relationship between chronic kidney disease and SYNTAX score. *Angiology* **2011**, *62*, 504–508. [CrossRef] [PubMed]
105. Herzog, C.A.; Ma, J.Z.; Collins, A.J. Poor long-term survival after acute myocardial infarction among patients on long-term dialysis. *N. Engl. J. Med.* **1998**, *339*, 799–805. [CrossRef] [PubMed]
106. Anavekar, N.S.; McMurray, J.J.V.; Velazquez, E.J.; Solomon, S.D.; Kober, L.; Rouleau, J.-L.; White, H.D.; Nordlander, R.; Maggioni, A.P.; Dickstein, K.; et al. Relation between renal dysfunction and cardiovascular outcomes after myocardial infarction. *N. Engl. J. Med.* **2004**, *351*, 1285–1295. [CrossRef] [PubMed]
107. Szummer, K.; Lundman, P.; Jacobson, S.H.; Schön, S.; Lindbäck, J.; Stenestrand, U.; Wallentin, L.; Jernberg, T. Relation between renal function, presentation, use of therapies and in-hospital complications in acute coronary syndrome: Data from the Swedeheart register. *J. Intern. Med.* **2010**, *268*, 40–49. [CrossRef]
108. Ezekowitz, J.; McAlister, F.A.; Humphries, K.H.; Norris, C.; Tonelli, M.; Ghali, W.A.; Knudtson, M.L. The association among renal insufficiency, pharmacotherapy, and outcomes in 6427 patients with heart failure and coronary artery disease. *J. Am. Coll. Cardiol.* **2004**, *44*, 1587–1592. [CrossRef]
109. Konstantinidis, I.; Patel, S.; Camargo, M.; Patel, A.; Poojary, P.; Coca, S.G.; Nadkarni, G.N. Repres.sentation and reporting of kidney disease in cerebrovascular disease: A systematic review of randomized controlled trials. *PLoS ONE* **2017**, *12*, e0176145. [CrossRef]
110. Baber, U.; Stone, G.W.; Weisz, G.; Moreno, P.; Dangas, G.; Maehara, A.; Mintz, G.S.; Cristea, E.; Fahy, M.; Xu, K.; et al. Coronary plaque composition, morphology, and outcomes in patients with and without chronic kidney disease presenting with acute coronary syndromes. *JACC Cardiovasc. Imaging* **2012**, *5*, S53–S61. [CrossRef]
111. Park, D.-W.; Kim, Y.-H.; Yun, S.-C.; Ahn, J.-M.; Lee, J.-Y.; Kim, W.-J.; Kang, S.-J.; Lee, S.-W.; Lee, C.W.; Park, S.-W. Frequency, causes, predictors, and clinical significance of peri-procedural myocardial infarction following percutaneous coronary intervention. *Eur. Heart J.* **2013**, *34*, 1662–1669. [CrossRef]
112. Zeitouni, M.; Silvain, J.; Guedeney, P.; Kerneis, M.; Yan, Y.; Overtchouk, P.; Barthelemy, O.; Hauguel-Moreau, M.; Choussat, R.; Helft, G.; et al. Periprocedural myocardial infarction and injury in elective coronary stenting. *Eur. Heart J.* **2018**, *39*, 1100–1109. [CrossRef] [PubMed]
113. Valgimigli, M.; Patialiakas, A.; Thury, A.; McFadden, E.; Colangelo, S.; Campo, G.; Tebaldi, M.; Ungi, I.; Tondi, S.; Roffi, M.; et al. Zotarolimus-Eluting Versus Bare-Metal Stents in Uncertain Drug-Eluting Stent Candidates. *J. Am. Coll. Cardiol.* **2015**, *65*, 805–815. [CrossRef] [PubMed]
114. Ariotti, S.; Adamo, M.; Costa, F.; Patialiakas, A.; Briguori, C.; Thury, A.; Colangelo, S.; Campo, G.; Tebaldi, M.; Ungi, I.; et al. Is Bare-Metal Stent Implantation Still Justifiable in High Bleeding Risk Patients Undergoing Percutaneous Coronary Intervention? A Pre-Specified Analysis from the ZEUS Trial. *JACC Cardiovasc. Interv.* **2016**, *9*, 426–436. [CrossRef] [PubMed]
115. Crimi, G.; Leonardi, S.; Costa, F.; Adamo, M.; Ariotti, S.; Valgimigli, M. Role of stent type and of duration of dual antiplatelet therapy in patients with chronic kidney disease undergoing percutaneous coronary interventions. Is bare metal stent implantation still a justifiable choice? A post-hoc analysis of the all comer PRODIGY trial. *Int. J. Cardiol.* **2016**, *212*, 110–117. [CrossRef] [PubMed]
116. Bangalore, S.; Guo, Y.; Samadashvili, Z.; Blecker, S.; Xu, J.; Hannan, E.L. Revascularization in Patients With Multivessel Coronary Artery Disease and Chronic Kidney Disease: Everolimus-Eluting Stents Versus Coronary Artery Bypass Graft Surgery. *J. Am. Coll. Cardiol.* **2015**, *66*, 1209–1220. [CrossRef] [PubMed]
117. Wiviott, S.D.; Braunwald, E.; McCabe, C.H.; Montalescot, G.; Ruzyllo, W.; Gottlieb, S.; Neumann, F.-J.; Ardissino, D.; De Servi, S.; Murphy, S.A.; et al. Prasugrel versus Clopidogrel in Patients with Acute Coronary Syndromes. *N. Engl. J. Med.* **2007**, *357*, 2001–2015. [CrossRef] [PubMed]
118. Wallentin, L.; Becker, R.C.; Budaj, A.; Cannon, C.P.; Emanuelsson, H.; Held, C.; Horrow, J.; Husted, S.; James, S.; Katus, H.; et al. Ticagrelor versus Clopidogrel in Patients with Acute Coronary Syndromes. *N. Engl. J. Med.* **2009**, *361*, 1045–1057. [CrossRef]
119. Giustino, G.; Costa, F. Characterization of the Individual Patient Risk After Percutaneous Coronary Intervention: At the Crossroads of Bleeding and Thrombosis. *JACC Cardiovasc. Interv.* **2019**, *12*, 831–834. [CrossRef]
120. Matsuo, T.; Koide, M.; Kario, K.; Suzuki, S.; Matsuo, M. Extrinsic Coagulation Factors and Tissue Factor Pathway Inhibitor in End-Stage Chronic Renal Failure. *Pathophysiol. Haemost. Thromb.* **1997**, *27*, 163–167. [CrossRef]

121. Landray, M.J.; Wheeler, D.C.; Lip, G.Y.; Newman, D.J.; Blann, A.D.; McGlynn, F.J.; Ball, S.; Townend, J.; Baigent, C. Inflammation, endothelial dysfunction, and platelet activation in patients with chronic kidney disease: The chronic renal impairment in Birmingham (CRIB) study. *Am. J. Kidney Dis.* **2004**, *43*, 244–253. [CrossRef]
122. Eknoyan, G., III; Brown, I.C.H. Biochemical Abnormallities of Platelets in Renal Failure. *Am. J. Nephrol.* **1981**, *1*, 17–23. [CrossRef] [PubMed]
123. Benigni, A.; Boccardo, P.; Galbusera, M.; Monteagudo, J.; De Marco, L.; Remuzzi, G.; Ruggeri, Z.M. Reversible Activation Defect of the Platelet Glycoprotein IIb-IIIa Complex in Patients With Uremia. *Am. J. Kidney Dis.* **1993**, *22*, 668–676. [CrossRef]
124. Park, S.H.; Kim, W.; Park, C.S.; Kang, W.Y.; Hwang, S.H.; Kim, W. A Comparison of Clopidogrel Responsiveness in Patients With Versus Without Chronic Renal Failure. *Am. J. Cardiol.* **2009**, *104*, 1292–1295. [CrossRef] [PubMed]
125. Franchi, F.; James, S.K.; Lakic, T.G.; Budaj, A.J.; Cornel, J.H.; Katus, H.A.; Keltai, M.; Kontny, F.; Lewis, B.S.; Storey, R.F.; et al. Impact of Diabetes Mellitus and Chronic Kidney Disease on Cardiovascular Outcomes and Platelet P2Y12 Receptor Antagonist Effects in Patients With Acute Coronary Syndromes: Insights From the PLATO Trial. *J. Am. Heart Assoc.* **2019**, *8*, e011139. [CrossRef] [PubMed]
126. Baber, U.; Mehran, R.; Kirtane, A.J.; Gurbel, P.A.; Christodoulidis, G.; Maehara, A.; Witzenbichler, B.; Weisz, G.; Rinaldi, M.J.; Metzger, D.C.; et al. Prevalence and Impact of High Platelet Reactivity in Chronic Kidney Disease. *Circ. Cardiovasc. Interv.* **2015**, *8*, e001683. [CrossRef]
127. Rollini, F.; Cho, J.R.; DeGroat, C.; Bhatti, M.; Alobaidi, Z.; Ferrante, E.; Jakubowski, J.A.; Sugidachi, A.; Zenni, M.M.; Bass, T.A.; et al. Impact of chronic kidney disease on platelet P2Y12 receptor signalling in patients with type 2 diabetes mellitus. *Thromb. Haemost.* **2017**, *117*, 201–203. [CrossRef]
128. Tantry, U.S.; Bonello, L.; Aradi, D.; Price, M.J.; Jeong, Y.-H.; Angiolillo, D.J.; Stone, G.W.; Curzen, N.; Geisler, T.; ten Berg, J.; et al. Consensus and Update on the Definition of On-Treatment Platelet Reactivity to Adenosine Diphosphate Associated With Ischemia and Bleeding. *J. Am. Coll. Cardiol.* **2013**, *62*, 2261–2273. [CrossRef]
129. Morel, O.; El Ghannudi, S.; Jesel, L.; Radulescu, B.; Meyer, N.; Wiesel, M.-L.; Caillard, S.; Campia, U.; Moulin, B.; Gachet, C.; et al. Cardiovascular Mortality in Chronic Kidney Disease Patients Undergoing Percutaneous Coronary Intervention Is Mainly Related to Impaired P2Y12 Inhibition by Clopidogrel. *J. Am. Coll. Cardiol.* **2011**, *57*, 399–408. [CrossRef]
130. Best, P.J.; Steinhubl, S.R.; Berger, P.B.; Dasgupta, A.; Brennan, D.M.; Szczech, L.A.; Califf, R.M.; Topol, E. The efficacy and safety of short- and long-term dual antiplatelet therapy in patients with mild or moderate chronic kidney disease: Results from the Clopidogrel for the Reduction of Events During Observation (CREDO) Trial. *Am. Heart J.* **2008**, *155*, 687–693. [CrossRef]
131. Wang, H.; Qi, J.; Li, Y.; Tang, Y.; Li, C.; Li, J.; Han, Y. Pharmacodynamics and pharmacokinetics of ticagrelor vs. clopidogrel in patients with acute coronary syndromes and chronic kidney disease. *Br. J. Clin. Pharmacol.* **2018**, *84*, 88–96. [CrossRef]
132. Small, D.S.; Wrishko, R.E.; Ii, C.S.E.; Ni, L.; Winters, K.J.; Farid, N.A.; Li, Y.G.; Brandt, J.T.; Salazar, D.E.; Borel, A.G.; et al. Prasugrel pharmacokinetics and pharmacodynamics in subjects with moderate renal impairment and end-stage renal disease. *J. Clin. Pharm. Ther.* **2009**, *34*, 585–594. [CrossRef] [PubMed]
133. Nishi, T.; Ariyoshi, N.; Nakayama, T.; Fujimoto, Y.; Sugimoto, K.; Wakabayashi, S.; Hanaoka, H.; Kobayashi, Y. Impact of chronic kidney disease on platelet inhibition of clopidogrel and prasugrel in Japanese patients. *J. Cardiol.* **2017**, *69*, 752–755. [CrossRef] [PubMed]
134. Cannon, C.P.; A Harrington, R.; James, S.; Ardissino, D.; Becker, R.C.; Emanuelsson, H.; Husted, S.; Katus, H.; Keltai, M.; Khurmi, N.S.; et al. Comparison of ticagrelor with clopidogrel in patients with a planned invasive strategy for acute coronary syndromes (PLATO): A randomised double-blind study. *Lancet* **2010**, *375*, 283–293. [CrossRef]
135. Edfors, R.; Sahlén, A.; Szummer, K.; Renlund, H.; Evans, M.; Carrero, J.-J.; Spaak, J.; James, S.K.; Lagerqvist, B.; Varenhorst, C.; et al. Outcomes in patients treated with ticagrelor versus clopidogrel after acute myocardial infarction stratified by renal function. *Heart* **2018**, *104*, 1575–1582. [CrossRef]
136. Melloni, C.; Cornel, J.; Hafley, G.; Neely, M.L.; Clemmensen, P.; Zamoryakhin, D.; Prabhakaran, D.; White, H.D.; Fox, K.; Ohman, E.M.; et al. Impact of chronic kidney disease on long-term ischemic and bleeding outcomes in medically managed patients with acute coronary syndromes: Insights from the TRILOGY ACS Trial. *Eur. Heart J. Acute Cardiovasc. Care* **2016**, *5*, 443–454. [CrossRef]
137. Collet, J.-P.; Roffi, M.; Byrne, R.A.; Costa, F.; Valgimigli, M.; Bueno, H.; Jeppsson, A.; Jüni, P.; Kastrati, A.; Kolh, P.; et al. Case-based implementation of the 2017 ESC Focused Update on Dual Antiplatelet Therapy in Coronary Artery Disease. *Eur. Heart J.* **2018**, *39*, e1–e33. [CrossRef]
138. Costa, F.; Adamo, M.; Ariotti, S.; Ferrante, G.; Navarese, E.P.; Leonardi, S.; Garcia-Garcia, H.; Vranckx, P.; Valgimigli, M. Left main or proximal left anterior descending coronary artery disease location identifies high-risk patients deriving potentially greater benefit from prolonged dual antiplatelet therapy duration. *EuroIntervention* **2016**, *11*, e1222–e1230. [CrossRef]
139. Costa, F.; van Klaveren, D.; James, S.; Heg, D.; Räber, L.; Feres, F.; Pilgrim, T.; Hong, M.-K.; Kim, H.-S.; Colombo, A.; et al. Derivation and validation of the predicting bleeding complications in patients undergoing stent implantation and subsequent dual antiplatelet therapy (PRECISE-DAPT) score: A pooled analysis of individual-patient datasets from clinical trials. *Lancet* **2017**, *389*, 1025–1034. [CrossRef]
140. Gargiulo, G.; Santucci, A.; Piccolo, R.; Franzone, A.; Ariotti, S.; Baldo, A.; Esposito, G.; Moschovitis, A.; Windecker, S.; Valgimigli, M. Impact of chronic kidney disease on 2-year clinical outcomes in patients treated with 6-month or 24-month DAPT duration: An analysis from the PRODIGY trial. *Catheter. Cardiovasc. Interv.* **2017**, *90*, E73–E84. [CrossRef]

141. Costa, F.; Van Klaveren, D.; Feres, F.; James, S.; Räber, L.; Pilgrim, T.; Hong, M.-K.; Kim, H.-S.; Colombo, A.; Steg, P.G.; et al. Dual Antiplatelet Therapy Duration Based on Ischemic and Bleeding Risks After Coronary Stenting. *J. Am. Coll. Cardiol.* **2019**, *73*, 741–754. [CrossRef]
142. Gargiulo, G.; Costa, F.; Ariotti, S.; Biscaglia, S.; Campo, G.; Esposito, G.; Leonardi, S.; Vranckx, P.; Windecker, S.; Valgimigli, M. Impact of proton pump inhibitors on clinical outcomes in patients treated with a 6- or 24-month dual-antiplatelet therapy duration: Insights from the PROlonging Dual-antiplatelet treatment after Grading stent-induced Intimal hyperplasia studY trial. *Am. Heart J.* **2016**, *174*, 95–102. [CrossRef] [PubMed]
143. Reinecke, H.; Brand, E.; Mesters, R.; Schäbitz, W.-R.; Fisher, M.; Pavenstädt, H.; Breithardt, G. Dilemmas in the management of atrial fibrillation in chronic kidney disease. *J. Am. Soc. Nephrol.* **2009**, *20*, 705–711. [CrossRef] [PubMed]
144. Andò, G.; Costa, F. Double or triple antithrombotic therapy after coronary stenting and atrial fibrillation: A systematic review and meta-analysis of randomized clinical trials. *Int. J. Cardiol.* **2020**, *302*, 95–102. [CrossRef] [PubMed]
145. Costa, F.; Valgimigli, M.; Steg, P.G.; Bhatt, D.L.; Hohnloser, S.H.; Ten Berg, J.M.; Miede, C.; Nordaby, M.; Lip, G.Y.; Oldgren, J.; et al. Antithrombotic Therapy according to Baseline Bleeding Risk in Patients with Atrial Fibrillation Undergoing Percutaneous Coronary Intervention: Applying the PRECISE-DAPT Score in RE-DUAL PCI. *Eur. Heart J.* **2020**. Available online: https://academic.oup.com/ehjcvp/advance-article/doi/10.1093/ehjcvp/pvaa135/6015238 (accessed on 16 April 2022).
146. Hijazi, Z.; Alexander, J.H.; Li, Z.; Wojdyla, D.M.; Mehran, R.; Granger, C.B.; Parkhomenko, A.; Bahit, M.C.; Windecker, S.; Aronson, R.; et al. Apixaban or Vitam.min K Antagonists and Aspirin or Placebo according to Kidney Function in Patients with Atrial Fibrillation after Acute Coronary Syndrome or Percutaneous Coronary Intervention: Insights from the AUGUSTUS Trial. *Circulation.* **2021**, *143*, 1215–1223. [CrossRef] [PubMed]
147. Hohnloser, S.H.; Steg, P.G.; Oldgren, J.; Nickenig, G.; Kiss, R.G.; Ongen, Z.; Estrada, J.L.N.; Ophuis, T.O.; Lip, G.Y.; Nordaby, M.; et al. Renal Function and Outcomes With Dabigatran Dual Antithrombotic Therapy in Atrial Fibrillation Patients After PCI. *JACC Cardiovasc. Interv.* **2019**, *12*, 1553–1561. [CrossRef]
148. Jamrozik, K. Age-specific relevance of usual blood pressure to vascular mortality: A meta-analysis of individual data for one million adults in 61 prospective studies. *Lancet* **2002**, *360*, 1903–1913. [CrossRef]
149. Sim, J.J.; Shi, J.; Kovesdy, C.P.; Kalantar-Zadeh, K.; Jacobsen, S.J. Impact of achieved blood pressures on mortality risk and end-stage renal disease among a large, diverse hypertension population. *J. Am. Coll. Cardiol.* **2014**, *64*, 588–597. [CrossRef]
150. Upadhyay, A.; Earley, A.; Haynes, S.M.; Uhlig, K. Systematic review: Blood pressure target in chronic kidney disease and proteinuria as an effect modifier. *Ann. Intern. Med.* **2011**, *154*, 541–548. [CrossRef]
151. Cheung, A.K.; Rahman, M.; Reboussin, D.M.; Craven, T.E.; Greene, T.; Kimmel, P.L.; Cushman, W.C.; Hawfield, A.T.; Johnson, K.C.; Lewis, C.E.; et al. Effects of Intensive BP Control in CKD. *J. Am. Soc. Nephrol.* **2017**, *28*, 2812–2823. [CrossRef]
152. Bakris, G.L.; A Sarafidis, P.; Weir, M.R.; Dahlöf, B.; Pitt, B.; Jamerson, K.; Velazquez, E.J.; Staikos-Byrne, L.; Kelly, R.Y.; Shi, V.; et al. Renal outcomes with different fixed-dose combination therapies in patients with hypertension at high risk for cardiovascular events (ACCOMPLISH): A prespecified secondary analysis of a randomised controlled trial. *Lancet Lond. Engl.* **2010**, *375*, 1173–1181. [CrossRef]
153. Mancia, G.; Fagard, R.; Narkiewicz, K.; Redon, J.; Zanchetti, A.; Böhm, M.; Christiaens, T.; Cifkova, R.; De Backer, G.; Dominiczak, A.; et al. 2013 ESH/ESC Guidelines for the management of arterial hypertension: The Task Force for the management of arterial hypertension of the European Society of Hypertension (ESH) and of the European Society of Cardiology (ESC). *Eur. Heart J.* **2013**, *34*, 2159–2219. [CrossRef] [PubMed]
154. Authors/Task Force Members, ESC Committee for Practice Guidelines (CPG), ESC National Cardiac Societies. 2019 ESC/EAS guidelines for the management of dyslipidaemias: Lipid modification to reduce cardiovascular risk. *Atherosclerosis* **2019**, *290*, 140–205. [CrossRef] [PubMed]
155. Wanner, C.; Tonelli, M. Kidney Disease: Improving Global Outcomes Lipid Guideline Development Work Group Members. KDIGO Clinical Practice Guideline for Lipid Management in CKD: Summary of recommendation statements and clinical approach to the patient. *Kidney Int.* **2014**, *85*, 1303–1309. [CrossRef] [PubMed]
156. Mach, F.; Ray, K.K.; Wiklund, O.; Corsini, A.; Catapano, A.L.; Bruckert, E.; De Backer, G.; A Hegele, R.; Hovingh, G.K.; A Jacobson, T.; et al. Adverse effects of statin therapy: Perception vs. the evidence—Focus on glucose homeostasis, cognitive, renal and hepatic function, haemorrhagic stroke and cataract. *Eur. Heart J.* **2018**, *39*, 2526–2539. [CrossRef] [PubMed]

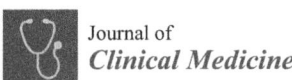

Article

Hospital-Acquired Functional Decline and Clinical Outcomes in Older Cardiac Surgical Patients: A Multicenter Prospective Cohort Study

Tomoyuki Morisawa [1,*], Masakazu Saitoh [1], Shota Otsuka [2], Go Takamura [3], Masayuki Tahara [4], Yusuke Ochi [5], Yo Takahashi [6], Kentaro Iwata [7], Keisuke Oura [8], Koji Sakurada [9] and Tetsuya Takahashi [1]

[1] Faculty of Health Science, Juntendo University, 3-2-12 Hongo, Bunkyo-ku, Ochanomizu Center Building 5F, Tokyo 113-0033, Japan; m.saito.tl@juntendo.ac.jp (M.S.); te-takahashi@juntendo.ac.jp (T.T.)
[2] Department of Rehabilitation, The Sakakibara Heart Institute of Okayama, 2-5-1 Nakai-Cho, Kita-ku, Okayama 700-0804, Japan; qqqz3sm9k@gmail.com
[3] Department of Rehabilitation, Tsuchiya General Hospital, 3-30 Nakajima-Cho, Hiroshima 730-8655, Japan; reha-pt@tsuchiya-hp.jp
[4] Department of Physical Therapy, Higashi Takarazuka Satoh Hospital, 2-1 Nagao-Cho, Takarazuka-shi 665-0873, Japan; m-tahara@mail.hts-hsp.com
[5] Department of Rehabilitation, Fukuyama Cardiovascular Hospital, 2-39 Midori-Cho, Fukuyama-shi 720-0804, Japan; fch_reha@yahoo.co.jp
[6] Department of Rehabilitation, Yuuai Medical Center, 50-5 Azayone, Tomishiro, Okinawa 901-0224, Japan; yo.takahashi7448@gmail.com
[7] Department of Rehabilitation, Kobe City Medical Center General Hospital, 1-1-2 Minatojimaminami-Cho, Chuo-ku, Kobe-shi 650-0047, Japan; iwaken@kcho.jp
[8] Department of Rehabilitation, Nozomi Heart Clinic, 3-5-36 Miyahara, Yodogawa-ku, Osaka-shi 532-0003, Japan; oura30155@gmail.com
[9] Department of Rehabilitation, The Cardiovascular Institute, 3-2-19 Nishiazabu, Minato-ku, Tokyo 106-0031, Japan; sakura282517@gmail.com
* Correspondence: t.morisawa.ul@juntendo.ac.jp; Tel.: +81-3-3813-3111

Abstract: This study aimed to determine the effect of hospital-acquired functional decline (HAFD) on prognosis, 1-year post-hospital discharge, of older patients who had undergone cardiac surgery in seven Japanese hospitals between June 2017 and June 2018. This multicenter prospective cohort study involved 247 patients with cardiac disease aged ≥ 65 years. HAFD was defined as a decrease in the short physical performance battery at hospital discharge compared with before surgery. Primary outcomes included a composite outcome of frailty severity, total mortality, and cardiovascular readmission 1-year post-hospital discharge. Secondary outcomes were changes in the total score and sub-item scores in the Ki-hon Checklist (KCL), assessed pre- and 1-year postoperatively. Poor prognostic outcomes were observed in 33% of patients, and multivariate analysis identified HAFD (odds ratio [OR] 3.43, 95% confidence interval [CI] 1.75–6.72, $p < 0.001$) and low preoperative gait speed (OR 2.47, 95% CI 1.18–5.17, $p = 0.016$) as independent predictors of poor prognosis. Patients with HAFD had significantly worse total KCL scores and subscale scores for instrumental activities of daily living, mobility, oral function, and depression at 1-year post-hospital discharge. HAFD is a powerful predictor of prognosis in older patients who have undergone cardiac surgery.

Keywords: outcome assessment; functional decline; cardiovascular disease; cardiac surgery

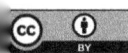

1. Introduction

It is important to assess the physical function of older cardiac surgical patients before surgery because poor physical function, which includes preoperative gait speed [1–3], frailty [4,5], and sarcopenia [6], is an independent poor prognostic factor. In particular, the gait speed is a simple and powerful assessment of physical function in older adults and is also used as a diagnostic criterion for frailty and sarcopenia [7–9]. In fact, previous studies have demonstrated that there is an association between gait speed and poor short-term prognosis in patients undergoing coronary artery bypass grafting or valvular surgery, suggesting that it is a crucial assessment tool in predicting the prognosis of older cardiac surgical patients [2,3].

Recently, hospital-acquired functional decline (HAFD) has garnered attention as a novel predictor of poor prognosis for hospitalized older patients. HAFD, which refers to the functional decline that develops in at least 20–40% of hospitalized older patients, can either be newly developed or a pre-existent condition that worsened during hospitalization [10–13]. HAFD is assessed by whether pre-hospital activities of daily living (ADL), instrumental ADL (IADL), or physical function have recovered at discharge, and it is reported to be related to in-hospital mobility and nutritional intake [11]. HAFD is a powerful poor prognostic predictor for hospitalized older patients [12–15], and the occurrence of HAFD in older cardiac surgical patients may be a prognostic predictor independent of preoperative low gait speed. However, the incidence of HAFD in older cardiac surgical patients, and the effect of HAFD occurrence on prognosis, are unclear.

Therefore, the purpose of this study was to determine the frequency of HAFD in older cardiac surgical patients and to examine whether the occurrence of HAFD is associated with a composite poor prognosis (severity of frailty, death, and cardiovascular readmission) one year after discharge.

2. Materials and Methods

This was a multicenter, prospective cohort study. A total of 281 patients with heart disease, aged ≥65 years, underwent elective cardiac surgery (coronary artery bypass graft, valvular disease surgery, or combined surgery) in seven Japanese hospitals between June 2017 and June 2018. The following exclusion criteria were applied: (1) a diagnosis of dementia; (2) an inability to walk independently or having bed rest due to severe preoperative heart failure; (3) in-hospital death; (4) data loss; (5) missing follow-up data.

2.1. Progression of Postoperative Rehabilitation

All patients started rehabilitation, under the guidance of a physiotherapist, the day after surgery. The postoperative rehabilitation protocol used for this study followed the Japanese Circulation Society Guidelines for the Rehabilitation of Patients with Cardiovascular Disease [16]. The rehabilitation started with active and passive movements in bed, with the ADL being extended gradually to sitting on the edge of the bed, standing, walking, aerobic exercise, and resistance training. Rehabilitation was performed five times per week for 60 min/day until the day before discharge.

2.2. Clinical Outcomes

The primary outcome included the composite outcomes of the severity of frailty, death, and cardiovascular readmission one year after hospital discharge. The severity of frailty is defined as a progression in the frailty category, during the one year after hospital discharge, compared with the preoperative status. The severity of frailty was assessed using the Kihon Checklist [17]. The KCL is a questionnaire that consists of 25 questions that can be answered with a yes/no. Overall scores can be stratified into three levels: robust (0–3 points), pre-frail (4–7 points), and frail (≥8 points) [18].

The secondary outcome was the change in the total scores and the scores of the seven domains of the KCL, administered preoperatively and one year postoperatively, in both groups (HAFD group vs. non-HAFD group). The 25 questions of the KCL are categorized into seven domains: IADL, mobility, nutrition, oral function, social, cognitive, and depression, enabling the analysis for each domain. This was important, as it allowed the problematic domains to be identified.

2.3. Definition of HAFD

HAFD was defined as a decrease in at least one point on the short physical performance battery (SPPB) before discharge compared to the score obtained before cardiac surgery [12,19]. The SPPB is a highly standardized geriatric physical functioning test that consists of assessments for balance, gait, strength, and endurance [20], and it is the highest recommended index in terms of validity, reliability, and responsiveness among the various physical function assessments used clinically in older adults [21]. Guralnik et al. reported that a 1-point change in the SPPB score results in a meaningful difference in mortality and risk of nursing home admission [20], with a minimal clinically important difference of one point [22]. Since the minimal clinically important difference in older cardiac patients who undergo rehabilitation during the hospitalization period is approximately one point, the HAFD in this study was defined as a decrease in the SPPB at discharge of at least one point from the preoperative level [23,24].

2.4. Clinical Characteristics and Measurements of Physical Function

The age, sex, body mass index (BMI), New York Heart Association cardiac function classification, comorbidity, and data from previous medical histories, as well as the results of investigations (left ventricular ejection fraction, hemoglobin, albumin, and estimated glomerular filtration ratio) were obtained from the medical records. All the preoperative clinical data were measured or obtained between the day before the surgery and the day of the surgery. Preoperative frailty was defined as a total KCL score of ≥ 8 points [18]. Data regarding surgical procedure, operation time, and intraoperative bleeding were collected from the surgical records. The postoperative course of the patients was recorded as the number of days spent in the intensive care unit, the postoperative day on which rehabilitation started, the postoperative day on which ambulation started and when ambulation independence was achieved, and the duration of the hospital stay.

The physical function was assessed using the SPPB, grip strength, and gait speed before surgery and at discharge. The SPPB was assessed using the SPPB manual [20]. The grip strength was measured with a Jamar hand grip dynamometer (Nihon Medix, Chiba, Japan), with the patients seated on a chair, their knees bent at 90° flexion, and the forearms in a neutral position. The gait speed was measured using a 4-m course, with the patients instructed to walk from the start to finish at their normal pace, while a stopwatch measured the time it took for them to finish the course. This test was performed twice, and the shortest time taken was used for the analysis.

The Asian Working Group for Sarcopenia specified the cut-off values for diagnosing sarcopenia as a grip strength of 26 kg for men, 18 kg for women and a gait speed of 0.8 m/s [8]. Preoperative grip strength and gait speeds below the cut-off values were defined as "low preoperative gait speed" and "low preoperative grip strength."

2.5. One-Year Follow-Up Data

One year after discharge from the hospital, follow-up surveys were conducted by mail to determine patient survival, cardiovascular-related readmissions, and the KCL score.

Statistical Analysis

Continuous variables were expressed as median (interquartile range [IQR]), because they were not normally distributed, and categorical variables were expressed as number and percentage. The two groups (HAFD and non-HAFD groups) were compared using the chi-square test, for categorical covariates, or the Mann–Whitney U-test. A 2-sided p-value < 0.05 was considered statistically significant. Univariate and multivariate analyses were used to determine the odds ratio for each factor, to extract factors involved in the primary outcome of poor prognosis, one year after hospital discharge in an exploratory manner. To determine the influence of the relationship between the outcomes, variables with p-values <0.05 in the univariate analysis, and those deemed to be clinically important, were entered into a multivariate analysis. To avoid collinearity, the correlation coefficients between each parameter were determined and confirmed as not highly correlated. In a sub-analysis examining the interaction between HAFD and low preoperative gait speed, which increases the risk of poor prognosis, the patients were divided into four groups, according to HAFD and low preoperative gait speed, and logistic regression analysis was performed with poor prognosis as the dependent variable. A two-way analysis of variance was used for the secondary outcome and the change in preoperative and postoperative KCL scores between the two groups. All analyses were performed using IBM SPSS Statistics for Windows, Version 21.0 (IBM Corp., Armonk, NY, USA).

3. Results

3.1. Study Population and Incidence of HAFD

Among the 281 patients who were enrolled in the study initially, 34 patients were excluded, including 2 patients who died in-hospital, 10 patients whose data was lost, and 22 who had missing follow-up data. The baseline demographics and characteristics of the study population are shown in Tables 1 and 2. By definition, 52 of 247 patients (21%) experienced HAFD after cardiac surgery.

The HAFD group had a significantly higher percentage of females, higher rates of chronic obstructive pulmonary disease (COPD), and lower preoperative hemoglobin levels, as well as grip strength, compared to the non-HAFD group. The HAFD group also had a significantly lower SPPB at discharge compared to the non-HAFD group.

3.2. Association between HAFD and the Primary Outcome

The primary outcome, poor prognosis, was observed in 82 patients (33%), severity of frailty in 57 patients (23%), death in four patients (2%), and cardiovascular-related rehospitalization in 21 patients (9%). After performing the univariate analysis, the age, sex, BMI, left ventricular ejection fraction, hemoglobin level, low preoperative gait speed, operative time, and HAFD were included in the multivariate regression analysis (Table 2). The results showed that HAFD (OR 3.437, 95% CI 1.756–6.729, $p < 0.001$), and low preoperative gait speed (OR 2.477, 95% CI 1.185–5.176, $p = 0.016$) were associated independently with poor prognosis.

Figure 1 shows the risk of poor prognosis for the interaction between low preoperative gait speed and HAFD. The combination of both low preoperative gait speed and HAFD (OR 12.84, 95% CI 2.61–63.08) showed a greater increase in the incidence of poor prognostic outcomes compared to low preoperative gait speed (OR 2.14, 95% CI 0.99–4.61) or HAFD (OR 3.21, 95% CI 1.59–6.50) alone.

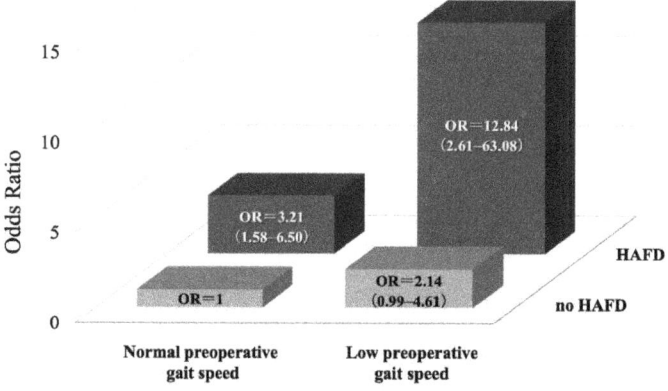

Figure 1. The interplay between low preoperative gait speed and HAFD increases the risk of poor prognosis. OR, odds ratio; HAFD, hospitalization-acquired functional decline.

Table 1. Patient clinical characteristics.

	All (n = 247)	HAFD Group (n = 52)	Non-HAFD Group (n = 195)	p-Value
Age, years	74.0 (69, 79)	75.0 (69, 80)	75.0 (68, 80)	0.231
Sex, female, % (n)	38 (95)	50 (26)	35 (69)	0.040 *
Body mass index, kg/m^2	23.1 (21.0, 25.3)	23.1 (19.8, 25.4)	23.6 (21.8, 25.6)	0.222
NYHA class, % (n) Class I/ Class II/ Class III/ Class IV	38 (94)/52 (129)/9 (21)/1 (3)	44 (23)/46 (24)/10 (5)/0 (0)	37 (71)/54 (105)/8 (16)/1 (3)	0.568
LVEF, %	63 (55, 70)	64 (55, 71)	64 (56, 71)	0.640
Comorbidity				
Diabetes mellitus, % (n)	34 (84)	44 (23)	31 (61)	0.058
Chronic kidney disease, % (n)	22 (55)	25 (13)	18 (35)	0.323
Chronic heart failure, % (n)	39 (95)	35 (18)	40 (77)	0.631
Chronic obstructive pulmonary disease, % (%(n)	6 (14)	14 (7)	4 (7)	0.013 *
Cerebrovascular disease, % (n)	15 (32)	14 (7)	13 (25)	0.530
Hemoglobin, g/dL	12.9 (11.6, 14.1)	12.5 (11.6, 13.6)	13.3 (11.7, 14.5)	0.025*
Albumin, g/dl	4.0 (3.7, 4.2)	4.1 (3.8, 4.2)	4.0 (3.7, 4.2)	0.787
eGFR, ml/min/1.73 m^2	59.3 (44.3, 70.1)	56.0 (38.6, 65.9)	59.3 (45.7, 70.8)	0.117
Preoperative SPPB score, points	12 (10, 12)	12 (11, 12)	12 (11, 12)	0.199
Postoperative SPPB score, points	12 (10, 12)	10 (9, 11)	12 (11, 12)	<0.001 *
Preoperative gait speed, m/s	0.98 (0.83, 1.13)	0.97 (0.82, 1.04)	1.03 (0.88, 1.16)	0.152
Preoperative grip strength, kg	23.7 (17.9, 31.0)	20.2 (16.3, 26.7)	25.0 (18.5, 32.1)	0.002 *
Preoperative frailty, % (n)	25 (61)	29 (15)	24 (46)	0.470
Type of Operation, % (n) CABG/Valve surgery/ Multiple valve surgery/ CABG + valve surgery	26 (64)/32 (80) 23 (56) 19 (47)	27 (14)/31 (16) 17 (9) 25 (13)	26 (50)/33 (64) 24 (47) 17 (34)	0.441
Operation time, min	300 (251, 351)	288 (245, 332)	302 (243, 365)	0.691
Bleeding, mL	570 (320, 1218)	471 (320, 970)	610 (260, 1350)	0.732
Length of ICU stay, days	4.0 (3.0, 5.0)	4.0 (3.0, 5.0)	3.0 (2, 4)	0.142
Postoperative day that rehabilitation was started, days	1.0 (1.0, 1.0)	1.0 (1.0, 1.0)	1.0 (1, 1)	0.370
Postoperative day that ambulation was started, days	3.0 (2.0, 4.0)	3.0 (2.0, 4.0)	3.0 (2, 4)	0.229
Postoperative day when ambulation independence was achieved, days	5.0 (4.0, 6.3)	5.0 (5.0, 7.0)	5.0 (4, 7)	0.180
Length of hospital stay, days	19.0 (16.0, 25.0)	22.0 (15.0, 27.0)	19.0 (16, 24)	0.132

Note. HAFD, hospital-acquired functional decline; LVEF, left ventricular ejection fraction; NYHA, New York Heart Association; eGFR, estimated glomerular filtration ratio; SPPB, short physical performance battery; CABG, coronary arterial bypass graft; ICU, intensive care unit. Values are presented as median (interquartile range) or n (%). * $p < 0.05$.

Table 2. Predictors of all-cause mortality, readmission, and frailty severity, according to the univariate and multivariate regression analyses.

	Univariate Analysis				Multivariate Analysis			
	OR	95% CI		p-Value	OR	95% CI		p-Value
Age (every 1-year increase)	1.035	0.989	1.084	0.137	1.027	0.975	1.082	0.317
Female	1.153	0.670	1.986	0.607	1.173	0.609	2.256	0.634
BMI (every 1-kg/m^2 increase)	0.966	0.895	1.043	0.378	1.002	0.917	1.095	0.964
NYHA class $\geq$ III (every degree increase)	1.529	0.648	3.610	0.333				
LVEF (every 1% increase)	0.977	0.957	0.998	0.031 *	0.982	0.959	1.005	0.129
Diabetes mellitus	1.220	0.700	2.127	0.483				
CKD	1.448	0.755	2.778	0.266				
Hemoglobin	0.805	0.687	0.942	0.007 *	0.847	0.701	1.023	0.085
Albumin	0.670	0.349	1.285	0.228				
Low preoperative gait speed	2.318	1.200	4.479	0.012 *	2.477	1.185	5.176	0.016 *
Low preoperative grip strength	1.046	0.598	1.828	0.875				
Preoperative SPPB score	0.937	0.816	1.077	0.361				
Bleeding	1.000	1.000	1.000	0.357				
Operative time	1.003	1.000	1.006	0.093	1.004	1.000	1.007	0.051
Postoperative ICU stay	1.120	0.980	1.282	0.097				
Postoperative hospital stay	0.994	0.967	1.023	0.690				
Hospital-acquired functional decline	3.467	1.842	6.528	<0.001 **	3.437	1.756	6.729	<0.001 **

Note. BMI, body mass index; NYHA, New York Heart Association; LVEF, left ventricular ejection fraction; CKD, chronic kidney disease; SPPB, short physical performance battery; ICU, intensive care unit; OR, odds ratio; CI, confidence interval. * $p < 0.05$; ** $p < 0.001$.

3.3. Changes in the Kihon Checklist Score among the HAFD and Non-HAFD Groups

Figure 2 show the changes in the KCL score in the HAFD and non-HAFD groups before surgery and one year after hospital discharge. The two groups showed a significant main effect and an interaction between the two groups on the total KCL scores (F = 10.55, $p < 0.001$) and IADL (F = 4.29, $p < 0.05$), mobility (F = 10.44, $p < 0.001$), oral function (F = 7.27, $p < 0.01$), and depression (F = 6.11, $p < 0.05$).

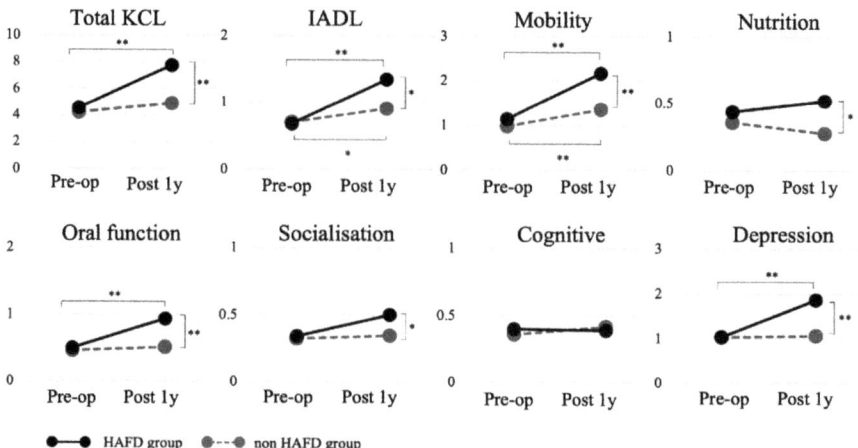

Figure 2. Changes in the Kihon Checklist score between the HAFD and non-HAFD groups. HAFD, hospitalization-acquired functional decline; KCL, Kihon Checklist; IADL, instrumental activities of daily living; Pre-op, preoperative; Post 1y, 1 year post hospital discharge. ** $p < 0.01$, * $p < 0.05$.

4. Discussion

This study clarified the effect of HAFD on poor prognosis, one year after discharge, in older cardiac surgical patients. To the best of our knowledge, this is the first study to report on older cardiac surgical patients who have undergone standard open-heart surgery, although there have been previous studies on patients who have undergone minimally invasive transcatheter aortic valve implantation [12].

We found that the incidence of HAFD in older cardiac surgery patients was 21%. This was consistent with the findings of previous studies that reported that the incidence of HAFD was approximately 20–40% [10–12]. HAFD has also been shown to be related to in-hospital mobility, nutrition intake, and continence care, as well as to the length of hospital stay and the condition of the patient before hospitalization [11]. In this study, we found a significantly higher proportion of patients with COPD, significantly lower hemoglobin levels, and preoperative grip strength, as well as a higher proportion of females in the HAFD group compared to the non-HAFD group. It has been reported that patients with COPD, and those with a low preoperative forced expiratory volume in one second, had a prolonged duration of postoperative ventilator use, a higher incidence of postoperative respiratory complications, and in-hospital mortality [25,26]. Preoperative abnormalities in lung function, due to COPD, may delay the recovery of physical function after surgery. A recent meta-analysis of studies concluded that preoperative anemia was associated with poor outcomes after surgery [27]. Since preoperative anemia was associated with an increased amount of red blood cell transfusions [27], we speculated that the high degree of postoperative anemia was associated with a lower rate of physical inactivity and a higher incidence of HAFD. Although there was no significant difference in the progression of postoperative rehabilitation between the HAFD and non-HAFD groups, we speculated that the HAFD group tended to have a lower preoperative reserve capacity and did not fully recover their physical function at the time of discharge from the hospital due to the surgical invasion.

The total KCL score in the HAFD group, one year after discharge, was significantly higher than both the preoperative scores and that of the non-HAFD group, which was interpreted as an increase in the severity of frailty. The total KCL score of the HAFD group one year after discharge was 7.7 points, and considering that a total score of eight points or more corresponds to frailty [18], many in the HAFD group were likely to be in a frail state. A higher total KCL score has been associated with increased mortality and a higher risk of requiring long-term care insurance services [18,28–30]. In particular, increases in the severity of frailty stratification scores have been found to be associated with increases in the mortality rate [31] and in the rate of new forms of long-term care service and support required [18]. Recently, a large multicenter study reported that multifaceted frailty (physical/social/cognitive), in older patients with cardiac disease, increased the risk of readmission and death [32]. An increase in the severity of frailty has also been shown to substantially increase healthcare costs [33,34] with major effects on society, including further poor prognosis and more healthcare professionals required to care for these patients. Therefore, the selection of frailty severity as a clinical outcome in this study, in addition to death and rehospitalization, appears to be an important and appropriate outcome measure of poor prognosis.

The KCL subtests of mobility, IADL, oral function, and depression were scored higher than the preoperative and non-HAFD groups. The occurrence of HAFD indicated that mobility had not recovered, even after 1 year of discharge, suggesting that the decline in motor function may have caused IADL and depression. In our study, 33% of patients had a poor prognosis. For example, Govers et al. reported that 38% of older cardiac surgical patients (aged 65–79 years) had decreased ADL scores one year after discharge [35], which was similar to previous studies.

HAFD was the most relevant predictor for poor prognosis one year after discharge. In previous studies, gait speed has been used, clinically, as an important prognostic predictor after cardiac surgery [1,2]. A previous multicenter study also reported that preoperative walking speed was an important predictor for postoperative functional recovery [36]. In the present study, preoperative gait speed was also identified as an independent predictor for poor prognosis in the multivariate analysis. However, in the present study, HAFD was found to be a more powerful predictor than the preoperative gait speed. This finding indicated that, even if the gait speed was normal preoperatively, the prognosis worsened when HAFD occurred postoperatively. Therefore, a prognostic prediction that considered the degree of recovery of physical function after surgery is important. Furthermore, considering that the prognosis of poor outcome is 12 times higher when low preoperative gait speed and HAFD occurred together (compared to no low preoperative gait speed or HAFD), the evaluation of HAFD is important in clinical practice.

In recent years, the advances in surgical techniques have expanded the scope of surgery to include older and severely ill patients, while acute care hospitals have shortened the length of hospital stays. Therefore, the number of patients with HAFD is expected to increase in the future, making the findings of this study significant. When considering surgical treatment for older patients, HAFD should be considered, and physical function should be monitored regularly by physiotherapists and nurses before and after surgery. Simple exercise (walking and chair stand) has been reported to reduce HAFD [37]. For patients with delayed recovery of postoperative physical function, the occurrence of HAFD may be prevented with an active improvement of physical activity and the incorporation of programs to increase the physical function in postoperative care.

Limitations

First, the sample size was small. Moreover, a number of patients in each group did not respond to the post-discharge survey, which may have affected the post-discharge survey results. While the first author did not participate in data analysis, the co-authors participated in the measurements at each site, so the possibility that they had some influence on the results cannot be ruled out completely. The median preoperative SPPB of patients in this study was 12 points, and many had a high preoperative physical function. In addition, the KCL is a self-administered questionnaire, and patients with obvious dementia before surgery were excluded from the study. Therefore, the results of this study are biased toward older cardiac surgery patients whose physical and cognitive functions are relatively well preserved. In addition, since this study aimed to investigate the composite outcome one year post-hospital discharge, the speed of occurrence of the outcomes of death and readmission was not examined. Further studies are required to examine the timing concerning the occurrence of disability in future. Furthermore, this study did not address the cause of HAFD. In the future, it is necessary to examine factors, such as delirium, that lead to HAFD. Finally, this study was carried out in Japan. Thus, the results of this study may not be applicable to patients from other countries.

5. Conclusions

HAFD occurred in 21% of older cardiac surgical patients and was an independent predictor for poor prognosis one year postoperatively. More importantly, HAFD was a more powerful prognostic predictor than low preoperative gait speed, and the combination of low preoperative gait speed and the occurrence of HAFD increased the odds ratio 12-fold. Since HAFD was the most relevant prognostic predictor in older cardiac surgical patients, the prognosis should include both preoperative and postoperative functional recovery.

Author Contributions: Conceptualization, T.M., M.S., K.S. and T.T.; methodology, T.M., M.S., K.S. and T.T.; software, T.M., M.S., K.S. and T.T.; validation, T.M., M.S. and T.T.; formal analysis, T.M.; investigation, S.O., G.T., M.T., Y.O., Y.T., K.I. and K.O.; resources, T.M. and T.T.; data curation, S.O., G.T., M.T., Y.O., Y.T., K.I. and K.O.; writing—original draft preparation, T.M., M.S., K.S. and T.T.; writing—review and editing, T.M., M.S., K.S. and T.T.; visualization, T.M.; supervision, T.T.; project administration, T.M. and T.T.; funding acquisition, T.M. All authors have read and agreed to the published version of the manuscript.

Funding: This work was supported by Japan Society for the Promotion of Science KAKENHI (grant number 17K01544).

Institutional Review Board Statement: This study was conducted in accordance with the Helsinki Declaration and was approved by the ethics committees of all participating hospitals and by the ethics review committee of faculty of hearth science Juntendo University (19-003). Written informed consent was obtained from all patients for participation in the study.

Informed Consent Statement: Informed consent was obtained from all subjects involved in the study.

Data Availability Statement: The dataset(s) supporting the conclusions of this article cannot be provided due to ethical restrictions.

Acknowledgments: We would like to thank all the staff members from the Sakakibara Heart Institute of Okayama, Tsuchiya General Hospital, Higashi Takarazuka Satoh Hospital, Tomishiro Central Hospital, Fukuyama Cardiovascular Hospital, Kansai Electronic Power Hospital, Kobe City Medical Center General Hospital, The Cardiovascular Institute, and Juntendo University involved in this study.

Conflicts of Interest: The authors declare no conflict of interest.

References

1. Afilalo, J.; Sharma, A.; Zhang, S.; Brennan, J.M.; Edwards, F.H.; Mack, M.J.; McClurken, J.B.; Cleveland, J.C.; Smith, P.K.; Shahian, D.M.; et al. Gait Speed and 1-Year Mortality Following Cardiac Surgery: A Landmark Analysis From the Society of Thoracic Surgeons Adult Cardiac Surgery Database. *J. Am. Heart Assoc.* **2018**, *7*, e010139. [CrossRef]
2. Afilalo, J.; Eisenberg, M.J.; Morin, J.F.; Bergman, H.; Monette, J.; Noiseux, N.; Perrault, L.P.; Alexander, K.P.; Langlois, Y.; Dendukuri, N.; et al. Gait Speed as an Incremental Predictor of Mortality and Major Morbidity in Elderly Patients Undergoing Cardiac Surgery. *J. Am. Coll. Cardiol.* **2010**, *56*, 1668–1676. [CrossRef]
3. Afilalo, J.; Kim, S.; O'Brien, S.; Brennan, J.M.; Edwards, F.H.; Mack, M.J.; McClurken, J.B.; Cleveland, J.C.; Smith, P.K.; Shahian, D.M.; et al. Gait Speed and Operative Mortality in Older Adults Following Cardiac Surgery. *JAMA Cardiol.* **2016**, *1*, 314–321. [CrossRef]
4. Yanagawa, B.; Graham, M.M.; Afilalo, J.; Hassan, A.; Arora, R.C. Frailty as a Risk Predictor in Cardiac Surgery: Beyond the Eyeball Test. *J. Thorac. Cardiovasc. Surg.* **2018**, *156*, 172–176.e2. [CrossRef]
5. Sepehri, A.; Beggs, T.; Hassan, A.; Rigatto, C.; Shaw-Daigle, C.; Tangri, N.; Arora, R.C. The Impact of Frailty on Outcomes after Cardiac Surgery: A Systematic Review. *J. Thorac. Cardiovasc. Surg.* **2014**, *148*, 3110–3117. [CrossRef]
6. Okamura, H.; Kimura, N.; Tanno, K.; Mieno, M.; Matsumoto, H.; Yamaguchi, A.; Adachi, H. The Impact of Preoperative Sarcopenia, Defined Based on Psoas Muscle Area, on Long-Term Outcomes of Heart Valve Surgery. *J. Thorac. Cardiovasc. Surg.* **2019**, *157*, 1071–1079.e3. [CrossRef]
7. Satake, S.; Arai, H. The Revised Japanese Version of the Cardiovascular Health Study Criteria (Revised J-CHS Criteria). *Geriatr. Gerontol. Int.* **2020**, *20*, 992–993. [CrossRef]
8. Chen, L.K.; Liu, L.K.; Woo, J.; Assantachai, P.; Auyeung, T.W.; Bahyah, K.S.; Chou, M.Y.; Chen, L.Y.; Hsu, P.S.; Krairit, O.; et al. Sarcopenia in Asia: Consensus Report of the Asian Working Group for Sarcopenia. *J. Am. Med. Dir. Assoc.* **2014**, *15*, 95–101. [CrossRef]
9. Chen, L.K.; Woo, J.; Assantachai, P.; Auyeung, T.W.; Chou, M.Y.; Iijima, K.; Jang, H.C.; Kang, L.; Kim, M.; Kim, S.; et al. Asian Working Group for Sarcopenia: 2019 Consensus Update on Sarcopenia Diagnosis and Treatment. *J. Am. Med. Dir. Assoc.* **2020**, *21*, 300–307.e2. [CrossRef]
10. Hirsch, C.H.; Sommers, L.; Olsen, A.; Mullen, L.; Winograd, C.H. The Natural History of Functional Morbidity in Hospitalized Older Patients. *J. Am. Geriatr. Soc.* **1990**, *38*, 1296–1303. [CrossRef]
11. Zisberg, A.; Shadmi, E.; Gur-Yaish, N.; Tonkikh, O.; Sinoff, G. Hospital-Associated Functional Decline: The Role of Hospitalization Processes Beyond Individual Risk Factors. *J. Am. Geriatr. Soc.* **2015**, *63*, 55–62. [CrossRef] [PubMed]
12. Saitoh, M.; Saji, M.; Kozono-Ikeya, A.; Arimitsu, T.; Sakuyama, A.; Ueki, H.; Nagayama, M.; Isobe, M. Hospital-Acquired Functional Decline and Clinical Outcomes in Older Patients Undergoing Transcatheter Aortic Valve Implantation. *Circ. J.* **2020**, *84*, 1083–1089. [CrossRef] [PubMed]
13. Tasheva, P.; Vollenweider, P.; Kraege, V.; Roulet, G.; Lamy, O.; Marques-Vidal, P.; Méan, M. Association between Physical Activity Levels in the Hospital Setting and Hospital-Acquired Functional Decline in Elderly Patients. *JAMA Netw. Open* **2020**, *3*, e1920185. [CrossRef] [PubMed]
14. Sleiman, I.; Rozzini, R.; Barbisoni, P.; Morandi, A.; Ricci, A.; Giordano, A.; Trabucchi, M. Functional Trajectories during Hospitalization: A Prognostic Sign for Elderly Patients. *J. Gerontol. Ser. A Biol. Sci. Med. Sci.* **2009**, *64*, 659–663. [CrossRef] [PubMed]
15. Fortinsky, R.H.; Covinsky, K.E.; Palmer, R.M.; Landefeld, C.S. Effects of Functional Status Changes before and during Hospitalization on Nursing Home Admission of Older Adults. *J. Gerontol. Ser. A Biol. Sci. Med. Sci.* **1999**, *54*, M521–M526. [CrossRef] [PubMed]
16. JCS Joint Working Group. Guidelines for Rehabilitation in Patients With Cardiovascular Disease (JCS 2012). *Circ. J.* **2014**, *78*, 2022–2093. [CrossRef] [PubMed]

17. Arai, H.; Satake, S. English Translation of the Kihon Checklist. *Geriatr. Gerontol. Int.* **2015**, *15*, 518–519. [CrossRef]
18. Satake, S.; Shimokata, H.; Senda, K.; Kondo, I.; Toba, K. Validity of Total Kihon Checklist Score for Predicting the Incidence of 3-Year Dependency and Mortality in a Community-Dwelling Older Population. *J. Am. Med. Dir. Assoc.* **2017**, *18*, 552.e1–552.e6. [CrossRef]
19. Yamada, M.; Arai, H. Predictive Value of Frailty Scores for Healthy Life Expectancy in Community-Dwelling Older Japanese Adults. *J. Am. Med. Dir. Assoc.* **2015**, *16*, 1002.e7–1002.e11. [CrossRef]
20. Kojima, G.; Taniguchi, Y.; Kitamura, A.; Shinkai, S. Are the Kihon Checklist and the Kaigo-Yobo Checklist Compatible With the Frailty Index? *J. Am. Med. Dir. Assoc.* **2018**, *19*, 797–800.e2. [CrossRef]
21. Satake, S.; Shimokata, H.; Senda, K.; Kondo, I.; Arai, H.; Toba, K. Predictive Ability of Seven Domains of the Kihon Checklist for Incident Dependency and Mortality. *J. Frailty Aging.* **2019**, *8*, 85–87. [CrossRef] [PubMed]
22. Kamiya, K.; Sato, Y.; Takahashi, T.; Tsuchihashi-Makaya, M.; Kotooka, N.; Ikegame, T.; Takura, T.; Yamamoto, T.; Nagayama, M.; Goto, Y.; et al. Multidisciplinary Cardiac Rehabilitation and Long-Term Prognosis in Patients With Heart Failure. *Circ. Heart Fail.* **2020**, *13*, e006798. [CrossRef]
23. Matsue, Y.; Kamiya, K.; Saito, H.; Saito, K.; Ogasahara, Y.; Maekawa, E.; Konishi, M.; Kitai, T.; Iwata, K.; Jujo, K.; et al. Prevalence and Prognostic Impact of the Coexistence of Multiple Frailty Domains in Elderly Patients With Heart Failure: The FRAGILE-HF Cohort Study. *Eur. J. Heart Fail.* **2020**, *22*, 2112–2119. [CrossRef] [PubMed]
24. Bock, J.O.; König, H.H.; Brenner, H.; Haefeli, W.E.; Quinzler, R.; Matschinger, H.; Saum, K.U.; Schöttker, B.; Heider, D. Associations of Frailty With Health Care Costs—Results of the Esther Cohort Study. *BMC Health Serv. Res.* **2016**, *16*, 128. [CrossRef] [PubMed]
25. Goldfarb, M.; Bendayan, M.; Rudski, L.G.; Morin, J.F.; Langlois, Y.; Ma, F.; Lachapelle, K.; Cecere, R.; DeVarennes, B.; Tchervenkov, C.I.; et al. Cost of Cardiac Surgery in Frail Compared with Nonfrail Older Adults. *Can. J. Cardiol.* **2017**, *33*, 1020–1026. [CrossRef] [PubMed]
26. Morisawa, T.; Saitoh, M.; Takahashi, T.; Watanabe, H.; Mochizuki, M.; Kitahara, E.; Fujiwara, T.; Fujiwara, K.; Nishitani-Yokoyama, M.; Minamino, T.; et al. Association of Phase Angle With Hospital-Acquired Functional Decline in Older Patients Undergoing Cardiovascular Surgery. *Nutrition.* **2021**, *91–92*, 111402. [CrossRef]
27. Guralnik, J.M.; Simonsick, E.M.; Ferrucci, L.; Glynn, R.J.; Berkman, L.F.; Blazer, D.G.; Scherr, P.A.; Wallace, R.B. A Short Physical Performance Battery Assessing Lower Extremity Function: Association With Self-Reported Disability and Prediction of Mortality and Nursing Home Admission. *J. Gerontol.* **1994**, *49*, M85–M94. [CrossRef] [PubMed]
28. Freiberger, E.; de Vreede, P.; Schoene, D.; Rydwik, E.; Mueller, V.; Frändin, K.; Hopman-Rock, M. Performance-Based Physical Function in Older Community-Dwelling Persons: A Systematic Review of Instruments. *Age Ageing.* **2012**, *41*, 712–721. [CrossRef]
29. Puthoff, M.L. Outcome Measures in Cardiopulmonary Physical Therapy: Short Physical Performance Battery. *Cardiopulm. Phys. Ther. J.* **2008**, *19*, 17–22. [CrossRef]
30. Rinaldo, L.; Caligari, M.; Acquati, C.; Nicolazzi, S.; Paracchini, G.; Sardano, D.; Giordano, A.; Marcassa, C.; Corrà, U. Functional Capacity Assessment and Minimal Clinically Important Difference in Post-Acute Cardiac Patients: The Role of Short Physical Performance Battery. *Eur. J. Prev. Cardiol.* **2021**, zwab044. [CrossRef]
31. Katijjahbe, M.A.; Granger, C.L.; Denehy, L.; Royse, A.; Royse, C.; Clarke, S.; El-Ansary, D. Short Physical Performance Battery Can Be Utilized to Evaluate Physical Function in Patients after Cardiac Surgery. *Cardiopulm. Phys. Ther. J.* **2018**, *29*, 88–96. [CrossRef]
32. Rutten, E.P.; Spruit, M.A.; McDonald, M.L.; Rennard, S.; Agusti, A.; Celli, B.; Miller, B.E.; Crim, C.; Calverley, P.M.; Hanson, C.; et al. Continuous Fat-Free Mass Decline in COPD: Fact or Fiction? *Eur. Respir. J.* **2015**, *46*, 1496–1498. [CrossRef] [PubMed]
33. McAllister, D.A.; Wild, S.H.; MacLay, J.D.; Robson, A.; Newby, D.E.; MacNee, W.; Innes, J.A.; Zamvar, V.; Mills, N.L. Forced Expiratory Volume in One Second Predicts Length of Stay and in-Hospital Mortality in Patients Undergoing Cardiac Surgery: A Retrospective Cohort Study. *PLoS ONE* **2013**, *8*, e64565. [CrossRef] [PubMed]
34. Fowler, A.J.; Ahmad, T.; Phull, M.K.; Allard, S.; Gillies, M.A.; Pearse, R.M. Meta-Analysis of the Association between Preoperative Anaemia and Mortality after Surgery. *Br. J. Surg.* **2015**, *102*, 1314–1324. [CrossRef]
35. Govers, A.C.; Buurman, B.M.; Jue, P.; de Mol, B.A.; Dongelmans, D.A.; de Rooij, S.E. Functional Decline of Older Patients 1 Year after Cardiothoracic Surgery Followed by Intensive Care Admission: A Prospective Longitudinal Cohort Study. *Age Ageing.* **2014**, *43*, 575–580. [CrossRef]
36. Itagaki, A.; Saitoh, M.; Okamura, D.; Kawamura, T.; Otsuka, S.; Tahara, M.; Mori, Y.; Kamisaka, K.; Ochi, Y.; Yuguchi, S.; et al. Factors Related to Physical Functioning Decline after Cardiac Surgery in Older Patients: A Multicenter Retrospective Study. *J. Cardiol.* **2019**, *74*, 279–283. [CrossRef]
37. Ortiz-Alonso, J.; Bustamante-Ara, N.; Valenzuela, P.L.; Vidán-Astiz, M.; Rodríguez-Romo, G.; Mayordomo-Cava, J.; Javier-González, M.; Hidalgo-Gamarra, M.; Lopéz-Tatis, M.; Valades-Malagón, M.I.; et al. Effect of a Simple Exercise Program on Hospitalization-Associated Disability in Older Patients: A Randomized Controlled Trial. *J. Am. Med. Dir. Assoc.* **2020**, *21*, 531–537.e1. [CrossRef]

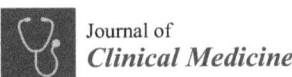

Article

Kidney Function According to Different Equations in Patients Admitted to a Cardiology Unit and Impact on Outcome

Vincenzo Livio Malavasi [1], Anna Chiara Valenti [1], Sara Ruggerini [1], Marcella Manicardi [1], Carlotta Orlandi [1], Daria Sgreccia [1], Marco Vitolo [1,2,3], Marco Proietti [3,4,5], Gregory Y. H. Lip [3,6] and Giuseppe Boriani [1,*]

1. Cardiology Division, Department of Biomedical, Metabolic and Neural Sciences, University of Modena and Reggio Emilia, Policlinico di Modena, 41125 Modena, Italy; nanni.malavasi@gmail.com (V.L.M.); annachiaravalenti@gmail.com (A.C.V.); sara.ruggerini@yahoo.it (S.R.); marcella.manicardi@gmail.com (M.M.); orlandi_carlotta@libero.it (C.O.); daria.sgreccia@gmail.com (D.S.); marco.vitolo90@gmail.com (M.V.)
2. Clinical and Experimental Medicine PhD Program, University of Modena and Reggio Emilia, Policlinico di Modena, 41125 Modena, Italy
3. Liverpool Centre for Cardiovascular Science, University of Liverpool and Liverpool Heart & Chest Hospital, Liverpool L14 3PE, UK; marco.proietti@unimi.it (M.P.); gregory.lip@liverpool.ac.uk (G.Y.H.L.)
4. Department of Clinical Sciences and Community Health, University of Milan, 20122 Milan, Italy
5. Geriatric Unit, IRCCS Istituti Clinici Scientifici Maugeri, 20138 Milan, Italy
6. Aalborg Thrombosis Research Unit, Department of Clinical Medicine, Aalborg University, 9220 Aalborg, Denmark
* Correspondence: giuseppe.boriani@unimore.it

Abstract: Background: This paper aims to evaluate the concordance between the Chronic Kidney Disease Epidemiology Collaboration (CKD-EPI) formula and alternative equations and to assess their predictive power for all-cause mortality in unselected patients discharged alive from a cardiology ward. Methods: We retrospectively included patients admitted to our Cardiology Division independently of their diagnosis. The total population was classified according to Kidney Disease: Improving Global Outcomes (KDIGO) categories, as follows: G1 (estimated glomerular filtration rate (eGFR) $\geq$90 mL/min/1.73 m^2); G2 (eGFR 89–60 mL/min/1.73 m^2); G3a (eGFR 59–45 mL/min/1.73 m^2); G3b (eGFR 44–30 mL/min/1.73 m^2); G4 (eGFR 29–15 mL/min/1.73 m^2); G5 (eGFR <15 mL/min/1.73 m^2). Cockcroft-Gault (CG), CG adjusted for body surface area (CG-BSA), Modification of Diet in Renal Disease (MDRD), Berlin Initiative Study (BIS-1), and Full Age Spectrum (FAS) equations were also assessed. Results: A total of 806 patients were included. Good agreement was found between the CKD-EPI formula and CG-BSA, MDRD, BIS-1, and FAS equations. In subjects younger than 65 years or aged $\geq$85 years, CKD-EPI and MDRD showed the highest agreement (Cohen's kappa (K) 0.881 and 0.588, respectively) while CG showed the lowest. After a median follow-up of 407 days, overall mortality was 8.2%. The risk of death was higher in lower eGFR classes (G3b HR4.35; 95%CI 1.05–17.80; G4 HR7.13; 95%CI 1.63–31.23; G5 HR25.91; 95%CI 6.63–101.21). The discriminant capability of death prediction tested with ROC curves showed the best results for BIS-1 and FAS equations. Conclusion: In our cohort, the concordance between CKD-EPI and other equations decreased with age, with the MDRD formula showing the best agreement in both younger and older patients. Overall, mortality rates increased with the renal function decreasing. In patients aged $\geq$75 years, the best discriminant capability for death prediction was found for BIS-1 and FAS equations.

Keywords: chronic kidney disease; glomerular filtration rate; CKD-EPI; elderly; cardiovascular disease

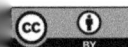

1. Introduction

Chronic kidney disease (CKD) is defined as kidney damage lasting for at least 3 months, with or without a decrease in Glomerular Filtration Rate (GFR), and assessed by circulating markers of kidney damage or renal biopsy, or as a reduction in GFR <60 mL/min per 1.73 m^2 for 3 months, with or without kidney damage [1,2]. CKD is a frequent condition among hospitalized patients due to its close association with increasing age and various co-morbidities. This relation is particularly strong in patients with cardiovascular diseases (CVD), including acute and chronic coronary syndrome (ACS and CCS), heart failure (HF), or atrial fibrillation (AF) [3–19]. Several studies emphasized the bidirectional relation between renal function and cardiovascular outcomes [5,20–22] as CVD is responsible for 40–50% of all deaths in nephropathic patients [5,23,24], and CKD, even in early stages, has been related to fatal and nonfatal cardiovascular events, regardless of traditional cardiovascular risk factors [25–32]. Thus, an accurate assessment of renal function is crucial in clinical decision-making processes and may affect prognostic stratification. Since the diagnostic standard to directly measure GFR (inulin clearance) is not easily practicable in daily clinical life, several formulas have been proposed to estimate GFR. In 1976, Cockcroft and Gault (CG) analyzed data from 249 patients (96% male) and developed a simple formula to estimate creatinine clearance (CCr) from serum creatinine (SCr) [33]. To reduce shortcomings, Rostoker et al. [34] proposed a modified CG formula adjusted for body surface area (CG-BSA). However, BSA indexation per se might be misleading in individuals with extreme BMI. More recently, the Modification of Diet in Renal Disease (MDRD) study, a multi-center trial based on a sample of 1628 patients with CKD, published a simplified 4-variables equation (age, gender, SCr, race) [35,36]. Since the MDRD equation tends to underestimate renal function in healthy individuals, in 2009, the Chronic Kidney Disease Epidemiology Collaboration (CKD-EPI) proposed a new equation that resulted in more accurate values for higher eGFR [37]. Remarkably, none of these formulas was developed in geriatric populations, and their reliability in estimating GFR in the elderly has been questioned [38,39]. In 2012, a new formula was developed by Berlin Initiative Study (BIS-1) and validated in a population-based cohort study of subjects >70 years [40]. Even more recently, the Full Age Spectrum (FAS) formula for GFR estimation was derived and validated by Pottel et al. to be used across the full age spectrum [41–44]. Because SCr is influenced by several variables—creatinine filtration [45], variations in tubular secretion [46,47], muscle mass [48,49], diet [50]—the estimation of GFR based on SCr is recommended and widely used for the initial assessment of renal function [51]. Actually, the latest Clinical Practice Guidelines delivered by the Kidney Disease: Improving Global Outcomes (KDIGO) group recommend the use of the CKD-EPI equation for CKD assessment and management [1,31]. The aim of our study was to assess the concordance between the CKD-EPI formula and the above-mentioned different equations in a real-world, unselected population admitted to our Cardiology Division. In addition, we aimed to evaluate how these different formulas perform in terms of all-cause mortality prediction.

2. Materials and Methods

We retrospectively reviewed patients consecutively admitted to the Cardiology Department of the Modena University Hospital during a 6-month period, between January and October 2016.

Patients were qualified independently of the type of CVD and according to the diagnosis at discharge. Selected patients received a diagnosis of acute coronary syndrome (ACS), chronic coronary syndrome (CCS), acute or chronic heart failure (HF), atrial fibrillation (AF), or other arrhythmias. Other diagnoses were classified as miscellaneous. Chronic coronary syndromes were defined as a history of prior ACS, including ST-segment elevation myocardial infarction, non-ST-segment elevation myocardial infarction, unstable angina, or a previous percutaneous or surgical revascularization. Valvular heart disease was considered when at least moderate valvular regurgitation or stenosis was the reason for hospitalization. Dyslipidemia was defined by a history of hypercholesterolemia, hypertriglyceridemia, or mixed hyperlipemia on diet or pharmacological therapy. A smoking habit was considered as present if a patient was a former or current smoker.

Parameters of interest were collected from the last available assessment before hospital discharge and included individual cardiac risk factors, serum creatinine, body height, and weight. Estimated GFR was then individually calculated according to the CKD-

EPI formula and the study population was classified according to the five KDIGO categories [1] as follows: G1 (eGFR ≥90 mL/min/1.73 m^2); G2 (eGFR between 89 and 60 mL/min/1.73 m^2); G3a (eGFR between 59 and 45 mL/min/1.73 m^2); G3b (eGFR between 44 and 30 mL/min/1.73 m^2); G4 (eGFR between 29 and 15 mL/min/1.73 m^2); G5 (eGFR <15 mL/min/1.73 m^2).

Furthermore, estimated GFR was individually assessed using CG, CG-BSA, MDRD, BIS-1, and FAS equations.

For the purpose of the present analysis, we included patients alive at the time of discharge and living in our geographical region. Patients who died during the in-hospital stay or with missing follow-up data were not included. No other exclusion criteria were applied.

All data were collected from Hospital Information System, and follow-up data were updated on the basis of ISTAT (Italian National Institute of Statistics, Rome, Italy) death notifications in which the status of all Italian citizens is complete and constantly updated.

2.1. Endpoint

The aim of our study was to assess the concordance between the CKD-EPI formula (reference) and the above-mentioned five equations. Moreover, we aimed to evaluate how these different formulas perform in predicting all-cause mortality compared to the CKD-EPI equation.

The study was approved by the local ethics committee, and the research was performed in accordance with the ethical standards laid down in the 1964 Declaration of Helsinki and its later amendments. Informed consent was obtained from all the subjects involved in the study.

2.2. Statistical Analysis

Continuous variables, when not-normally distributed, were reported as median [interquartile range (IQR)], and among groups, comparisons were made using a non-parametric analysis of variance (Kruskal-Wallis test). Categorical variables were reported as percentages, among groups, comparisons were made using χ^2 or Fisher exact tests if any expected cell count was less than five.

Weighted Cohen's kappa coefficient was used to assess the agreement in the classification of patients among KDIGO categories of eGFR with the six equations used for eGFR. Concordance was defined as follows: K < 0.20 poor; 0.20–0.40 modest; 0.41–0.60 moderate; 0.61–0.80 good; >0.80 excellent [52]. Moreover, to evaluate if each formula tends to over-or under-estimate the GFR when compared with CKD-EPI, we plotted the difference between CKD-EPI and the value of each formula against the CKD-EPI. We did not perform the same analysis for the CG formula because it measures creatinine clearance and not GFR.

Kaplan-Meier curves for survival according to CKD-EPI groups were performed and then compared using the log-rank test. A multivariable Cox regression analysis adjusted for age, gender, and diagnosis at discharge was also built to evaluate the effect of CKD-EPI groups on mortality.

The relationship between eGFR and death prediction was evaluated through the area under the curves (AUCs) of the receiver operating characteristic (ROC) curves for every eGFR formula, and ROC curves were then compared according to the De Long method [53].

Considering the CKD-EPI equation as a reference (cut-off value 60 mL/min/1.73 m^2), prediction model performance was assessed using the measure of model reclassification (Integrated Discrimination Improvement [IDI]) [54], matching one-on-one the result of every equation against the CKD-EPI formula.

All statistical analyses were performed using SPSS 23.0 (SPSS Statistics for Mac, Version (Armonk, NY, USA: IBM Corp) and R version 3.5.0 ((R Core Team, Vienna, Austria, (2021). R: A language and environment for statistical computing. R Foundation for Statistical Computing, Vienna, Austria, URL https://www.R-project.org/, accessed on 10 August 2021) with the package PredictABEL [55].

3. Results

A total of 806 patients were included in the present study (median age 71 years (IQR 61–79); 510 (63.3%) males), with a median follow-up of 407 days. The 20 patients who died during the in-hospital stay were excluded. The total cohort was grouped according to KDIGO classes of renal function, and its characteristics are summarized in Table 1.

Table 1. Patients' clinical characteristics according to KDIGO classes.

		KDIGO Categories According to CKD-EPI eGFR (mL/min/1.73 m^2)							
	Overall (n = 806)	G1 eGFR ≥ 90 (n = 203)	G2 eGFR 89–60 (n = 368)	G3a eGFR 59–45 (n = 99)	G3b eGFR 44–30 (n = 78)	G4 eGFR 29–15 (n = 38)	G5 eGFR < 15 (n = 20)	p
		Clinical features							
F-U days, median (IQR)	407 (284–473)	430 (365–478)	414 (277–478)	382 (269–474)	330 (243–433)	325 (223–359)	283 (145–378)	<0.001
Males, n (%)	510 (63.3)	137 (67.5)	247 (67.1)	56 (56.6)	37 (47.4)	21 (55.3)	12 (60)	0.009
Age, yrs median (IQR)	71 (61–79)	58 (50–65)	73 (66–79)	77 (72–83)	81 (76–85)	83 (80–86)	63 (58–71)	<0.001
Hypertension, n (%)	551 (68.4)	105 (51.7)	258 (70.1)	84 (84.8)	63 (80.8)	32 (84.2)	9 (45)	<0.001
Diabetes, n (%)	198 (24.6)	41 (20.2)	84 (22.8)	33 (33.3)	24 (30.8)	12 (31.6)	4 (20)	0.086
Dyslipidemia, n (%)	414 (51.4)	95 (46.8)	203 (55.2)	57 (57.6)	38 (48.7)	15 (39.5)	6 (30)	0.044
Smoking, n (%)	220 (27.3)	78 (38.4)	101 (27.4)	21 (21.2)	10 (12.8)	5 (13.2)	5 (25)	<0.001
Family history of CVD, n (%)	108 (13.4)	48 (23.6)	45 (12.2)	6 (6.1)	6 (7.7)	0	3 (15)	<0.001
History of CKD, n (%)	107 (13.3)	0	10 (2.7)	20 (20.2)	37 (47.4)	22 (57.9)	18 (90)	<0.001
BMI, median (IQR)	26.6 (24–29.4)	26.7 (23.7–30.1)	26.6 (24.2–29.4)	26.8 (23.6–29.3)	27 (23.4–30.8)	25.5 (23.5–27.8)	25.7 (21.2–29.9)	0.690
SCr mg/dl median (IQR)	0.94 (0.71–1.20)	0.71 (0.62–0.86)	0.91 (0.82–1.03)	1.20 (1.01–1.33)	1.50 (1.32–1.71)	2.21 (2.01–2.52)	5.85 (4.31–7.02)	<0.001
		Age groups							<0.001
Age < 65 yrs, n (%)	241 (29.9)	149 (73.4)	64 (17.4)	9 (9.1)	6 (7.7)	2 (5.3)	11 (55)	
Age 65–74 yrs, n (%)	221 (27.4)	47 (23.2)	134 (36.4)	22 (22.2)	10 (12.8)	3 (7.9)	5 (25)	
Age 75–84 yrs, n (%)	258 (32)	7 (3.4)	142 (38.6)	52 (52.5)	37 (47.4)	17 (44.7)	3 (15)	
Age ≥ 85 yrs, n (%)	86 (10.7)	0	28 (7.6)	16 (16.2)	25 (32.1)	16 (42.1)	1 (5)	
Diagnosis at discharge								<0.001
CCS n (%)	108 (13.4)	37 (18.2)	48 (13)	13 (13.1)	6 (7.7)	2 (5.3)	2 (10)	
ACS n (%)	345 (42.8)	102 (50.2)	163 (44.3)	35 (35.4)	24 (30.8)	9 (23.7)	12 (60)	
HF n (%)	110 (13.6)	13 (6.4)	38 (10.3)	21 (21.2)	27 (34.6)	8 (21.1)	3 (15)	
VHD n (%)	17 (2.1)	1 (0.5)	9 (2.5)	4 (4)	3 (3.8)	0	0	
AF n (%)	14 (1.7)	2 (1)	6 (1.6)	1 (1)	1 (1.3)	4 (10.5)	0	
Other arrhythmias n (%)	127 (15.8)	23 (11.4)	61 (16.6)	18 (18.2)	14 (17.9)	9 (23.7)	2 (10)	
Miscellaneous n (%)	85 (10.5)	25 (12.3)	43 (11.7)	7 (7.1)	3 (3.8)	6 (15.8)	1 (5)	
Outcome								
Deaths n (%)	66 (8.2)	3 (1.5)	18 (4.9)	11 (11.1)	15 (19.2)	11 (28.9)	8 (40)	<0.001

Legend: AF: atrial fibrillation; ACS: acute coronary syndrome; BMI: body mass index; CCS: chronic coronary disease; CKD: chronic kidney disease; CVD: cardiovascular disease; F-U: follow-up; HF: heart failure; IQR: interquartile range; SCr: serum creatinine; VHD: valvular heart disease; yrs: years.

The population characteristics according to age groups are shown in Supplementary Table S1. Patients were discharged with the following diagnosis: ACS (42.8%), CCS (13.4%), HF (13.6%), VHD (2.1%), AF (1.7%), other arrhythmias (15.8%), and other causes (10.5%). CCS and ACS were more common in patients younger than 75 years (76 (16.5%) in patients

<75 years vs. 32 (9.3%) in those ≥75 years for CCS ($p = 0.003$); 226 (48.9%) in patients <75 years vs. 119 (34.6%) ≥75 years for ACS ($p < 0.001$)), while HF and arrhythmias other than AF were more frequent in older ages (39 (8.4%) in patients <75 years vs. 69 (20.1%) in patients ≥75 years, for HF ($p < 0.001$); 51 (11%) in patients <75 years vs. 76 (22.1%) in patients ≥75 years, for other arrhythmias ($p < 0.001$)). Renal function, as assessed by all the equations considered, significantly decreased over increasing age groups (see Supplementary Table S1).

3.1. eGFR with CG, CG-BSA, MDRD, CKD-EPI, BIS1 and FAS Equations, Concordance Analysis

Using Cohen's weighted K test for the concordance of attribution to each class of eGFR and considering the CKD-EPI equation as the reference method, we found good agreement between CKD-EPI and CG-BSA, MDRD, BIS-1, and FAS formulas (weighted K coefficient 0.659, 0.751, 0.660 and 0.663, respectively) and moderate agreement with CG equation (weighted K coefficient 0.535) (Table 2).

Table 2. Concordance in head-to-head comparison among formulas estimating GFR according to weighted Cohen's kappa coefficients [K (95% CI)]. Concordance was defined as follows: K < 0.20 poor; 0.20–0.40 modest; 0.41–0.60 moderate; 0.61–0.80 good; >0.80 excellent. We show comparisons with moderate concordance in bold, in italicization with good concordance, in bold and italics those with excellent concordance.

	CG	CG-BSA	MDRD	BIS-1	FAS
CKD-EPI	**0.535** (**0.699–0.761**)	*0.659* (*0.575–0.743*)	*0.751* (*0.651–0.851*)	*0.660* (*0.560–0.760*)	*0.663* (*0.563–0.763*)
CG		*0.717* (*0.650–0.783*)	**0.460** (**0.393–0.527**)	**0.514** (**0.447–0.581**)	**0.505** (**0.438–0.572**)
CG-BSA			**0.499** (**0.432–0.566**)	*0.732* (*0.665–0.799*)	*0.739* (*0.672–0.806*)
MDRD				**0.477** (**0.410–0.544**)	**0.470** (**0.403–0.537**)
BIS-1					***0.896*** (***0.829–0.962***)

Legend: CKD-EPI: Chronic Kidney Disease Epidemiology Collaboration; CG: Cockcroft-Gault; CG-BSA: CG adjusted for body surface area; MDRD: The Modification of Diet in Renal Disease; BIS-1: Berlin Initiative Study; FAS: Full age spectrum. We show comparisons with moderate concordance in bold, in italicization with good concordance, in bold and italics those with excellent concordance.

When performing the concordance analysis among age groups (Table 3), using CKD-EPI as the reference, the highest agreement was found between the CKD-EPI and MDRD, particularly in the age group <65 years (weighted K coefficient 0.881). In patients aged ≥ 85 years, MDRD and BIS1 showed the best agreement with CKD-EPI (weighted K coefficient 0.588 and 0.568, respectively) compared to other equations. The agreement between attributions based on CKD-EPI and CG was moderate in all age groups. As shown in Table 3, an inverse relationship was observed between concordance and age, with the weighted K coefficient consistently decreasing with increasing age.

Of note, compared to CKD-EPI, all formulas overestimated the renal function for GFR values higher than 100 mL/min/m^2 (Supplementary Figures S1–S4). Under this cut-off, MDRD and BIS-1 showed a better concordance compared to CKD-EPI (Supplementary Figure S2 and Figure S3, respectively). The FAS equation overestimated renal function for extreme values (under 15 mL/min/m^2 and above 100 mL/min/m^2) and underestimated values in the middle range (Supplementary Figure S4).

Table 3. Concordance of eGFR evaluated with Cohen's weighted K test assessed by different equations among age groups. Concordance was defined as follows: K < 0.20 poor; 0.20–0.40 modest; 0.41–0.60 moderate; 0.61–0.80 good; >0.80 excellent. Comparisons with moderate concordance are labeled with (*), the ones with good concordance with (**), and the ones with excellent concordance with (***).

	CG	CG-BSA	MDRD	BIS-1	FAS
CKD-EPI in pts <65 y	0.523 (0.456–0.589) *	0.762 (0.695–0.829) *	0.881 (0.814–0.947) ***	0.688 (0.621–0.754) **	0.747 (0.680–0.814) **
CKD-EPI in pts 65–74 y	0.396 (0.329–0.462)	0.727 (0.660–0.793) **	0.717 (0.650–0.784) **	0.646 (0.579–0.712) **	0.671 (0.604–0.738)**
CKD-EPI in pts 75–84 y	0.486 (0.410–0.553) *	0.512 (0.445–0.578) *	0.652 (0.585–0.719) **	0.557 (0.490–0.623) *	0.560 (0.593–0.627) *
CKD-EPI in pts ≥85 y	0.413 (0.346–0.480) *	0.350 (0.283–0.417)	0.588 (0.501–0.635) *	0.568 (0.501–0.634) *	0.422 (0.355–0.489) *

Legend: CKD-EPI: Chronic Kidney Disease Epidemiology Collaboration; CG: Cockcroft-Gault; CG-BSA: CG adjusted for body surface area; MDRD: The Modification of Diet in Renal Disease; BIS-1: Berlin Initiative Study; FAS: Full age spectrum; y: years.

3.2. Survival Analysis

During a median follow-up of 407 days (IQR 284–473), overall mortality was 8.2% (66 deaths). There were 3 deaths (1.5%) in the CKD-EPI group G1, 18 (4.9%) in G2, 11 (11.1%) in G3a, 15 (19.2%) in G3b, 11 (28.9%) in G4, and 8 (40%) in G5 (p for trend < 0.0001).

As highlighted in Kaplan-Meier curves of survival according to KDIGO stages (Figure 1), patients with advanced CKD had the worst survival rates compared to those with early stages of CKD (Log Rank test, p < 0.0001).

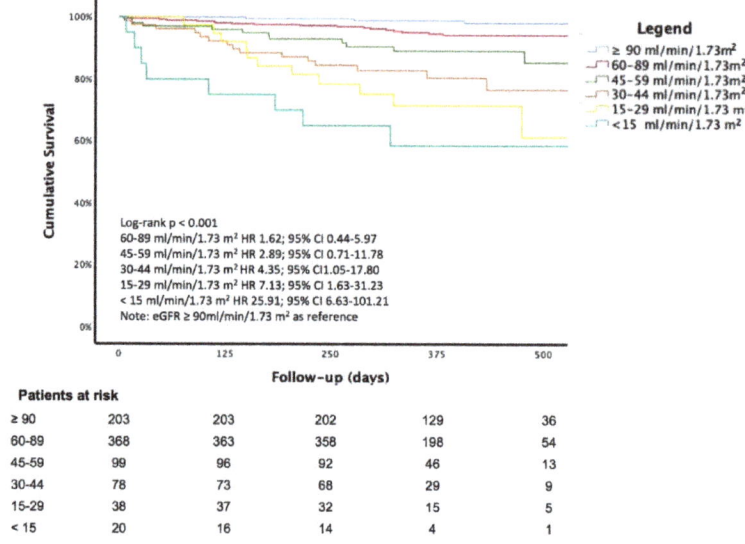

Figure 1. Kaplan-Meier curve of survival according to stages of renal function (eGFR with CKD-EPI equation). Note that the hazard ratio for each group was adjusted for age, sex, and diagnosis at discharge. Legend: Chronic Kidney Disease Epidemiology Collaboration; CG: Cockcroft-Gault; CG-BSA: CG adjusted for body surface area; MDRD: The Modification of Diet in Renal Disease; BIS-1: Berlin Initiative Study; FAS: Full age spectrum.

The multivariable Cox regression analysis, adjusted for age, gender, and diagnosis at discharge, showed a significant increase in mortality for decreasing eGFR values; the KDIGO class G5 had an almost 25-fold increased risk in mortality compared to KDIGO class G1 (HR 25.91; 95% CI, 6.63–101.21, p < 0.0001) (Figure 1).

According to AUCs of the ROC curves, the best discriminant capability for death prediction was found for BIS-1 (AUC = 0.782; 95% CI 0.752–0.810) followed by FAS

(AUC = 0.776; 95% CI 0.746–0.804), CG-BSA equation (AUC = 0.779; 95%CI 0.748–0.807), CG (AUC = 0.778; 95%CI 0.747–0.806), CKD-EPI (AUC = 0.769; 95%CI 0.738–0.797), and MDRD (AUC = 0.750; 95%CI 0.719–0.780) (Figure 2). A pairwise comparison of ROC curves shows that BIS-1 and FAS formulas perform significantly better compared with CKD-EPI ($p = 0.035$ and $p = 0.001$, respectively) while MDRD is significantly worst ($p = 0.005$). Moreover CG-BSA, BIS-1 and FAS are significantly better than MDRD (respectively, $p = 0.028$, $p = 0.001$, and $p = 0.001$). When matched, BIS-1 and FAS are significantly different ($p = 0.005$). Other comparisons of AUC's do not reach statistical significance.

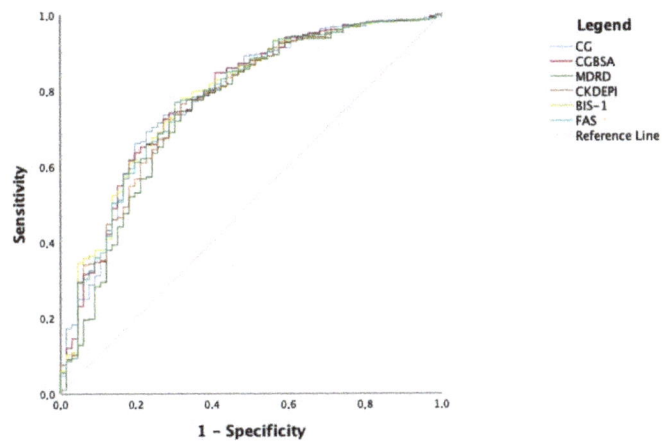

CG 0.778	CG/BSA 0.779	MDRD 0.750	CKD-EPI 0.769	FAS 0.779	BIS-1 0.782
p= 0.4785	p=0.2559	p=0.0052	ref	p=0.0353	p=0.0012

Figure 2. ROC curves and AUCs for death prediction according to eGFR values with different equations of eGFR in the whole cohort. The table below reports p-values of each formula compared with CKD-EPI considered as reference. Legend: BIS-1: Berlin Initiative Study; CKD-EPI: Chronic Kidney Disease Epidemiology Collaboration; CG: Cockcroft-Gault; CG-BSA: CG adjusted for body surface area; FAS: Full age spectrum; MDRD: The Modification of Diet in Renal Disease.

BIS-1 and FAS, when compared with CKD-EPI, IDI is significantly different in the whole group of patients as well as in patients $\geq$75 years (Table 4), giving a better discrimination power of about 1.5% in the whole cohort and about 3% in older ($\geq$75 years) patients.

Table 4. Summary of risk classification of eGFR equations by means of different tests.

	Whole Population (n 806)					
	Deaths n (%)	HR (95% CI)	AUC	p	IDI%	p
CKD-EPI <60 mL/min/1.73 m²	45 (68.2)	3.97 (2.24–7.04)	0.769	ref	ref	NA
CG <60 mL/min	50 (75.8)	4.62 (2.40–8.91)	0.778	0.479	−0.23 (−1.54–1.08)	0.733
CG-BSA <60 mL/min/1.73 m²	49 (74.2)	3.30 (1.72–6.32)	0.779	0.256	0.54 (−0.8–1.88)	0.431
MDRD <60 mL/min/1.73 m²	41 (62.1)	3.82 (2.22–6.59)	0.750	0.005	−0.43 (−1.14–0.28)	0.232
BIS-1 <60 mL/min/1.73 m²	51 (77.3)	3.43 (1.75–6.71)	0.782	0.035	1.63 (0.51–2.75)	0.004
FAS <60 mL/min/1.73 m²	51 (77.3)	3.70 (1.90–7.17)	0.776	0.001	1.40 (0.28–2.51)	0.014

Table 4. *Cont.*

	Patients aged ≥75 years (n 344)					
	Deaths n (%)	HR (95% CI)	AUC	p	IDI%	p
CKD-EPI <60 mL/min/1.73 m²	36 (76.6)	3.18 (1.58–6.40)	0.705	ref	ref	NA
CG <60 mL/min	42 (89.4)	4.61 (1.78–11.96)	0.725	0.261	0.79 (−0.89–2.47)	0.358
CG-BSA <60 mL/min/1.73 m²	41 (87.2)	2.69 (1.11–6.51)	0.717	0.255	0.94 (−0.93–2.81)	0.326
MDRD <60 mL/min/1.73 m²	32 (68.1)	2.84 (1.49–5.42)	0.698	0.023	−0.82 (−1.92–0.28)	0.145
BIS-1 <60 mL/min/1.73 m²	41 (87.2)	2.30 (0.95–5.57)	0.707	0.553	**3.26 (1.65–4.87)**	**<0.001**
FAS <60 mL/min/1.73 m²	41 (87.2)	2.67 (1.10–6.51)	0.706	0.692	**2.73 (1.16–4.31)**	**<0.001**

Legend: AUC: area under the curve; BIS-1: Berlin Initiative Study; CG: Cockcroft-Gault; CG-BSA: CG adjusted for body surface area; CKD-EPI: Chronic Kidney Disease Epidemiology Collaboration; FAS: full age spectrum; HR: hazard ratio; IDI: integrated discrimination improvement; MDRD: The Modification of Diet in Renal Disease. Statistical significance is highlighted in bold. Note that AUC was calculated considering the variables as continuous ones.

4. Discussion

The main findings of our study are that the concordance between CKD-EPI and other equations decreases with age, with the best agreement highlighted for the MDRD formula in both younger and older patients. Overall, mortality rates increased with the renal function decreasing. In patients aged ≥ 75 years, the best discriminant capability for death prediction was found for BIS-1 and FAS equations.

4.1. Concordance between CKD-EPI and Different eGFR Equations

Our concordance analysis has important clinical implications considering that, besides the recommended adoption of the CKD-EPI formula for estimating GFR, other equations are currently used for specific purposes (i.e., CG in NOACs prescription [31,56]) and in different scenarios (i.e., many laboratories still adopt the MDRD equation).

Irrespectively of age, in a relatively unselected cohort of patients admitted to a cardiology ward for various cardiovascular diseases, we found the highest agreement between CKD-EPI and MDRD (weighted K coefficient 0.751) and only moderate agreement with the CG equation (weighted K coefficient 0.533).

This finding is in line with previous data exploring the correlation between CKD-EPI and MDRD in different populations such as renal transplant recipients, advanced renal failure, and the elderly [57–59]. In a cohort of 1992 nephrology patients, Torreggiani et al. found that the highest heterogeneity was observed with BIS-1. [60] We could not confirm that observation since, according to our results, MDRD and BIS-1 showed the most similar estimation curve when compared with CKD-EPI (Figures S1–S4). Different clinical settings and the distribution of elderly patients may explain the difference.

Similar results were highlighted by Boriani et al. [32], considering CKD-EPI, MDRD, CG, and CG-BSA formulas. However, the present study considered two more equations (BIS-1 and FAS) that revealed good concordance with the CKD-EPI equation.

4.2. eGFR Estimates and Patient's Age

Our results underline that the concordance between eGFR assessed by the CKD-EPI formula and the other five equations decreases consistently with increasing age. Of note, for patients aged 85 years or more, MDRD had the greatest agreement with CKD-EPI (weighted K coefficient 0.588) followed by BIS-1 (weighted K coefficient 0.568), while CG showed the worst concordance (weighted K coefficient 0.348).

In a cohort of 1992 patients, Torreggiani et al. [60] found that estimated glomerular filtration rate (eGFR) decreased with age regardless of which equation was used. Analyzing the correlations between CKD-EPI and other eGFR equations, the highest heterogeneity was observed with BIS-1; the revised Lund-Malmo tended to underestimate eGFR while MDRD overestimated it. Compared to the reference CKD-EPI, FAS tended to classify patients with CKD in lower stages. Considering an eGFR threshold limit of 45 mL/min for defining significant CKD in patients over 65 years of age, the variability in CKD staging was 10%, no matter which equation was used.

Remarkably, estimation of GFR in the elderly is still a matter of debate as all equations integrate age with different mathematical models. Many studies have shown that distinct GFR estimations give different results in very old patients, raising concerns about which equation should be most appropriately used in this population [38,61–63].

Flamant et al. compared CG, MDRD, and CKD-EPI equations in 782 patients aged 65 years or more. In the entire population, the CG equation significantly underestimated measured GFR and had the lowest overall accuracy, whereas the estimation of GFR through the MDRD and CKD-EPI formulas did not significantly differ from the measured value. Moreover, in age subgroup analysis, biases significantly varied with age when considering the CG formula, but not with the MDRD and CKD-EPI equations.

As the CG equation considers a linear decrease of GFR with increasing age, its biases are emphasized in older subjects. On the contrary, the MDRD and CKD-EPI equations predict a slighter impact of age on renal function, thus preserving their overall performance even in old and very old patients [64].

However, in other cases, no difference was found among these equations in the elderly. In one large study on 1297 renal transplanted recipients undergoing inulin clearance measurement, Buron et al. evaluated the performance of four SCr-based formulas (CG, MDRD simplified, CKD-EPI, and Kankivell formula). The MDRD formula provided the best estimate of GFR with a mean bias of -0.5 mL/min/1.73 m^2, a standard deviation of bias of 12 mL/min/1.73 m^2, and a 30% accuracy. According to their results, gender and age did not modify the MDRD estimation of GFR, which remained superior to other formulas in each subgroup, except for patients older than 60 years, where the CG formula yielded equivalent results to the MDRD formula [65].

Kilbride et al. [66] studied 394 individuals with a median age of 80 years. The authors compared the accuracy of the MDRD, CKD-EPI creatinine, CKD-EPI cystatin C, and CKD-EPI combined equations with direct measurement of GFR. Considering the accuracy (the percentage of estimates within 30% of mGFR) of the equations, the creatinine-based equations in the elderly were similar to that observed in younger people (~80–85%).

4.3. eGFR and Cardiovascular Outcomes

Despite the KIDGO 2012 guidelines for the evaluation and management of CKD recommending the use of CKD-EPI [1], it is still unknown which equation would be better to use according to different clinical scenarios. Recently Rivera-Carvaca et al. [67], in a multi-center prospective registry on 1699 patients with acute coronary syndrome (ACS), showed that the CG equation has a superior predictive ability for major adverse cardiovascular events, major bleeding, and all-cause mortality compared with MDRD. A superior predictive ability for major bleeding was found even in comparison with CKD-EPI.

More recently, a study on 3985 patients with ACS [68] found similar results: CG and European Kidney Function Consortium equations were better than MDRD and CKD-EPI equations for risk discrimination for all-cause-mortality and bleeding, suggesting that in patients with ACS, the CG equation could be the most appropriate equation.

However, in elderly patients, CG often underestimates the GFR. In a recent cross-sectional study on 2247 participants aged 65 to 90 years who underwent inulin GFR measurements, none of the four equations considered for eGFR calculation (CKD-EPI, Lund-Malmö Revised, (LMR), full age spectrum (FAS), and Berlin Initiative Study 1) had superior diagnostic performance, while each had limitations regarding accuracy [69].

In the specific setting of atrial fibrillation, the use of different equations instead of the CG formula may significantly influence NOACs prescription and patient management [13].

An accurate assessment of renal function is critical as it may have relevant implications on prognostic stratification. As highlighted in our study, the survival rate significantly declines from G1 to G5 KDIGO categories, and the risk of all-cause death significantly increases in G3b, G4, G5 KDIGO classes (Figure 1).

In AF in- or outpatients enrolled in the EORP-AF pilot registry, the renal function, assessed by CKD-EPI formula, showed a crucial prognostic relevance. Besides the cut-off points that differed from those suggested by KDIGO, results showed that as renal function declines, patients' prognosis progressively worsens [32].

A large amount of literature previously investigated the association between CKD and outcomes [3]. A systematic review involving 39 studies and 1,371,990 patients showed that non-dialysis-dependent CKD is related to an increased risk for all-cause and cardiovascular death independently of potential confounders and CKD definitions and despite differences in studies' design and population.

The relation between CKD and all-cause mortality remained significant even in the general population, considering that younger patients and groups with a lower prevalence of known CVD had a significantly higher predicted relative risk for death associated with CKD [24]. This latest finding was shown in our analysis, considering that an estimated GFR lower than 60 mL/min/1.73 m^2 was related to higher hazard ratios for all-cause mortality in younger patients (<75 years) and without a known history of CVD (Figure 2).

Our results suggest that the assessment of eGFR may support clinicians in identifying those patients with a worse prognosis that may benefit from stricter surveillance and stronger control of associated conditions (diabetes, hypertension, coronary disease) to avoid further deterioration of renal function [70].

Moreover, the prognostic implications of reduced renal function have a specific impact on cardiologists' daily decision-making processes when prescribing contrast-based diagnostic or interventional procedures [71], for the infective risk stratification in CIED procedures [72], or when considering the appropriateness of a defibrillator for primary prevention of sudden cardiac death [73].

4.4. Strengths and Limitations

The retrospective nature of our study represents an intrinsic limitation. Our population was relatively unselected and enrolled in a single center. Specific data on cardiovascular mortality were missing, so we could not assess the performance of different formulas on it. Moreover, since in-hospital deaths were excluded, our results can only apply to stable, pre-discharge patients. However, our study highlights how differently formulas perform in a "real-world" population and the implication of their use in long-term prognostic stratification.

Given the availability of different formulas for eGFR, there is the need to define the most appropriate approach for kidney function assessment, as well as for outcome prediction, to be used in a wide range of individuals, including the elderly.

Supplementary Materials: The following supporting information can be downloaded at: https://www.mdpi.com/article/10.3390/jcm11030891/s1, Figure S1: renal function estimation of body surface area adjusted Cockroft-Gault equation (CGBSA) plotted against the difference between CKD-EPI equation and CG-BSA values; Figure S2: renal function estimation of MDRD equation plotted against the difference between CKD-EPI equation and MDRD values; Figure S3: renal function estimation of BIS-1 equation plotted against the difference between CKDEPI equation and BIS-1 values; Figure S4: renal function estimation of FAS equation plotted against the difference between CKDEPI equation and FAS values.

Author Contributions: Made substantial contributions to conception and design of the study and performed data analysis and interpretation: V.L.M., A.C.V., M.M., D.S., M.V., M.P., G.Y.H.L. and G.B. Performed data acquisition, as well as provided administrative, technical, and material support: S.R., M.M. and C.O. All authors have read and agreed to the published version of the manuscript.

Funding: This research received no external funding.

Institutional Review Board Statement: The study was approved by the local ethics committee (reference number 911, data of approval 14 March 2017), and the research was performed in accordance with the ethical standards laid down in the 1964 Declaration of Helsinki and its later amendments.

Informed Consent Statement: Informed consent was obtained from all the subjects involved in the study.

Data Availability Statement: Not applicable.

Conflicts of Interest: Boriani G received small speaker fees from Medtronic, Boston, Biotronik, Boehringer, and Bayer, outside of the submitted work. The other authors declare no conflict of interest.

References

1. KDIGO. 2012 clinical practice guideline for the evaluation and management of chronic kidney disease. *Kidney Int.* **2013**, *3*, 1–150.
2. Foundation NK. K/DOQI clinical practice guidelines for chronic kidney disease: Evaluation, classification, and stratification. *Am. J. Kidney Dis.* **2002**, *39* (Suppl. 1), S1–S266.
3. Go, A.S.; Chertow, G.M.; Fan, D.; McCulloch, C.E.; Hsu, C.Y. Chronic kidney disease and the risks of death, cardiovascular events, and hospitalization. *N. Engl. J. Med.* **2004**, *351*, 1296–1305. [CrossRef] [PubMed]
4. Sarnak, M.J.; Levey, A.S.; Schoolwerth, A.C.; Coresh, J.; Culleton, B.; Hamm, L.L.; McCullough, P.A.; Kasiske, B.L.; Kelepouris, E.; Klag, M.J.; et al. Kidney disease as a risk factor for development of cardiovascular disease: A statement from the American Heart Association Councils on Kidney in Cardiovascular Disease, High Blood Pressure Research, Clinical Cardiology, and Epidemiology and Prevention. *Hypertension* **2003**, *42*, 1050–1065. [CrossRef]
5. Thompson, S.; James, M.; Wiebe, N.; Hemmelgarn, B.; Manns, B.; Klarenbach, S.; Tonelli, M. Alberta Kidney Disease Network. Cause of Death in Patients with Reduced Kidney Function. *J. Am. Soc. Nephrol.* **2015**, *26*, 2504–2511. [CrossRef]
6. Su, G.; Xu, Y.; Xu, X.; Xu, H.; Lu, L.; Marrone, G.; Lindholm, B.; Wen, Z.; Liu, X.; Johnson, D.W.; et al. Association between reduced renal function and cardiovascular mortality in patients hospitalized with infection: A multi-center cohort study. *Eur. J. Intern. Med.* **2018**, *57*, 32–38. [CrossRef]
7. Gallo, P.; De Vincentis, A.; Pedone, C.; Nobili, A.; Tettamanti, M.; Gentilucci, U.V.; Picardi, A.; Mannucci, P.M.; Incalzi, R.A. REPOSI Investigators. Prognostic relevance of glomerular filtration rate estimation obtained through different equations in hospitalized elderly patients. *Eur. J. Intern. Med.* **2018**, *54*, 60–64. [CrossRef]
8. Topaz, G.; Gharra, W.; Eisen, A.; Hershko, A.Y.; Shilo, L.; Beeri, G.; Kitay-Cohen, Y.; Pereg, D. Impaired renal function is associated with adverse outcomes in patients with chest pain discharged from internal medicine wards. *Eur. J. Intern. Med.* **2018**, *53*, 57–61. [CrossRef]
9. Bozzano, V.; Abati, E. (GrAM) GdAM. Fluid intake and chronic kidney disease: Effect of coaching an increase in fluid intake on kidney function decline. *Intern. Emerg Med.* **2018**, *13*, 1283–1285. [CrossRef]
10. Riva, N.; Ageno, W.; Gatt, A. Estimating renal function in patients with atrial fibrillation: Which dose of direct oral anticoagulants? *Intern. Emerg. Med.* **2018**, *13*, 1001–1004. [CrossRef]
11. Boriani, G.; Vitolo, M.; Diemberger, I.; Proietti, M.; Valenti, A.C.; Malavasi, V.L.; Lip, G.Y.H. Optimizing indices of AF susceptibility and burden to evaluate AF severity, risk and outcomes. *Cardiovasc. Res.* **2021**, *117*, 1–21. [CrossRef] [PubMed]
12. Sgura, F.A.; Arrotti, S.; Magnavacchi, P.; Monopoli, D.; Gabbieri, D.; Banchelli, F.; Tondi, S.; Denegri, A.; D'Amico, R.; Guiducci, V.; et al. Kidney dysfunction and short term all-cause mortality after transcatheter aortic valve implantation. *Eur. J. Intern. Med.* **2020**, *81*, 32–37. [CrossRef] [PubMed]
13. Malavasi, V.L.; Pettorelli, D.; Fantecchi, E.; Zoccali, C.; Laronga, G.; Trenti, T.; Lip, G.Y.H.; Boriani, G. Variations in clinical management of non-vitamin K antagonist oral anticoagulants in patients with atrial fibrillation according to different equations for estimating renal function: Post hoc analysis of a prospective cohort. *Intern. Emerg. Med.* **2018**, *13*, 1059–1067. [CrossRef] [PubMed]
14. Pugliese, N.R.; Fabiani, I.; Conte, L.; Nesti, L.; Masi, S.; Natali, A.; Colombo, P.C.; Pedrinelli, R.; Dini, F.L. Persistent congestion, renal dysfunction and inflammatory cytokines in acute heart failure: A prognosis study. *J. Cardiovasc. Med.* **2020**, *21*, 494–502. [CrossRef] [PubMed]
15. Campanile, A.; Castellani, C.; Santucci, A.; Annunziata, R.; Tutarini, C.; Reccia, M.R.; Del Pinto, M.; Verdecchia, P.; Cavallini, C. Predictors of in-hospital and long-term mortality in unselected patients admitted to a modern coronary care unit. *J. Cardiovasc. Med.* **2019**, *20*, 327–334. [CrossRef]
16. Shetty, S.; Malik, A.H.; Ali, A.; Yang, Y.C.; Aronow, W.S.; Briasoulis, A. Impact of acute kidney injury on in-hospital outcomes among patients hospitalized with acute heart failure—A propensity-score matched analysis. *Eur. J. Intern. Med.* **2020**, *79*, 76–80. [CrossRef]
17. Sanchez-Serna, J.; Hernandez-Vicente, A.; Garrido-Bravo, I.P.; Pastor-Perez, F.; Noguera-Velasco, J.A.; Casas-Pina, T.; Rodriguez-Serrano, A.I.; Núñez, J.; Pascual-Figal, D. Impact of pre-hospital renal function on the detection of acute kidney injury in acute decompensated heart failure. *Eur. J. Intern. Med.* **2020**, *77*, 66–72. [CrossRef]

18. Correale, M.; Paolillo, S.; Mercurio, V.; Limongelli, G.; Barillà, F.; Ruocco, G.; Palazzuoli, A.; Scrutinio, D.; Lagioia, R.; Lombardi, C.; et al. Co-morbidities in chronic heart failure: An update from Italian Society of Cardiology (SIC) Working Group on Heart Failure. *Eur. J. Intern. Med.* **2020**, *71*, 23–31. [CrossRef]
19. Kashani, K.; Rosner, M.H.; Ostermann, M. Creatinine: From physiology to clinical application. *Eur. J. Intern. Med.* **2020**, *72*, 9–14. [CrossRef]
20. Fox, C.S.; Matsushita, K.; Woodward, M.; Bilo, H.J.; Chalmers, J.; Heerspink, H.J.; Lee, B.J.; Perkins, R.M.; Rossing, P.; Sairenchi, T.; et al. Associations of kidney disease measures with mortality and end-stage renal disease in individuals with and without diabetes: A meta-analysis. *Lancet* **2012**, *380*, 1662–1673. [CrossRef]
21. Lokhandwala, S.; McCague, N.; Chahin, A.; Escobar, B.; Feng, M.; Ghassemi, M.M.; Stone, D.J.; Celi, L.A. One-year mortality after recovery from critical illness: A retrospective cohort study. *PLoS ONE* **2018**, *13*, e0197226. [CrossRef] [PubMed]
22. Tonelli, M.; Muntner, P.; Lloyd, A.; Manns, B.J.; Klarenbach, S.; Pannu, N.; James, M.T.; Hemmelgarn, B.R. Alberta Kidney Disease Network. Risk of coronary events in people with chronic kidney disease compared with those with diabetes: A population-level cohort study. *Lancet* **2012**, *380*, 807–814. [CrossRef]
23. Vanholder, R.; Massy, Z.; Argiles, A.; Spasovski, G.; Verbeke, F.; Lameire, N. European Uremic Toxin Work Group. Chronic kidney disease as cause of cardiovascular morbidity and mortality. *Nephrol. Dial. Transplant.* **2005**, *20*, 1048–1056. [CrossRef] [PubMed]
24. Tonelli, M.; Wiebe, N.; Culleton, B.; House, A.; Rabbat, C.; Fok, M.; McAlister, F.; Garg, A.X. Chronic kidney disease and mortality risk: A systematic review. *J. Am. Soc. Nephrol.* **2006**, *17*, 2034–2047. [CrossRef]
25. Manjunath, G.; Tighiouart, H.; Ibrahim, H.; MacLeod, B.; Salem, D.N.; Griffith, J.L.; Coresh, J.; Levey, A.S.; Sarnak, M.J. Level of kidney function as a risk factor for atherosclerotic cardiovascular outcomes in the community. *J. Am. Coll. Cardiol.* **2003**, *41*, 47–55. [CrossRef]
26. Anavekar, N.S.; McMurray, J.J.; Velazquez, E.J.; Solomon, S.D.; Kober, L.; Rouleau, J.L.; White, H.D.; Nordlander, R.; Maggioni, A.; Dickstein, K.; et al. Relation between renal dysfunction and cardiovascular outcomes after myocardial infarction. *N. Engl. J. Med.* **2004**, *351*, 1285–1295. [CrossRef]
27. Gibson, C.M.; Dumaine, R.L.; Gelfand, E.V.; Murphy, S.A.; Morrow, D.A.; Wiviott, S.D.; Giugliano, R.P.; Cannon, C.P.; Antman, E.M.; Braunwald, E. TIMI Study Group. Association of glomerular filtration rate on presentation with subsequent mortality in non-ST-segment elevation acute coronary syndrome; observations in 13,307 patients in five TIMI trials. *Eur. Heart J.* **2004**, *25*, 1998–2005. [CrossRef]
28. Kpaeyeh, J.A., Jr.; Divoky, L.; Hyer, J.M.; Daly, D.D., Jr.; Maran, A.; Waring, A.; Gold, M.R. Impact of Renal Function on Survival After Cardiac Resynchronization Therapy. *Am. J. Cardiol.* **2017**, *120*, 262–266. [CrossRef]
29. García-Gil, M.; Parramon, D.; Comas-Cufí, M.; Martí, R.; Ponjoan, A.; Alves-Cabratosa, L.; Blanch, J.; Petersen, I.; Elosua, R.; Grau, M.; et al. Role of renal function in cardiovascular risk assessment: A retrospective cohort study in a population with low incidence of coronary heart disease. *Prev Med.* **2016**, *89*, 200–206. [CrossRef]
30. Edfors, R.; Sahlén, A.; Szummer, K.; Renlund, H.; Evans, M.; Carrero, J.J.; Spaak, J.; James, S.K.; Lagerqvist, B.; Varenhorst, C.; et al. Outcomes in patients treated with ticagrelor versus clopidogrel after acute myocardial infarction stratified by renal function. *Heart* **2018**, *104*, 1575–1582. [CrossRef]
31. Boriani, G.; Savelieva, I.; Dan, G.A.; Deharo, J.C.; Ferro, C.; Israel, C.W.; Lane, D.A.; La Manna, G.; Morton, J.; Mitjans, A.M.; et al. Chronic kidney disease in patients with cardiac rhythm disturbances or implantable electrical devices: Clinical significance and implications for decision making-a position paper of the European Heart Rhythm Association endorsed by the Heart Rhythm Society and the Asia Pacific Heart Rhythm Society. *Europace* **2015**, *17*, 1169–1196. [PubMed]
32. Boriani, G.; Laroche, C.; Diemberger, I.; Popescu, M.I.; Rasmussen, L.H.; Petrescu, L.; Crijns, H.J.G.M.; Tavazzi, L.; Maggioni, A.P.; Lip, G.Y.H. Glomerular filtration rate in patients with atrial fibrillation and 1-year outcomes. *Sci. Rep.* **2016**, *6*, 30271. [CrossRef] [PubMed]
33. Cockcroft, D.W.; Gault, M.H. Prediction of creatinine clearance from serum creatinine. *Nephron* **1976**, *16*, 31–41. [CrossRef] [PubMed]
34. Rostoker, G.; Andrivet, P.; Pham, I.; Griuncelli, M.; Adnot, S. A modified Cockcroft-Gault formula taking into account the body surface area gives a more accurate estimation of the glomerular filtration rate. *J. Nephrol.* **2007**, *20*, 576–585. [PubMed]
35. Levey, A.S.; Bosch, J.P.; Lewis, J.B.; Greene, T.; Rogers, N.; Roth, D. A more accurate method to estimate glomerular filtration rate from serum creatinine: A new prediction equation. Modification of Diet in Renal Disease Study Group. *Ann. Intern. Med.* **1999**, *130*, 461–470. [CrossRef]
36. Levey, A.S.; Coresh, J.; Greene, T.; Marsh, J.; Stevens, L.A.; Kusek, J.W.; Van Lente, F.; Chronic Kidney Disease Epidemiology Collaboration. Expressing the Modification of Diet in Renal Disease Study equation for estimating glomerular filtration rate with standardized serum creatinine values. *Clin. Chem.* **2007**, *53*, 766–772. [CrossRef]
37. Levey, A.S.; Stevens, L.A.; Schmid, C.H.; Zhang, Y.L.; Castro, A.F., 3rd; Feldman, H.I.; Kusek, J.W.; Eggers, P.; Van Lente, F.; Greene, T.; et al. A new equation to estimate glomerular filtration rate. *Ann. Intern. Med.* **2009**, *150*, 604–612. [CrossRef]
38. Gill, J.; Malyuk, R.; Djurdjev, O.; Levin, A. Use of GFR equations to adjust drug doses in an elderly multi-ethnic group—a cautionary tale. *Nephrol Dial. Transplant.* **2007**, *22*, 2894–2899. [CrossRef]
39. Garasto, S.; Fusco, S.; Corica, F.; Rosignuolo, M.; Marino, A.; Montesanto, A.; De Rango, F.; Maggio, M.; Mari, V.; Corsonello, A.; et al. Estimating glomerular filtration rate in older people. *Biomed. Res. Int.* **2014**, *2014*, 916542. [CrossRef]

40. Schaeffner, E.S.; Ebert, N.; Delanaye, P.; Frei, U.; Gaedeke, J.; Jakob, O.; Kuhlmann, M.K.; Schuchardt, M.; Tölle, M.; Ziebig, R.; et al. Two novel equations to estimate kidney function in persons aged 70 years or older. *Ann. Intern. Med.* **2012**, *157*, 471–481. [CrossRef]
41. Pottel, H.; Mottaghy, F.M.; Zaman, Z.; Martens, F. On the relationship between glomerular filtration rate and serum creatinine in children. *Pediatr Nephrol.* **2010**, *25*, 927–934. [CrossRef] [PubMed]
42. Pottel, H.; Hoste, L.; Martens, F. A simple height-independent equation for estimating glomerular filtration rate in children. *Pediatr Nephrol.* **2012**, *27*, 973–979. [CrossRef] [PubMed]
43. Pottel, H.; Vrydags, N.; Mahieu, B.; Vandewynckele, E.; Croes, K.; Martens, F. Establishing age/sex related serum creatinine reference intervals from hospital laboratory data based on different statistical methods. *Clin. Chim Acta.* **2008**, *396*, 49–55. [CrossRef]
44. Pottel, H.; Hoste, L.; Dubourg, L.; Ebert, N.; Schaeffner, E.; Eriksen, B.O.; Melsom, T.; Lamb, E.J.; Rule, A.D.; Turner, S.T.; et al. An estimated glomerular filtration rate equation for the full age spectrum. *Nephrol Dial. Transplant.* **2016**, *31*, 798–806. [CrossRef]
45. Levey, A.S. Measurement of renal function in chronic renal disease. *Kidney Int.* **1990**, *38*, 167–184. [CrossRef] [PubMed]
46. Miller, B.F.; Winkler, A.W. The renal excretion of endogenous creatinine in man. comparison with exogenous creatinine and inulin. *J. Clin. Invest.* **1938**, *17*, 31–40. [CrossRef]
47. Shemesh, O.; Golbetz, H.; Kriss, J.P.; Myers, B.D. Limitations of creatinine as a filtration marker in glomerulopathic patients. *Kidney Int.* **1985**, *28*, 830–838. [CrossRef]
48. Perrone, R.D.; Madias, N.E.; Levey, A.S. Serum creatinine as an index of renal function: New insights into old concepts. *Clin. Chem.* **1992**, *38*, 1933–1953. [CrossRef] [PubMed]
49. Heymsfield, S.B.; Arteaga, C.; McManus, C.; Smith, J.; Moffitt, S. Measurement of muscle mass in humans: Validity of the 24-h urinary creatinine method. *Am. J. Clin. Nutr.* **1983**, *37*, 478–494. [CrossRef]
50. Preiss, D.J.; Godber, I.M.; Lamb, E.J.; Dalton, R.N.; Gunn, I.R. The influence of a cooked-meat meal on estimated glomerular filtration rate. *Ann. Clin. Biochem.* **2007**, *44 Pt 1*, 35–42. [CrossRef]
51. Levey, A.S.; Inker, L.A.; Coresh, J. GFR estimation: From physiology to public health. *Am. J. Kidney Dis.* **2014**, *63*, 820–834. [CrossRef] [PubMed]
52. Viera, A.J.; Garrett, J.M. Understanding interobserver agreement: The kappa statistic. *Fam Med.* **2005**, *37*, 360–363. [PubMed]
53. DeLong, E.R.; DeLong, D.M.; Clarke-Pearson, D.L. Comparing the areas under two or more correlated receiver operating characteristic curves: A non-parametric approach. *Biometrics* **1988**, *44*, 837–845. [CrossRef] [PubMed]
54. Pencina, M.J.; D'Agostino, R.B.; Vasan, R.S. Evaluating the added predictive ability of a new marker: From area under the ROC curve to reclassification and beyond. *Stat. Med.* **2008**, *27*, 157–172; discussion 207-12. [CrossRef] [PubMed]
55. Kundu, S.; Aulchenko, Y.S.; van Duijn, C.M.; Janssens, A.C. PredictABEL: An R package for the assessment of risk prediction models. *Eur. J. Epidemiol.* **2011**, *26*, 261–264. [CrossRef] [PubMed]
56. January, C.T.; Wann, L.S.; Alpert, J.S.; Calkins, H.; Cigarroa, J.E.; Cleveland, J.C.; Ellinor, P.T.; Ezekowitz, M.D.; Field, M.E.; Furie , K.L.; et al. 2014 AHA/ACC/HRS guideline for the management of patients with atrial fibrillation: A report of the American College of Cardiology/American Heart Association Task Force on Practice Guidelines and the Heart Rhythm Society. *J. Am. Coll Cardiol.* **2014**, *64*, e1–e76. [CrossRef]
57. Ruiz-Esteban, P.; López, V.; García-Frías, P.; Cabello, M.; González-Molina, M.; Vozmediano, C.; Hernandez, D. Concordance of estimated glomerular filtration rates using Cockcroft-Gault modification of diet in renal disease, and chronic kidney disease epidemiology in renal transplant recipients. *Transplant. Proc.* **2012**, *44*, 2561–2563. [CrossRef] [PubMed]
58. Esteve Poblador, S.; Gorriz Pintado, S.; Ortuño Alonso, M. Comparison between two equations to estimated glomerular filtration rate. *Rev. Clin. Esp.* **2012**, *212*, 75–80. [CrossRef]
59. Teruel, J.L.; Rexach, L.; Burguera, V.; Gomis, A.; Rodríguez-Mendiola, N.; Díaz, A.; Collazo, S.; Quereda, C. Home care programme for patients with advanced chronic kidney disease. A two-year experience. *Nefrologia.* **2014**, *34*, 611–616.
60. Torreggiani, M.; Chatrenet, A.; Fois, A.; Moio, M.R.; Mazé, B.; Coindre, J.P.; Crochette, R.; Sigogne, M.; Wacrenier, S.; Lecointre, L.; et al. Elderly Patients in a Large Nephrology Unit: Who Are Our Old, Old-Old and Oldest-Old Patients? *J. Clin. Med.* **2021**, *10*, 1168. [CrossRef] [PubMed]
61. Stevens, L.A.; Levey, A.S. Use of the MDRD study equation to estimate kidney function for drug dosing. *Clin. Pharmacol Ther.* **2009**, *86*, 465–467. [CrossRef] [PubMed]
62. Michels, W.M.; Grootendorst, D.C.; Verduijn, M.; Elliott, E.G.; Dekker, F.W.; Krediet, R.T. Performance of the Cockcroft-Gault, MDRD, and new CKD-EPI formulas in relation to GFR, age, and body size. *Clin. J. Am. Soc. Nephrol.* **2010**, *5*, 1003–1009. [CrossRef] [PubMed]
63. Mandelli, S.; Riva, E.; Tettamanti, M.; Detoma, P.; Giacomin, A.; Lucca, U. Mortality Prediction in the Oldest Old with Five Different Equations to Estimate Glomerular Filtration Rate: The Health and Anemia Population-based Study. *PLoS ONE* **2015**, *10*, e0136039. [CrossRef] [PubMed]
64. Flamant, M.; Haymann, J.P.; Vidal-Petiot, E.; Letavernier, E.; Clerici, C.; Boffa, J.J.; Vrtovsnik, F. GFR estimation using the Cockcroft-Gault, MDRD study, and CKD-EPI equations in the elderly. *Am. J. Kidney Dis.* **2012**, *60*, 847–849. [CrossRef] [PubMed]
65. Buron, F.; Hadj-Aissa, A.; Dubourg, L.; Morelon, E.; Steghens, J.P.; Ducher, M.; Fauvel, J.P. Estimating glomerular filtration rate in kidney transplant recipients: Performance over time of four creatinine-based formulas. *Transplantation* **2011**, *92*, 1005–1011. [CrossRef] [PubMed]

66. Kilbride, H.S.; Stevens, P.E.; Eaglestone, G.; Knight, S.; Carter, J.L.; Delaney, M.P.; Farmer, C.K.; Irving, J.; O'Riordan, S.E.; Dalton, R.N.; et al. Accuracy of the MDRD (Modification of Diet in Renal Disease) study and CKD-EPI (CKD Epidemiology Collaboration) equations for estimation of GFR in the elderly. *Am. J. Kidney Dis.* **2013**, *61*, 57–66. [CrossRef]
67. Rivera-Caravaca, J.M.; Ruiz-Nodar, J.M.; Tello-Montoliu, A.; Esteve-Pastor, M.A.; Quintana-Giner, M.; Véliz-Martínez, A.; Orenes-Piñero, E.; Romero-Aniorte, A.I.; Vicente-Ibarra, N.; Pernias-Escrig, V.; et al. Disparities in the Estimation of Glomerular Filtration Rate According to Cockcroft-Gault, Modification of Diet in Renal Disease-4, and Chronic Kidney Disease Epidemiology Collaboration Equations and Relation With Outcomes in Patients With Acute Coronary Syndrome. *J. Am. Heart Assoc.* **2018**, *7*, e008725.
68. Ndrepepa, G.; Holdenrieder, S.; Neumann, F.J.; Lahu, S.; Cassese, S.; Joner, M.; Xhepa, E.; Kufner, S.; Wiebe, J.; Laugwitz, K.L.; et al. Prognostic value of glomerular function estimated by Cockcroft-Gault creatinine clearance, MDRD-4, CKD-EPI and European Kidney Function Consortium equations in patients with acute coronary syndromes. *Clin. Chim Acta.* **2021**, *523*, 106–113. [CrossRef]
69. Da Silva Selistre, L.; Rech, D.L.; de Souza, V.; Iwaz, J.; Lemoine, S.; Dubourg, L. Diagnostic Performance of Creatinine-Based Equations for Estimating Glomerular Filtration Rate in Adults 65 Years and Older. *JAMA Intern. Med.* **2019**, *179*, 796–804. [CrossRef] [PubMed]
70. Cherney, D.Z.I.; Lytvyn, Y.; McCullough, P.A. Cardiovascular Risk Reduction in Patients With Chronic Kidney Disease: Potential for Targeting Inflammation With Canakinumab. *J. Am. Coll Cardiol.* **2018**, *71*, 2415–2418. [CrossRef] [PubMed]
71. Kuo, P.H.; Kanal, E.; Abu-Alfa, A.K.; Cowper, S.E. Gadolinium-based MR contrast agents and nephrogenic systemic fibrosis. *Radiology.* **2007**, *242*, 647–649. [CrossRef] [PubMed]
72. Polyzos, K.A.; Konstantelias, A.A.; Falagas, M.E. Risk factors for cardiac implantable electronic device infection: A systematic review and meta-analysis. *Europace* **2015**, *17*, 767–777. [CrossRef] [PubMed]
73. Boriani, G.; Malavasi, V.L. Patient outcome after implant of a cardioverter defibrillator in the 'real world': The key role of co-morbidities. *Eur. J. Heart Fail.* **2017**, *19*, 387–390. [CrossRef] [PubMed]

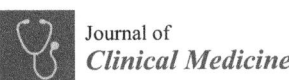

Article

Heart Transplantation of the Elderly—Old Donors for Old Recipients: Can We Still Achieve Acceptable Results?

Moritz Benjamin Immohr [1], Hug Aubin [1], Ralf Westenfeld [2], Sophiko Erbel-Khurtsidze [1], Igor Tudorache [1], Payam Akhyari [1], Artur Lichtenberg [1] and Udo Boeken [1,*]

[1] Department of Cardiac Surgery, Medical Faculty and University Hospital Düsseldorf, Heinrich-Heine-University Düsseldorf, 40225 Düsseldorf, Germany; Moritz.Immohr@med.uni-duesseldorf.de (M.B.I.); Hug.Aubin@med.uni-duesseldorf.de (H.A.); Sophiko.Erbel-Khurtsidze@med.uni-duesseldorf.de (S.E.-K.); Igor.Tudorache@med.uni-duesseldorf.de (I.T.); Payam.Akhyari@med.uni-duesseldorf.de (P.A.); Artur.Lichtenberg@med.uni-duesseldorf.de (A.L.)

[2] Division of Cardiology, Medical Faculty and University Hospital Düsseldorf, Heinrich-Heine-University Düsseldorf, 40225 Düsseldorf, Germany; Ralf.Westenfeld@med.uni-duesseldorf.de

* Correspondence: Udo.Boeken@med.uni-duesseldorf.de; Tel.: +49-211-8118331

Abstract: As society is ageing, an increasing prevalence of elderly heart failure patients will be expected. In order to increase the donor pool, acceptance of older donors might be a reasonable choice. All patients undergoing heart transplantation between 2010 and 2021 at a single department were retrospectively reviewed and divided into different study groups with regard to recipient ($\leq$60 years (R^Y) or >60 years (R^O)) and donor age ($\leq$50 years (D^Y) or >50 years (D^O)). A total of n = 201 patients were included (D^Y/R^Y, n = 91; D^O/R^Y, n = 38; D^Y/R^O, n = 41; D^O/R^O, n = 31). Neither incidence of severe primary graft dysfunction (p = 0.64) nor adverse events, such as kidney failure (p = 0.27), neurological complications (p = 0.63), infections (p = 0.21) or acute graft rejection (p = 1.00), differed between the groups. However, one-year survival was impaired in the D^O/R^O group (56.0%) compared to the other groups (D^Y/R^Y: 86.1%, D^Y/R^O: 78.8%, D^O/R^Y: 74.2%, p = 0.02). Given the impaired one-year survival, acceptance of grafts from old donors for old recipients should be performed with caution and by experienced centres only. Nevertheless, because of the otherwise dismal prognosis of elderly heart failure patients, transplantation of patients may still improve the therapy outcome.

Keywords: heart transplantation; age; elderly; frailty; demographic change

Citation: Immohr, M.B.; Aubin, H.; Westenfeld, R.; Erbel-Khurtsidze, S.; Tudorache, I.; Akhyari, P.; Lichtenberg, A.; Boeken, U. Heart Transplantation of the Elderly—Old Donors for Old Recipients: Can We Still Achieve Acceptable Results? *J. Clin. Med.* **2022**, *11*, 929. https://doi.org/10.3390/jcm11040929

Academic Editor: Patrick De Boever

Received: 14 January 2022
Accepted: 9 February 2022
Published: 10 February 2022

Publisher's Note: MDPI stays neutral with regard to jurisdictional claims in published maps and institutional affiliations.

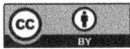

Copyright: © 2022 by the authors. Licensee MDPI, Basel, Switzerland. This article is an open access article distributed under the terms and conditions of the Creative Commons Attribution (CC BY) license (https://creativecommons.org/licenses/by/4.0/).

1. Introduction

Congestive heart failure is a global burden of disease affecting millions of people worldwide [1–3]. Among adults and the elderly, it is one of the leading causes for hospitalisation and origin of tremendous costs for health care systems [1–3]. Due to current demographic changes, numbers of heart failure patients are expected to further increase within the next decades [2]. By now, heart transplantation (HTx) is the standard of care for end-stage heart failure [4,5]. However, especially elderly heart failure patients often suffer from a variety of concomitant diseases and frailty, which has been reported to presently affect 45% of heart failure patients [6]. Transplanting these elderly and frail patients might be challenging [7]. To expand the donor pool for this increasing number of older patients on the transplant waiting list, accepting more and more old and marginal donors might be an option as it has been successfully performed for other donor organs [7–9]. However, cardiac grafts of old donors carry a risk for impaired long-term survival [10,11].

In order to investigate possible effects of donor and recipient age matching for the outcome after HTx, we aimed to analyse the postoperative outcome for young and old recipients of cardiac grafts from young and old donors. We therefore retrospectively reviewed our institutional data of the last decade and compared the outcome after HTx for different groups of donor and recipient age matching.

2. Materials and Methods

2.1. Patients and Study Design

All adult patients (n = 201) who underwent HTx between September 2010 and March 2021 in our department were prospectively enrolled in an institutional database. Patients were retrospectively reviewed and those who underwent cardiac re-transplantation were excluded. Afterwards, patients were divided into four study groups with regard to the recipient and donor age matching (Figure 1). Recipients aged 60 years or younger (n = 129) were declared as young recipients (R^Y). Correspondingly, recipients undergoing HTx over 60 years of age were declared as old recipients (R^O, n = 72). In line with the current literature [10,11], for donors, age limit was set at 50 years (donor age $\leq$ 50 years: young donors (D^Y, n = 132), donor age > 50 years: old donors (D^O, n = 69)). Accordingly, young recipients with young donors (D^Y/R^Y, n = 91) were compared to young recipients with old donors (D^O/R^Y, n = 38) as well as old recipients with young donors (D^Y/R^O, n = 41) and old recipients with old donors (D^O/R^O, n = 31).

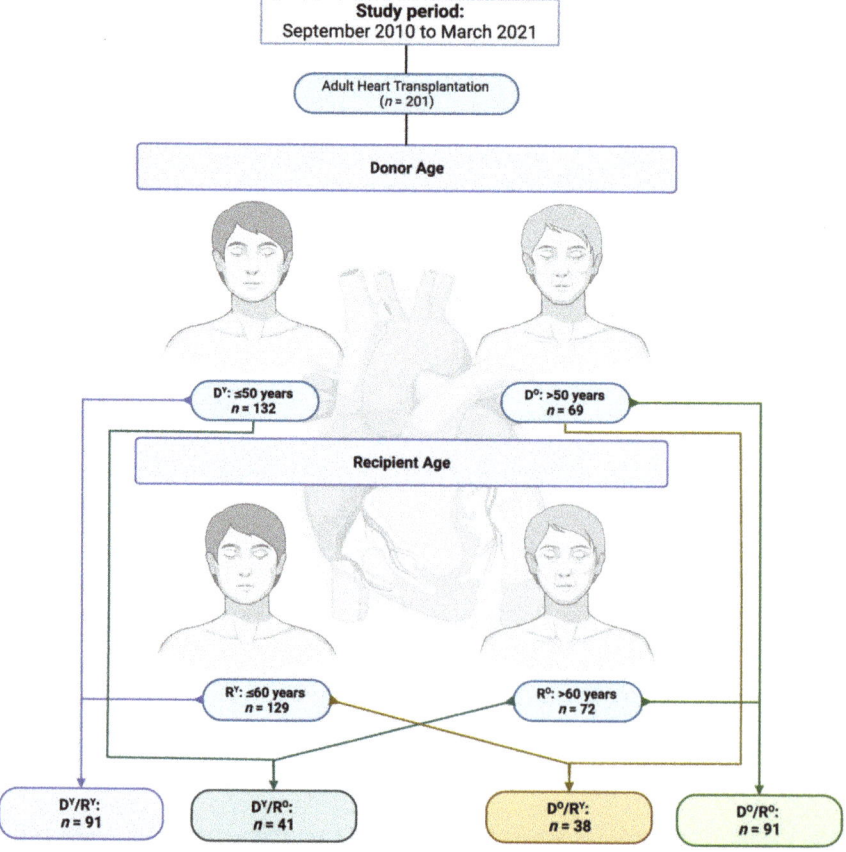

Figure 1. Study groups.

2.2. Study Objectives and Follow-Up Period

Relevant donor and recipient parameters were examined and impact of donor and recipient age matching on the postoperative morbidity and mortality was analysed. Patients were postoperatively followed-up every three to six months on a regular basis. Postoperative one-year survival was defined as the primary endpoint and impaired postoperative survival was hypothesised for old recipients with old donor organs. In addition, perioperative adverse events, such as acute kidney failure, neurological complications or bleeding complications, were defined as secondary endpoints of the study.

2.3. Surgical Procedure and Perioperative Management

HTx was performed with either orthotopic bicaval or biatrial technique. For immunosuppression a standardised institutional protocol consisting of tacrolimus, mycophenolate mofetil and prednisolone. Potential graft rejection was routinely examined by right ventricular endomyocardial biopsies and addressed with high-dose prednisolone therapy for at least three consecutive days. In case of antibody-mediated rejection, therapy was amended by immunoabsorption or plasmapheresis, anti-T-lymphocyte IgG and intravenous IgM-enriched human immunoglobulin. Patients suffering from primary graft dysfunction were treated following an institutional standard operating procedure covering adequate catecholamine therapy with epinephrine and norepinephrine and a relatively liberal regime of early implantation of veno-arterial extracorporeal membrane oxygenation (va-ECMO) and percutaneous microaxial pumps (Impella 5.0, Abiomed, Inc., Danvers, MA, USA).

2.4. Statistics

For statistical analyses SPSS Statistics 26 (IBM Corporation, Armonk, NY, USA) was used. All results are displayed as mean values with the standard deviation (SD) respectively percentage of the whole. Because of the small and unbalanced groups sizes, Gaussian distribution was not assumed, and variables were therefore compared by either nonparametric two-tailed Kruskal–Wallis tests or Fisher–Freeman–Halton tests. In case of statistically significant results ($p < 0.05$), additional post-hoc analyses were used by a Bonferroni correction. Postoperative survival after HTx was calculated by the Kaplan–Meier method and compared by log-rank test. Detailed information of the post-hoc tests are displayed in the Supplementary Table S1.

3. Results

3.1. Pre-Transplant Recipient Parameters

Detailed preoperative recipient parameters are displayed in Table 1. As given by the study protocol, there was a significant difference between the four groups with regard to the recipient age with a mean age of 48 years for D^Y/R^Y patients and 65 years in the D^O/R^O group. Recipient age ranged from 22 years (D^Y/R^Y) to 73 years (D^O/R^O). Younger recipients were much more often transplanted with high urgency wait list status compared to old recipients ($p < 0.01$). This was also underlined by the increased incidence of pre-transplant mechanical ventilation in the D^Y/R^Y and D^O/R^Y group compared to the other two groups. The same effect was also numerically observed for pre-transplant cardiopulmonary resuscitation. Interestingly, we did not observe any other differences with regard to the incidence of preoperative risk factors for impaired outcome or concomitant diseases. Especially, there was no difference in the incidence of previous mechanical circulatory support (ventricular assist devices or extracorporeal life support).

3.2. Pre-Transplant Donor Parameters

Detailed preoperative donor parameters are displayed in Table 2. Differences in demographic data of the four groups are once again given by the study protocol. Minimum donor age was 15 years (D^Y/R^Y) and maximum was 67 years (D^O/R^O). Although donor sex distribution and body mass index were inhomogeneous between the four groups, predicted heart mass ratio of the recipients and donors was comparable, indicating no relevant differences regarding organ size mismatch. Younger donors were much more likely to be resuscitated before recovery of the organs. Nevertheless, there were no differences regarding catecholamine therapy and concomitant diseases, indicating a similar distribution rate of marginal donors between the four groups.

Table 1. Preoperative recipient parameters.

Recipient Variables	D^Y/R^Y (n = 91)	D^O/R^Y (n = 38)	D^Y/R^O (n = 41)	D^O/R^O (n = 31)	p-Value
Age, y (SD)	48 (11)	52 (8)	64 (3)	65 (3)	<0.01
Female gender, n (%)	26 (28.6)	12 (31.6)	8 (19.5)	7 (22.6)	0.59
Height, cm (SD)	175 (8)	173 (11)	176 (7)	174 (7)	0.57
Weight, kg (SD)	78 (16)	75 (16)	79 (16)	79 (13)	0.52
Body mass index, kg/m^2 (SD)	25.7 (4.9)	25.2 (5.0)	25.5 (4.0)	26.2 (3.8)	0.64
Panel-reactive antibodies, % (SD)	3.1 (14.5)	1.3 (6.6)	3.1 (19.1)	0.2 (0.9)	0.66
High urgency wait list status, n (%)	52 (57.1)	19 (50.0)	19 (46.3)	7 (22.6)	0.01
Aetiology					
Ischemic cardiomyopathy, n (%)	24 (26.4)	18 (47.4)	23 (56.1)	16 (51.6)	
Dilated cardiomyopathy, n (%)	55 (60.4)	19 (50.0)	16 (39.0)	13 (41.9)	0.20
Other, n (%)	12 (13.2)	1 (2.6)	2 (4.8)	2 (6.4)	
Ventricular assist device, n (%)	50 (54.9)	17 (44.7)	23 (56.1)	18 (58.1)	0.66
Extracorporeal life support, n (%)	6 (6.7)	2 (5.3)	1 (2.4)	0 (0.0)	0.57
Concomitant diseases					
Diabetes mellitus, n (%)	17 (8.7)	9 (23.7)	9 (22.0)	6 (19.4)	0.58
Haemodialyis, n (%)	7 (7.8)	1 (2.6)	1 (2.6)	1 (3.2)	0.65
Smoking, n (%)	21 (23.1)	7 (18.4)	8 (19.5)	8 (25.8)	0.74
Arterial hypertension, n (%)	50 (54.9)	25 (65.8)	26 (63.4)	17 (54.8)	0.72
Pulmonary hypertension, n (%)	8 (8.8)	5 (13.2)	2 (4.9)	4 (12.9)	0.52
COPD, n (%)	7 (7.7)	2 (5.3)	2 (4.9)	4 (12.9)	0.60
Cardiopulmonary resuscitation, n (%)	13 (14.3)	5 (13.2)	5 (12.2)	0 (0.0)	0.17
Mechanical ventilation, n (%)	8 (8.8)	5 (13.2)	1 (2.4)	0 (0.0)	0.01
Blood transfusion, n (%)	8 (8.8)	1 (2.6)	2 (4.9)	1 (3.2)	0.58
Laboratory values					
Hemoglobin, g/dL (SD)	11.6 (2.4)	11.5 (2.3)	12.4 (1.9)	12.6 (2.4)	0.05
Bilirubin, mg/dL (SD)	1.0 (1.2)	0.8 (0.9)	0.8 (0.6)	1.4 (0.4)	0.83
Creatinine, mg/dL (SD)	1.4 (1.3)	1.3 (0.5)	1.5 (0.7)	1.4 (0.4)	0.19
AST, U/L (SD)	49 (87)	41 (34)	29 (15)	30 (12)	0.46
Lactate dehydrogenase, U/L (SD)	413 (460)	288 (142)	279 (108)	285 (86)	0.87

Preoperative recipient parameters. Patients were divided into four study groups with regard to the donor and recipient age (donor age $\leq$ 50 years and recipient age $\leq$ 60 years: D^Y/R^Y, n = 91; donor age > 50 years and recipient age $\leq$ 60 years: D^O/R^Y, n = 38; donor age $\leq$ 50 years and recipient age > 60 years: D^Y/R^O, n = 41; donor age > 50 years and recipient age > 60 years: D^O/R^O, n = 31). Detailed results for post-hoc analysis are displayed in Supplementary Table S1. COPD, chronic obstructive pulmonary disease; AST, aspartate aminotransferase; SD, standard deviation.

3.3. Operative Outcome

Table 3 shows the postoperative outcome of the patients. While warm ischemia did not differ between the groups, the average transport time was slightly prolonged in the groups with the younger donors compared to the corresponding groups of similar recipient age ($p = 0.02$). Consequently, total graft ischemic time was also slightly prolonged. There was a strong trend towards increased postoperative epinephrine doses in the D^O/R^O group with about 50% higher peak concentration compared to the D^Y/R^Y group ($p = 0.05$). Nevertheless, incidence of va-ECMO implantation and postoperative support duration was comparable between all groups. Perioperative severe adverse events were also comparable between all groups with no advantages for any of the four groups. In line with these results, duration of postoperative mechanical ventilation and hospital stay also did not differ.

Table 2. Donor parameters.

Donor Variables	D^Y/R^Y (n = 91)	D^O/R^Y (n = 38)	D^Y/R^O (n = 41)	D^O/R^O (n = 31)	p-Value
Age, y (SD)	35 (10)	56 (4)	38 (10)	58 (10)	<0.01
Female gender, n (%)	38 (41.8)	23 (60.5)	12 (29.3)	15 (48.4)	0.04
Height, cm (SD)	176 (9)	172 (8)	177 (6)	173 (8)	0.05
Weight, kg (SD)	80 (15)	79 (11)	79 (17)	81 (15)	0.81
Body mass index, kg/m² (SD)	25.6 (4.1)	26.7 (3.1)	25.2 (5.0)	27.9 (7.0)	0.01
Predicted Heart Mass Ratio, % (SD)	13.8 (10.4)	14.7 (13.4)	12.6 (9.7)	11.6 (7.9)	0.87
Cardiopulmonary resuscitation, n (%)	24 (26.4)	3 (7.9)	19 (46.3)	6 (19.4)	<0.01
Duration, min (SD)	18 (13)	13 (3)	17 (13)	22 (17)	0.92
Norepinephrine, µg/kg/min (SD)	0.12 (0.16)	0.14 (0.33)	0.14 (0.21)	0.10 (0.09)	0.68
Ejection fraction, % (SD)	61 (9)	62 (10)	57 (10)	62 (7)	0.28
Concomitant diseases					
Arterial hypertension, n (%)	14/41 (34.1)	18/25 (72.0)	10/22 (45.5)	16/20 (22.2)	<0.01
Diabetes mellitus, n (%)	6/37 (16.2)	2/11 (18.2)	0/15 (0.0)	5/10 (50.0)	0.02
Smoking, n (%)	49/76 (64.5)	16/30 (53.3)	21/39 (53.8)	14/26 (53.8)	0.56
Drug abuse, n (%)	8/75 (10.7)	1/31 (3.2)	8/34 (23.5)	0/24 (0.0)	0.02
Laboratory values					
Hemoglobin, g/dL (SD)	10.1 (2.8)	9.9 (1.9)	10.3 (2.9)	10.3 (2.4)	0.90
White blood cells, 1×10^9/L (SD)	15.1 (5.8)	14.9 (5.8)	14.3 (4.4)	21.0 (39.2)	0.89
Lactate dehydrogenase, U/L (SD)	510 (681)	352 (257)	525 (414)	347 (191)	0.04
Creatinine kinase, U/L (SD)	2029 (8139)	438 (643)	1068 (2326)	682 (1350)	0.11
C-reactive protein, mg/L (SD)	163 (232)	234 (416)	157 (110)	151 (96)	0.55

Donor parameters. Patients were divided into four study groups with regard to the donor and recipient age (donor age ≤ 50 years and recipient age ≤ 60 years: D^Y/R^Y, n = 91; donor age > 50 years and recipient age ≤ 60 years: D^O/R^Y, n = 38; donor age ≤ 50 years and recipient age > 60 years: D^Y/R^O, n = 41; donor age > 50 years and recipient age > 60 years: D^O/R^O, n = 31). Some data were not available or all donors. In this case altered group sizes are displayed within the corresponding line. Detailed results for post-hoc analysis are displayed in Supplementary Table S1. SD, standard deviation.

3.4. Postoperative Survival

Mean postoperative follow-up was about three years (991 days, SD: 1012 days) with a maximum of ten and a half years (3831 days). As shown in Table 3, 30-day survival was best for recipients of grafts from young donors (D^Y/R^Y = 94.4% and D^Y/R^O = 95.0% compared to D^O/R^Y = 84.2% and D^O/R^O = 80.6%, p = 0.05). The primary end-point of one-year survival was still best for D^Y/R^Y (86.1%), followed by comparable results for D^Y/R^O (78.8%) and D^O/R^Y (74.2%) but deeply impaired for D^O/R^O (56.0%) (p = 0.02). The cause of death within the first 30 days as well between 30 days and 1 year did not differ between the four groups. Within the first 30 days, multiple causes of death appeared; however, after 30 days, infective complications were the leading cause of death. Six patients died because of graft failure: three grafts from young and three grafts from old donors. In addition, the Kaplan–Meier survival curve is shown in Figure 2. Log-rank test (p = 0.10) identified no statistical significance between the four curves, but numerical differences indicated similar mid- to long-term results to those for short-term survival.

Table 3. Operative outcome.

Outcome Variables	D^Y/R^Y (n = 91)	D^O/R^Y (n = 38)	D^Y/R^O (n = 41)	D^O/R^O (n = 31)	p-Value
Total graft ischemic time, min (SD)	228 (55)	208 (45)	218 (48)	199 (37)	0.02
Transport time, min (SD)	162 (55)	142 (42)	151 (46)	134 (42)	0.02
Warm ischemia, min (SD)	66 (15)	66 (11)	67 (13)	65 (16)	0.71
Primary graft dysfunction					
Peak catecholamine					
Dobutamine, µg/kg/min (SD)	4.81 (2.16)	5.45 (2.84)	4.40 (2.29)	3.27 (2.43)	0.15
Epinephrine, µg/kg/min (SD)	0.21 (0.18)	0.27 (0.22)	0.20 (0.17)	0.32 (0.23)	0.05
Norepinephrine, µg/kg/min (SD)	0.35 (0.25)	0.37 (0.26)	0.35 (0.34)	0.37 (0.31)	0.94
va-ECMO, n (%)	27 (29.7)	10 (26.3)	16 (39.0)	9 (29.0)	0.64
Support duration, d (SD)	9.4 (9.3)	5.7 (5.1)	6.7 (3.6)	9.9 (4.9)	0.34
Deceased on support, n (%)	6/26 (23.1)	4/10 (40.0)	2/16 (12.5)	2/8 (25.0)	0.46
Postoperative morbidity					
Infective complications, n (%)	19/88 (21.6)	10/36 (27.8)	8/40 (20.0)	12/30 (40.0)	0.21
Acute graft rejection, n (%)	7/87 (8.0)	2/36 (5.6)	3/40 (7.5)	2/30 (6.7)	1.00
Hemodialysis on ICU, n (%)	43/89 (48.3)	23/37 (62.2)	25/40 (62.5)	19/30 (63.3)	0.27
Neurological complications, n (%)	17/88 (19.3)	5/36 (13.9)	7/40 (17.5)	8/30 (26.7)	0.63
Re-thoracotomy, n (%)	25/88 (28.4)	12/37 (32.4)	13/40 (32.5)	9/31 (29.0)	0.93
Postoperative hospital stay, d (SD)	42 (28)	41 (24)	51 (39)	54 (52)	0.68
Postoperative ICU/IMC stay, d (SD)	23 (27)	20 (20)	27 (31)	30 (31)	0.20
Mechanical ventilation, h (SD)	145 (197)	109 (141)	197 (210)	183 (232)	0.29
Blood transfusion					
Packed red blood cells, mL (SD)	3716 (5321)	3085 (3186)	3309 (2704)	4646 (5572)	0.70
Fresh frozen plasma, mL (SD)	5646 (8252)	3909 (3179)	6679 (5497)	8802 (8972)	0.09
Platelets, ml (SD)	1012 (2588)	833 (1198)	1106 (1308)	1775 (2719)	0.06
30-day survival, n (%)	85/90 (94.4)	32/38 (84.2)	38/40 (95.0)	25/31 (80.6)	0.05
Cause of death within 30 days					0.48
Graft failure	1 (20.0)	1 (16.7)	0 (0.0)	2 (33.3)	
Sepsis/MODS	2 (40.0)	0 (0.0)	0 (0.0)	2 (33.3)	
Coagulopathy	1 (20.0)	2 (33.3)	1 (50.0)	1 (16.7)	
Cerebral injury	1 (20.0)	0 (0.0)	0 (0.0)	0 (0.0)	
Visceral ischemia	0 (0.0)	0 (0.0)	1 (50.0)	0 (0.0)	
Other/unknown	0 (0.0)	3 (50.0)	0 (0.0)	1 (16.7)	
1-year survival, n (%)	62/72 (86.1)	23/31 (74.2)	26/33 (78.8)	14/25 (56.0)	0.02
Cause of death between 30 days and 1 year					0.52
Graft failure	0 (0.0)	0 (0.0)	2 (40.0)	0 (0.0)	
Sepsis/MODS	2 (40.0)	1 (50.0)	1 (20.0)	3 (60.0)	
Coagulopathy	1 (20.0)	0 (0.0)	0 (0.0)	0 (0.0)	
Cerebral injury	0 (0.0)	0 (0.0)	1 (20.0)	0 (0.0)	
Visceral ischemia	1 (20.0)	0 (0.0)	0 (0.0)	0 (0.0)	
Other/unknown	1 (20.0)	1 (50.0)	1 (20.0)	2 (40.0)	

Operative outcome. Patients were divided into four study groups with regard to the donor and recipient age (donor age ≤ 50 years and recipient age ≤ 60 years: D^Y/R^Y, n = 91; donor age > 50 years and recipient age ≤ 60 years: D^O/R^Y, n = 38; donor age ≤ 50 years and recipient age > 60 years: D^Y/R^O, n = 41; donor age > 50 years and recipient age > 60 years: D^O/R^O, n = 31). Detailed results for post-hoc analysis are displayed in Supplementary Table S1. ICU, intensive care unit; IMC, intermediate care unit; MODS, multiorgan dysfunction syndrome; SD, standard deviation; va-ECMO, veno-arterial extracorporeal life support.

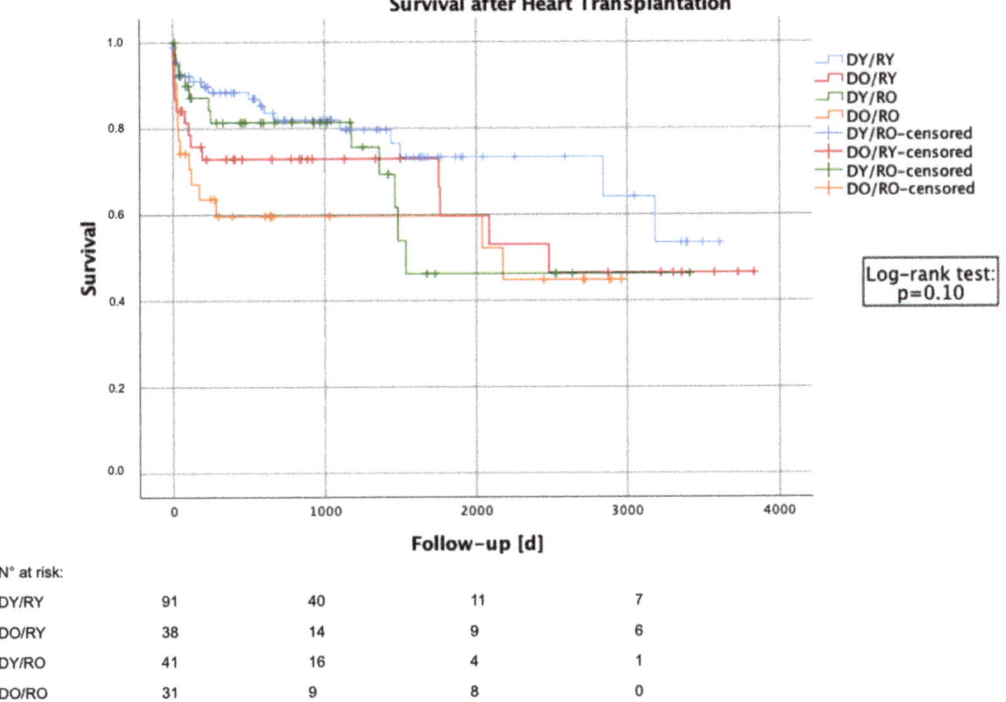

Figure 2. Estimated longer-term survival after heart transplantation by Kaplan–Meier method. Patients were divided into four study groups with regard to the donor and recipient age (donor age $\leq$ 50 years and recipient age $\leq$ 60 years: D^Y/R^Y, n = 91; donor age > 50 years and recipient age $\leq$ 60 years: D^O/R^Y, n = 38; donor age $\leq$ 50 years and recipient age > 60 years: D^Y/R^O, n = 41; donor age > 50 years and recipient age > 60 years: D^O/R^O, n = 31).

4. Discussion

In the coming years, there may be a rise in elderly end-stage heart failure patients due to a continuing demographic change leading to an ageing society. As HTx remains the gold standard of care, this rise will most likely also enter the transplant waiting list. In order to examine whether acceptance of older donors might be an option for those patients, we retrospectively analysed all of our transplant data from the last decade. Although we did not observe an increase in perioperative adverse events in the group of old recipients of organs from old donors, their postoperative survival was significantly impaired.

Except age, baseline characteristics of both the recipients as well as the donors were comparable between the groups. Therefore, the question arises as to why one-year survival of D^O/R^O was only 56%. Donor age is a known risk factor for impaired post-transplant long-term survival [10,11]. However, we already observed this for the very short-term survival. In addition, donor age is also a strong and independent risk factor for primary graft dysfunction, which we did not observe [12–15].

It was no surprise that patients of the D^Y/R^Y group had the best outcome as this has been reported in several previous studies [14–17]. In order to interpret our data of the D^O/R^O group, it is important to review the results of the D^Y/R^O and D^O/R^Y patients who had similar short-term survival. First, D^Y/R^Y patients had a better outcome than D^O/R^Y as well as D^Y/R^O patients. Secondly, D^O/R^Y patients had comparable outcome to D^Y/R^O patients. Finally, D^Y/R^O patients are superior to the D^O/R^O group. Similar results have recently been described in an Italian single-centre retrospective analysis as well as a retrospective review of the United Network for Organ Sharing (UNOS) registry [14,15].

Nevertheless, the implications of these results represent some kind of ethical dilemma. First, young donors should be allocated to every recipient, as this was best for all recipient ages. However, due to a continuous decline in organ donation, there is a lack of suitable donor organs in the Euro transplant region today [18,19]. Although D^O/R^Y were comparable to D^Y/R^O, allocating young donors primary to old recipients will still be questionable because donor age is a risk factor for impaired long-term outcome and these young recipients will then miss the even better outcome of the D^Y/R^Y group [10,11,18,19].

Implantation of left ventricular assist devices (LVAD) has gained increasingly more popularity in the elderly [20]. Unfortunately, risk for perioperative morbidity and mortality is also significantly increased compared to younger patients with reported in-hospital mortality of up to 50% in patients of 65 years and older [20–22]. Therefore, this is also a unsatisfying alternative to HTx for elderly patients.

Age itself is a strong and independent risk factor for mortality of heart failure patients [23,24]. In a large meta-analysis, Jones and colleagues reported a five-year survival after first diagnosis of heart failure of less than 50% for patients aged ≥ 75 years compared to about 80% for those aged ≤ 65 years [24]. This prognosis may be further impaired by frailty and concomitant diseases [6]. Therefore, in order to solve the mentioned ethical dilemma of missing suitable cardiac grafts from young donors for both groups of young and old recipients, individual consensus decisions with all related medical professions and the patient seemed to be crucial. First, individually shared decisions as to whether an elderly patient should be enrolled to stay on the HTx waiting list should be made in relation to their individual health status (urgency, frailty, concomitant diseases, suitability for LVAD implantation, etc.) and the predicted post-transplant survival [25]. Afterwards, the best offered donor organ should be accepted for elderly patients as with every patient on the waiting list.

The scientific value of our data is limited by the study's single-centre and retrospective design. The relatively small group sizes prohibited propensity score matching. In addition, the short follow-up period of the majority of patients combined with the known disproportionally high first-year mortality after HTx most likely underestimates the longer-term survival of the cohort assessed by the Kaplan–Meier method. The high number of censored patients led to a relatively small remaining follow-up cohort that may represent a bias for the longer-term follow-up. Furthermore, due to the retrospective character of the study, pretransplant frailty of the patients could unfortunately not be assessed.

5. Conclusions

Prevalence of heart failure will further increase within the next years due to an ageing society. Accordingly, an increasing number of elderly patients will enter the waiting list for heart transplantation. In order to increase the donor pool, accepting older donors can be performed without increasing the incidence of perioperative adverse events for both young and old recipients. However, donor age seems to be more important for the posttransplant survival than the recipient age. As we observed significantly impaired one-year survival for old recipients of grafts from old donors, organ acceptance should be performed with caution and by experienced centres only. However, given the otherwise often dismal prognosis of elderly and frail end-stage heart failure patients, transplantation of individual patients may still distinctly improve the therapy outcome of certain patients.

Supplementary Materials: The following supporting information can be downloaded at: https://www.mdpi.com/article/10.3390/jcm11040929/s1, Table S1: Results of post-hoc analysis.

Author Contributions: Conceptualisation, M.B.I. and U.B.; methodology, M.B.I.; validation, M.B.I., H.A., R.W., S.E.-K., I.T., P.A., A.L. and U.B.; formal analysis, M.B.I.; investigation, M.B.I.; resources, A.L. and U.B.; data curation, M.B.I., H.A., R.W., S.E.-K., I.T., P.A., A.L. and U.B.; writing—original draft preparation, M.B.I.; writing—review and editing, H.A., R.W., S.E.-K., I.T., P.A., A.L. and U.B.; visualisation, M.B.I.; supervision, P.A., A.L. and U.B.; project administration, A.L. and U.B. All authors have read and agreed to the published version of the manuscript.

Funding: This research received no external funding.

Institutional Review Board Statement: The study was conducted in accordance with the Declaration of Helsinki and approved by the Institutional Review Board (or Ethics Committee) of the Heinrich-Heine-University Düsseldorf (local study ID: 4567, approval date: 31 January 2014).

Informed Consent Statement: Informed consent was obtained from all subjects involved in the study.

Data Availability Statement: The data underlying this article will be shared on reasonable request to the corresponding author.

Acknowledgments: Figure 1 was created with Biorender.com.

Conflicts of Interest: The authors declare no conflict of interest.

References

1. Ziaeian, B.; Fonarow, G.C. Epidemiology and aetiology of heart failure. *Nat. Rev. Cardiol.* **2016**, *13*, 368–378. [CrossRef] [PubMed]
2. Mazurek, J.A.; Jessup, M. Understanding Heart Failure. *Heart Fail. Clin.* **2017**, *13*, 1–19. [CrossRef]
3. Dharmarajan, K.; Rich, M.W. Epidemiology, pathophysiology, and prognosis of heart failure in older adults. *Heart Fail. Clin.* **2017**, *13*, 417–426. [CrossRef] [PubMed]
4. Ponikowski, P.; Voors, A.A.; Anker, S.D.; Bueno, H.; Cleland, J.G.F.; Coats, A.J.S.; Falk, V.; Gonzalez-Juanatey, J.R.; Harjola, V.P.; Jankowska, E.A.; et al. 2016 ESC Guidelines for the diagnosis and treatment of acute and chronic heart failure: The Task Force for the diagnosis and treatment of acute and chronic heart failure of the European Society of Cardiology (ESC)Developed with the special contribution of the Heart Failure Association (HFA) of the ESC. *Eur. Heart J.* **2016**, *37*, 2129–2200. [CrossRef] [PubMed]
5. Yancy, C.W.; Jessup, M.; Bozkurt, B.; Butler, J.; Casey, D.E., Jr.; Drazner, M.H.; Fonarow, G.C.; Geraci, S.A.; Horwich, T.; Januzzi, J.L.; et al. 2013 ACCF/AHA guideline for the management of heart failure: A report of the American College of Cardiology Foundation/American Heart Association Task Force on Practice Guidelines. *J. Am. Coll. Cardiol.* **2013**, *62*, e147–e239. [CrossRef] [PubMed]
6. Vitale, C.; Jankowska, E.; Hill, L.; Piepoli, M.; Doehner, W.; Anker, S.D.; Lainscak, M.; Jaarsma, T.; Ponikowski, P.; Rosano, G.M.C.; et al. Heart Failure Association/European Society of Cardiology position paper on frailty in patients with heart failure. *Eur. J. Heart Fail.* **2019**, *21*, 1299–1305. [CrossRef] [PubMed]
7. Daneshvar, D.A.; Czer, L.S.; Phan, A.; Trento, A.; Schwarz, E.R. Heart transplantation in the elderly: Why cardiac transplantation does not need to be limited to younger patients but can be safely performed in patients above 65 years of age. *Ann. Transplant.* **2010**, *15*, 110–119.
8. Echterdiek, F.; Schwenger, V.; Döhler, B.; Latus, J.; Kitterer, D.; Heemann, U.; Süsal, C. Kidneys from elderly deceased donors-is 70 the new 60? *Front. Immunol.* **2019**, *10*, 2701. [CrossRef]
9. Schachtner, T.; Otto, N.M.; Reinke, P. Two decades of the Eurotransplant Senior Program: The gender gap in mortality impacts patient survival after kidney transplantation. *Clin. Kidney J.* **2019**, *13*, 1091–1100. [CrossRef]
10. Del Rizzo, D.F.; Menkis, A.H.; Pflugfelder, P.W.; Novick, R.J.; McKenzie, F.N.; Boyd, W.D.; Kostuk, W.J. The role of donor age and ischemic time on survival following orthotopic heart transplantation. *J. Heart Lung Transplant.* **1999**, *18*, 310–319. [CrossRef]
11. Immohr, M.B.; Akhyari, P.; Boettger, C.; Mehdiani, A.; Dalyanoglu, H.; Westenfeld, R.; Tudorache, I.; Aubin, H.; Lichtenberg, A.; Boeken, U. Effects of donor age and ischemia time on outcome after heart transplant: A 10-year single-center experience. *Exp. Clin. Transplant. Off. J. Middle East Soc. Organ Transplant.* **2021**, *19*, 351–358. [CrossRef]
12. Singh, S.S.A.; Dalzell, J.R.; Berry, C.; Al-Attar, N. Primary graft dysfunction after heart transplantation: A thorn amongst the roses. *Heart Fail. Rev.* **2019**, *24*, 805–820. [CrossRef]
13. Kobashigawa, J.; Zuckermann, A.; Macdonald, P.; Leprince, P.; Esmailian, F.; Luu, M.; Mancini, D.; Patel, J.; Razi, R.; Reichenspurner, H.; et al. Report from a consensus conference on primary graft dysfunction after cardiac transplantation. *J. Heart Lung Transplant.* **2014**, *33*, 327–340. [CrossRef] [PubMed]
14. Jawitz, O.K.; Raman, V.; Klapper, J.; Hartwig, M.; Patel, C.B.; Milano, C. Donor and recipient age matching in heart transplantation: Analysis of the UNOS Registry. *Transpl. Int.* **2019**, *32*, 1194–1202. [CrossRef] [PubMed]
15. Lechiancole, A.; Vendramin, I.; Sponga, S.; Guzzi, G.; Ferrara, V.; Nalli, C.; Di Nora, C.; Bortolotti, U.; Livi, U. Donor-recipient age interaction and the impact on clinical results after heart transplantation. *Clin. Transplant.* **2020**, *34*, e14043. [CrossRef] [PubMed]
16. López-Vilella, R.; González-Vílchez, F.; Crespo-Leiro, M.G.; Segovia-Cubero, J.; Cobo, M.; Delgado-Jiménez, J.; Arizón Del Prado, J.M.; Martínez-Sellés, M.; Sobrino Márquez, J.M.; Mirabet-Pérez, S.; et al. Impact of donor-recipient age on cardiac transplant survival. Subanalysis of the Spanish Heart Transplant Registry. *Rev. Esp. Cardiol.* **2021**, *74*, 393–401. [CrossRef] [PubMed]
17. Ram, E.; Lavee, J.; Kogan, A.; Kassif, Y.; Elian, D.; Freimark, D.; Peled, Y. Does donor-recipient age difference matter in outcome of heart transplantation? *Clin. Transplant.* **2019**, *33*, e13593. [CrossRef] [PubMed]
18. Eurotransplant, I.F. Eurotransplant International Foundation, Annual Report. 2018. Available online: https://www.eurotransplant.org/cms/mediaobject.php?file=ET_Jaarverslag_20181.pdf (accessed on 15 July 2019).
19. Fuchs, M.; Schibilsky, D.; Zeh, W.; Berchtold-Herz, M.; Beyersdorf, F.; Siepe, M. Does the heart transplant have a future? *Eur. J. Cardiothorac. Surg.* **2019**, *55*, i38–i48. [CrossRef] [PubMed]

20. Patel, P.C.; Sareyyupoglu, B.; Pham, S.M. Left ventricular assist devices in the elderly: Marching forward with cautions. *J. Card. Surg.* **2020**, *35*, 3409–3411. [CrossRef]
21. Lindvall, C.; Udelsman, B.; Malhotra, D.; Brovman, E.Y.; Urman, R.D.; D'Alessandro, D.A.; Tulsky, J.A. In-hospital mortality in older patients after ventricular assist device implantation: A national cohort study. *J. Thorac. Cardiovasc. Surg.* **2018**, *158*, 466–475.e464. [CrossRef]
22. Gazda, A.J.; Kwak, M.J.; Akkanti, B.; Nathan, S.; Kumar, S.; de Armas, I.S.; Baer, P.; Patel, B.; Kar, B.; Gregoric, I.D. Complications of LVAD utilization in older adults. *Heart Lung* **2020**, *50*, 75–79. [CrossRef] [PubMed]
23. Crespo-Leiro, M.G.; Anker, S.D.; Maggioni, A.P.; Coats, A.J.; Filippatos, G.; Ruschitzka, F.; Ferrari, R.; Piepoli, M.F.; Delgado Jimenez, J.F.; Metra, M.; et al. European Society of Cardiology Heart Failure Long-Term Registry (ESC-HF-LT): 1-year follow-up outcomes and differences across regions. *Eur. J. Heart Fail.* **2016**, *18*, 613–625. [CrossRef] [PubMed]
24. Jones, N.R.; Roalfe, A.K.; Adoki, I.; Hobbs, F.D.R.; Taylor, C.J. Survival of patients with chronic heart failure in the community: A systematic review and meta-analysis. *Eur. J. Heart Fail.* **2019**, *21*, 1306–1325. [CrossRef] [PubMed]
25. Claes, S.; Berchtold-Herz, M.; Zhou, Q.; Trummer, G.; Bock, M.; Zirlik, A.; Beyersdorf, F.; Bode, C.; Grundmann, S. Towards a cardiac allocation score: A retrospective calculation for 73 patients from a German transplant center. *J. Cardiothorac. Surg.* **2017**, *12*, 14. [CrossRef] [PubMed]

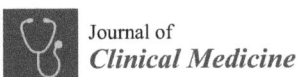

Article

Frailty Test Battery Development including Physical, Socio-Psychological and Cognitive Domains for Cardiovascular Disease Patients: A Preliminary Study

Nastasia Marinus [1,2,*], Carlo Vigorito [3], Francesco Giallauria [3,4], Paul Dendale [2,5], Raf Meesen [1], Kevin Bokken [1], Laura Haenen [1], Thomas Jansegers [1], Yenthe Vandenheuvel [1], Martijn Scherrenberg [2,5], Joke Spildooren [1,†] and Dominique Hansen [1,2,5,†]

1. REVAL-Rehabilitation Research Center, Faculty of Rehabilitation Sciences, Hasselt University, 3590 Diepenbeek, Belgium; raf.meesen@uhasselt.be (R.M.); kevin.bokken@student.uhasselt.be (K.B.); laura.haenen@student.uhasselt.be (L.H.); thomas.jansegers@student.uhasselt.be (T.J.); yenthe.vandenheuvel@student.uhasselt.be (Y.V.); joke.spildooren@uhasselt.be (J.S.); dominique.hansen@uhasselt.be (D.H.)
2. BIOMED-Biomedical Research Center, Hasselt University, 3590 Diepenbeek, Belgium; paul.dendale@jessazh.be (P.D.); martijn.scherrenberg@jessazh.be (M.S.)
3. Department of Translational Medical Sciences, Federico II University of Naples, 80131 Naples, Italy; vigorito@unina.it (C.V.); francesco.giallauria@unina.it (F.G.)
4. Faculty of Science and Technology, University of New England, Armidale, NSW 2350, Australia
5. Heart Centre Hasselt, Jessa Hospital, 3500 Hasselt, Belgium
* Correspondence: nastasia.marinus@uhasselt.be; Tel.: +32-(0)11-269203
† Shared last authors.

Abstract: Frailty is an age-related decline in physical, socio-psychological and cognitive function that results in extreme vulnerability to stressors. Therefore, this study aimed to elucidate which tests have to be selected to detect frailty in a comprehensive and feasible manner in cardiovascular disease (CVD) patients based on multivariate regression and sensitivity/specificity analyses. Patients (n = 133, mean age 78 ± 7 years) hospitalised for coronary revascularisation or heart failure (HF) were examined using the Fried and Vigorito criteria, together with some additional measurements. Moreover, to examine the association of frailty with 6-month clinical outcomes, hospitalisations and mortality up to 6 months after the initial hospital admission were examined. Some level of frailty was detected in 44% of the patients according to the Vigorito criteria and in 65% of the patients according to the Fried criteria. Frailty could best be detected by a score based on: sex, Mini Nutritional Assessment (MNA), Katz scale, timed up-and-go test (TUG), handgrip strength, Mini-Mental State Examination (MMSE), Geriatric Depression Scale (GDS-15) and total number of medications. Frailty and specific markers of frailty were significantly associated with mortality and six-month hospitalisations. We thus can conclude that, in patients with CVD, sex, MNA, Katz scale, TUG, handgrip strength, MMSE, GDS-15 and total number of medications play a key role in detecting frailty, assessed by a new time- and cost-efficient test battery.

Keywords: frailty; frailty assessment; cardiovascular disease; older adults

1. Introduction

Almost half of all (premature) deaths in Europe are caused by cardiovascular diseases (CVDs). As about 10% of Europeans currently suffer from CVD, a significant economic cost and burden are apparent [1–3]. Moreover, due to increasing prevalence rates of obesity, hypertension and diabetes mellitus, a 10% increase in the CVD prevalence rate is expected in the upcoming 10 years [4].

Fortunately, improvements in cardiac surgery [5] and rehabilitation [6–8], risk factor management [9] and cardioprotective medication [2] have considerably increased the

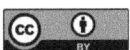

life expectancy of CVD patients [2,9]. However, ageing is commonly associated with the emergence of frailty [8]. Frailty is a progressive age-related decline in physiological systems that results in decreased reserves of intrinsic capacity, which confers extreme vulnerability to stressors [10]. This condition further increases the risk of adverse health outcomes, such as frequent hospitalisations and premature death, and therefore deserves great attention [1,11].

The prevalence rates of frailty in CVD patients can vary significantly according to the disease and treatment: from up to 19% in patients after percutaneous coronary intervention (PCI) to up to 76% in heart failure (HF) patients [12]. In these studies, the phenotype proposed by Fried [13] was the most frequently used frailty assessment tool. As mainly physical limitations are taken into account in this tool (i.e., weight loss, physical activity, walk time and handgrip strength), previous studies highlighted the need for a more comprehensive frailty assessment for better prediction of clinical outcomes in hospitalised older (CVD) patients [14–16].

For example, postoperative cognitive dysfunction (POCD), defined as the development of symptoms of cognitive dysfunction after surgery and anaesthesia in previously apparently cognitive healthy patients [17], occurs after cardiothoracic surgery in up to 43% of older patients [18–20] and can become a permanent disorder [21,22]. Moreover, depression (eventually in combination with anxiety), as well as a lack of social/emotional support in CVD patients, seems to be associated with adverse cardiovascular outcomes and mortality in a dose–response relationship [23]. Consequently, it is clear that besides the physical aspects of frailty, equal attention should be directed to the cognitive, social and psychological components of frailty as well, as already reiterated by the European Association of Preventive Cardiology [24,25] and more recently in the frailty score proposed by Vigorito [26]. In contrast to Fried et al. [13], this multidimensional frailty assessment tool takes into account not only the physical aspects of frailty (muscle strength, gait speed, mobility, comorbidities) but also nutritional, cognitive and psychosocial components with separate cut-off criteria for men vs. women. However, this Vigorito frailty assessment tool is not yet validated in CVD patients.

Therefore, if the Fried and Vigorito criteria and some other frequently used frailty assessment measurements were to be merged, the tests that should be selected to establish a comprehensive assessment that is feasible and low cost but sufficiently sensitive and specific (females vs. males) remain to be determined [12]. Such an assessment battery would then allow clinicians, working in different settings, to easily detect frailty and, moreover, predict hospitalisations and mortality in patients with CVD to initiate preventive strategies accordingly.

The aim of this study, therefore, was threefold: (1) to compare the frailty prevalence rates using Fried vs. the more comprehensive Vigorito criteria in CVD patients; (2) to establish which tests, from the physical, socio-psychological and cognitive domains, should be selected to be able to detect frailty in patients with CVD and (3) to establish a total score that may represent a valid measurement of frailty severity.

2. Materials and Methods

2.1. Subjects

Between October 2019 and April 2020, 133 unselected, consecutive participants were included in this cross-sectional study at the cardiology units of Jessa Hospital Hasselt, Belgium. Hospitalised participants were initially screened for inclusion and exclusion criteria based on their electronic patient file and, if necessary, based on additional information from the health staff (cardiologists, nurses) of the cardiology units of the hospital. After careful explanation of the study aims and methodology, written informed consent was obtained from all participants. This study was approved by the ethical committee of Jessa Hospital (19.81-REVA19.05) and registered at ClinicalTrials.gov (NCT04206904). The inclusion criteria were (i) men and women aged 65 years or older (ii) who were admitted to the hospital for mild vs. severe coronary revascularisation or surgery (PCI vs. (endo-)CABG) or for HF.

We preferred to include these different CVD pathologies based on previous literature confirming the variable frailty prevalence in these patient populations [12]. Participants were excluded if they refused to participate after receiving all study information or if they had a persistently unstable clinical condition that prevented them from safely participating, such as angina pectoris, advanced conduction disturbances, significant ventricular arrhythmias or decompensating HF. Participants were not excluded based on mental/cognitive state.

2.2. Study Design

In this cross-sectional study, the presence of frailty was initially assessed by two different frailty assessment tools. First, the presence/absence of frailty was examined according to the phenotype proposed by Fried [13]. Next, this frailty assessment was supplemented by the comprehensive multi-component and sex-specific frailty assessment tool proposed by Vigorito et al. [26], which was developed based on similar, previously published frailty assessment tools [14–16]. Furthermore, additional parameters were assessed, which could be of significant added value in the detection of frailty. The total test battery took 45 min to complete.

Patients undergoing coronarography, further defined as PCI patients (for coronary artery disease (CAD) patients undergoing a PCI) or as CORO patients (for CAD patients not undergoing PCI or CABG), were examined before or after their cardiac surgery, while CABG patients were all examined before surgery. HF patients were examined at any defined time during their hospital stay.

2.3. Baseline Characteristics

Baseline characteristics (age, body weight and length) were registered from the electronic file of the patients on the day of assessment.

2.4. Frailty Assessment

2.4.1. Fried Phenotype

The Fried frailty phenotype examines five components: involuntary weight loss, exhaustion, level of physical activity, walking time and grip strength. Based on these five criteria, subjects were considered to be pre-frail (fulfilling one or two criteria) or frail (fulfilling at least three criteria). A more detailed explanation of the different components can be found in Appendix A Table A1.

With regard to the walking time criteria, the walking time of the slowest participant was assigned to participants who were not able to execute the walking test due to, for example, walking difficulties or exhaustion. In this way, we were able to calculate a mean walking time for the total sample.

Furthermore, the Minnesota Leisure Time Activity questionnaire, which is used in the original Fried criteria, is largely inapplicable to hospitalised patients, as it examines participation in daily activities such as mowing the lawn, gardening, biking, dancing, swimming, etc. Therefore, we decided to use a modified version of the Fried phenotype by introducing the Katz scale. This scale has been used in previous studies to examine the level of physical activity according to the Fried phenotype [12,27–29]. It examines participation and level of (in)dependence in six activities (washing, dressing, mobility, toileting, level of (in)continence and eating) that are highly relevant for hospitalised patients. Based on this scale, subjects who were completely independent in 6 activities of daily living (ADL) (score 6: 1 point for each activity in which there was complete independence) were considered to be non-frail, while subjects with any dependence (score 0–5) were considered to be frail with regard to the level of physical activity.

2.4.2. Vigorito's Frailty Assessment Tool

The frailty assessment tool developed by Vigorito et al. [26] is composed of eight main components.

The Mini Nutritional Assessment (MNA) (long version) [30] was used to examine the nutritional status of the patient. To examine the level of (in)dependence in activities of daily living (ADL), the Katz scale was used. Mobility was evaluated by measuring the gait speed based on a 4.6 m walking test. A combination of mobility, balance and lower-extremity strength was assessed based on the timed up-and-go test (TUG). To be able to calculate the mean gait speed or TUG score for the total sample, the value of the slowest participant (i.e., lowest value for gait speed or highest value for TUG) of the total sample was assigned to participants who were not able to execute the mobility tests due to, for example, walking difficulties or exhaustion.

Handgrip strength (kg) of the dominant hand was examined with the Jamar handheld dynamometer® (Patterson Medical, Glossop, UK) [31]. However, when the dominant hand was medically unfeasible due to, for example, a PCI/stenting procedure on that hand, the non-dominant hand was tested. Moreover, to be able to calculate the mean handgrip strength of the total sample, the value of the weakest participant (i.e., lowest value) of the total sample was assigned to participants who were not able to squeeze with any hand due to, for example, exhaustion.

The Mini-Mental State Examination (MMSE) (Dutch version) [32] was used to examine the cognitive status of the patients. To detect the presence of a depressive mood, the Geriatric Depression Scale (GDS-15) (Dutch version) [33] was used. Finally, the use of cardioprotective and any other medications (except for vitamins, minerals and food supplements) was registered as a marker of comorbidities based on the electronic file of the patient at discharge from the hospital. Each component of the frailty assessment tool was scored separately to divide the patients into three frailty categories from not frail (score 0) to severe frailty (score 3). These eight sub-scores finally resulted in a total score ranging from not frail (score 0–6), minor frailty (7–12) and moderate frailty (score 13–18) to severe frailty (score 19–24) (see Appendix A Table A2).

2.4.3. Additional Frailty Measures

In addition to both frailty assessment tools, other measurements were executed to collect extra information regarding the functional status of the patient in an attempt to improve frailty assessment.

The International Physical Activity Questionnaire (IPAQ) [34] (long version) was used to examine the level of physical activity spent in the previous seven days. To examine the muscle strength (in kg) of the knee extensors (sitting position with hip and knee flexed 90°) and hip flexors (supine position with hip flexed 90°) of both legs, the MicroFET® dynamometer (Hoggan Health Industries Inc., West Jordan, UT, USA) [35] was used. Each measurement was repeated three times, and the highest value was used in the data analysis. Moreover, to examine the functional muscle strength of the lower limbs, the timed chair stand test was performed. The value of the weakest participant (lowest value (Microfet) and highest value (timed chair stand test)) of the total sample was assigned to participants who were not able to perform the muscle strength measurements due to, for example, exhaustion. Finally, the Falls Efficacy Scale International (FES-I) [36] was used, a questionnaire that examines the level of concern about falling (see Appendix A Table A3).

All frailty assessment tools were implemented by trained physiotherapists. The data analysis was performed by another blinded researcher.

2.5. Association of Frailty with 6-Month Clinical Outcomes

To examine the association of frailty with clinical outcomes, six months after the hospital admission in which the initial frailty assessment took place, the presence/absence of hospitalisations and mortality were examined based on records in the electronic patient file. A distinction was made between planned and urgent hospitalisations. Planned hospitalisations were considered to be hospital admissions that were planned in advance, such as a planned coronarography, PCI or valve surgery. Urgent hospitalisations were considered hospital admissions that were not planned in advance, such as hospitalisations via the emergency department of the hospital.

Patients were considered to be frail when fulfilling at least three out of five criteria (Fried) indicating the presence of mild, moderate or severe frailty (Vigorito) or based on the newly developed frailty cut-off score (new frailty assessment tool) (further explained in detail in Section 3.5).

2.6. Outcome Measures

The primary outcomes of this study were the frailty score and frailty characteristics based on the comprehensive frailty assessment battery developed by Vigorito (and additionally, according to the Fried phenotype). Secondary outcomes were hospitalisations and mortality 6 months after the initial frailty assessment.

2.7. Statistical Analysis

Statistical analyses were executed in SPSS v. 25.0 (IBM, Chicago, IL, USA) and JMP® Pro 14.1.0 (SAS Institute Inc., Buckinghamshire, UK). Shapiro–Wilk tests were used to test for normality, while Levene's tests for equality of variances were used to test for homoscedasticity. To compare two means, an independent samples t-test (in the case of normality) or a non-parametric Mann–Whitney U test (in the case of non-normally distributed data or sample size < 30) was used. Pearson chi-square or Fisher exact test (if cell number < 5) was performed to examine categorical data. To compare more than two means, one-way ANOVA (with Bonferroni test) (in the case of normality) or Kruskal–Wallis test (with pairwise comparisons) (in the case of non-normally distributed data) was used. A stepwise multivariate regression model was used in JMP to examine which specific components of frailty (age, sex, body length, body weight, BMI, MNA, calf circumference and upper arm circumference (which are part of the MNA), Katz scale, walking time, gait speed, TUG, handgrip strength, FES-I, MMSE, GDS-15, number of medications, muscle strength of knee extensors and hip flexors (left/right leg), timed chair stand test, CVD risk factors (hypertension, hypercholesterolemia, diabetes type 1, diabetes type 2, smoking), total number of risk factors and IPAQ) would predict the total frailty score the best and to develop a frailty assessment tool with the fewest assessments. In the case of correlating variables, such as gait speed and walking time, only one of the two variables was included in the analysis. To examine the association of frailty with 6-month clinical outcomes, chi-square analyses were performed between the presence/absence of planned/urgent hospitalisations or mortality and the frailty status of the patients (frail/not frail) according to Fried or Vigorito. Data are expressed as means ± standard deviation (SD) or as n (%). A p-value < 0.05 (2-tailed) was considered as statistically significant.

3. Results

3.1. Baseline Characteristics

This study included 133 participants (57 females) with a mean age of 78 ± 7 years, comprising 27 CORO patients, 30 PCI patients, 16 CABG patients and 60 HF patients. HF patients were significantly older compared to CORO (p = 0.002) and PCI patients (p = 0.002) (see Table 1).

Table 1. Baseline characteristics of the study population according to sex and CVD.

		Total	CORO	PCI	CABG	HF
n (%)	Total	133	27 (20.3)	30 (22.6)	16 (12.0)	60 (45.1)
	M	76 (57.1)	14 (51.9)	19 (63.3)	14 (87.5) †	29 (48.3)
	F	57 (42.9)	13 (48.1)	11 (36.7)	2 (12.5)	31 (51.7)

Table 1. Cont.

		Total	CORO	PCI	CABG	HF
Age (Years)	Total	78.1 ± 6.7	75.4 ± 5.3 *	75.5 ± 6.5 **	77.0 ± 7.6	80.9 ± 6.1
	M	77.2 ± 6.9	74.0 ± 4.1	75.9 ± 7.1	76.4 ± 7.9	79.9 ± 6.6
	F	79.4 ± 6.3	77.0 ± 6.1	74.8 ± 5.6	80.8 ± 5.1	81.9 ± 5.5
Body length (cm)	Total	166.3 ± 9.7	167.3 ± 10.1	166.9 ± 9.8	169.8 ± 6.5	164.7 ± 10.0
	M	172.4 ± 6.4 †	175.0 ± 6.3 †	172.3 ± 5.8 †	171.2 ± 5.5 †	171.8 ± 7.2 †
	F	158.2 ± 7.0	158.9 ± 5.6	157.7 ± 8.3	159.5 ± 0.7	158.0 ± 7.4
Body weight (kg)	Total	74.0 ± 13.4	78.2 ± 14.5	74.9 ± 12.1	76.0 ± 13.2	71.2 ± 13.2
	M	78.4 ± 12.1 †	82.3 ± 13.0	79.2 ± 12.2 †	77.4 ± 13.4	76.4 ± 11.0 †
	F	68.3 ± 12.8	73.8 ± 15.2	67.3 ± 7.5	66.1 ± 4.8	66.4 ± 13.3
BMI (kg/m^2)	Total	26.7 ± 4.2	27.9 ± 4.4	26.8 ± 3.2	26.3 ± 3.8	26.3 ± 4.6
	M	26.4 ± 3.6	26.9 ± 3.9	26.7 ± 3.5	26.4 ± 4.0	25.9 ± 3.3
	F	27.3 ± 4.9	29.1 ± 4.8	27.1 ± 2.8	26.0 ± 2.1	26.7 ± 5.5
Overweight % prevalence	Total	67 (50.4)	16 (59.3)	19 (63.3)	6 (37.5)	26 (43.3)
	M	40 (30.1)	8 (29.6)	12 (40.0)	5 (31.3)	15 (25.0)
	F	27 (20.3)	8 (29.6)	7 (23.3)	1 (6.3)	11 (18.3)
Obesity % prevalence	Total	22 (16.5)	6 (22.2)	4 (13.3)	2 (12.5)	10 (16.7)
	M	8 (6.0)	2 (7.4)	2 (6.7)	2 (12.5)	2 (3.3)
	F	14 (10.5)	4 (14.8)	2 (6.7)	0 (0.0)	8 (13.3)
Hypertension % prevalence	Total	120 (90.2)	21 (77.8)	23 (76.7)	16 (100)	60 (100)
	M	66 (49.6)	9 (33.3)	14 (46.7)	14 (87.5)	29 (48.3)
	F	54 (40.6)	12 (44.4)	9 (30.0)	2 (12.5)	31 (51.7)
Type 2 diabetes % prevalence	Total	36 (27.1)	6 (22.2)	5 (16.7)	3 (18.8)	22 (36.7)
	M	20 (15.0)	4 (14.8)	4 (13.3)	3 (18.8)	9 (15.0)
	F	16 (12.0)	2 (7.4)	1 (3.3)	0 (0.0)	13 (21.7)
Dyslipidaemia % prevalence	Total	102 (76.7)	19 (70.4)	27 (90.0)	15 (93.8)	41 (68.3)
	M	61 (45.9)	11 (40.7)	17 (56.7)	13 (81.3)	20 (33.3)
	F	41 (30.8)	8 (29.6)	10 (33.3)	2 (12.5)	21 (35.0)
NYHA						
Class I–II		-	-	-	-	1 (1.7)
Class II		-	-	-	-	13 (21.7)
Class II–III	Total	-	-	-	-	16 (26.7)
Class III		-	-	-	-	17 (28.3)
Class III–IV		-	-	-	-	3 (5.0)
Class IV		-	-	-	-	2 (3.3)
Unknown		-	-	-	-	8 (13.3)
		Total	CORO	PCI	CABG	HF
Cardioprotective medication						
Beta blockers		89 (66.9)	14 (51.9)	19 (63.3)	14 (87.5)	42 (70.0)
Calcium antagonists		37 (27.8)	10 (37.0)	5 (16.7)	3 (18.8)	19 (31.7)
ACE inhibitors		44 (33.1)	4 (14.8)	12 (40.0)	7 (43.8)	21 (35.0)
Angiotensin II receptor blockers		25 (18.8)	6 (22.2)	5 (16.7)	2 (12.5)	12 (20.0)

Table 1. Cont.

	Total	CORO	PCI	CABG	HF
Diuretics	78 (58.6)	5 (18.5)	10 (33.3)	10 (62.5)	53 (88.3)
Amiodarone	30 (22.6)	0 (0.0)	3 (10.0)	0 (0.0)	27 (45.0)
Sotalol	2 (1.5)	2 (7.4)	0 (0.0)	0 (0.0)	0 (0.0)
Flecainide	4 (3.0)	1 (3.7)	0 (0.0)	0 (0.0)	3 (5.0)
Anticoagulants	123 (92.5)	26 (96.3)	30 (100)	14 (87.5)	53 (88.3)
Ezetimibe	8 (6.0)	0 (0.0)	2 (6.7)	2 (12.5)	4 (6.7)
Statins	101 (75.9)	19 (70.4)	26 (86.7)	15 (93.8)	41 (68.3)
Nitrates	16 (12.0)	6 (22.2)	1 (3.3)	2 (12.5)	7 (11.7)
Sacubitril/Valsartan	4 (3.0)	0 (0.0)	0 (0.0)	0 (0.0)	4 (6.7)
Ivabradine	1 (0.8)	0 (0.0)	0 (0.0)	0 (0.0)	1 (1.7)
Molsidomine	12 (9.0)	4 (14.8)	3 (10.0)	4 (25.0)	1 (1.7)
Metformin	23 (17.3)	4 (14.8)	4 (13.3)	3 (18.8)	12 (20.0)
Sulphonylurea	4 (3.0)	1 (3.7)	1 (3.3)	1 (6.3)	1 (1.7)
Glinides/meglitinides	4 (3.0)	0 (0.0)	2 (6.7)	0 (0.0)	2 (3.3)
GLP1 analogues	1 (0.8)	0 (0.0)	0 (0.0)	0 (0.0)	1 (1.7)
DPP4 inhibitors	5 (3.8)	0 (0.0)	1 (3.3)	0 (0.0)	4 (6.7)
SGLT2 inhibitors	4 (3.0)	1 (3.7)	1 (3.3)	0 (0.0)	2 (3.3)
Insulin (ultrafast-acting)	3 (2.3)	1 (3.7)	0 (0.0)	0 (0.0)	2 (3.3)
Insulin (fast-acting)	2 (1.5)	0 (0.0)	0 (0.0)	0 (0.0)	2 (3.3)
Insulin (intermediate)	1 (0.8)	0 (0.0)	0 (0.0)	0 (0.0)	1 (1.7)
Insulin (slow-acting)	7 (5.3)	2 (7.4)	0 (0.0)	0 (0.0)	5 (8.3)
Opioids	10 (7.5)	2 (7.4)	0 (0.0)	0 (0.0)	8 (13.3)
Analgesics	29 (21.8)	3 (11.1)	0 (0.0)	8 (50.0)	18 (30.0)

BMI, body mass index; CABG, coronary artery bypass grafting; cm, centimetre; CORO, coronarography; CVD, cardiovascular disease; HF, heart failure; kg, kilogram; m, metre; n, number; NYHA, New York Heart Association; PCI, percutaneous coronary intervention; SD, standard deviation; $p < 0.05$ * CORO vs. HF; ** PCI vs. HF; † $p < 0.05$ between sexes. Results are expressed as mean ± SD or as n (% within CVD group) (for results per CVD) or as n (% within total population) (for results of the total population).

3.2. Prevalence of Frailty According to the Fried Phenotype

According to the Fried phenotype, 38% of the patients were categorised as being frail, while 26% of the patients were pre-frail (no significant difference, $p = 0.08$). The highest prevalence of frailty was detected in the HF patients (70%), with lower prevalence rates in CABG (19%), CORO (19%) and PCI (3%) patients. Major differences between HF patients and other patient populations were identified for nearly all outcomes ($p < 0.05$). Moreover, frailty was more prevalent in females than in males in the total population (46% vs. 33% respectively) and within each CVD individually because of significant differences in gait speed, handgrip strength and exhaustion ($p < 0.05$) (see Table 2 and Figure 1).

Table 2. Number of frail subjects according to CVD and sex and analysis of the frailty component scores based on the Fried frailty assessment tool.

			Total (n = 133)	CORO (n = 27) M (n = 14) F (n = 13)	PCI (n = 30) M (n = 19) F (n = 11)	CABG (n = 16) M (n = 14) F (n = 2)	HF (n = 60) M (n = 29) F (n = 31)
Weight loss	Total	Frail n (%)	20	1	3	4	12
	M		13 (17.1)	1 (7.1)	3 (15.8)	4 (28.6)	5 (17.2)
	F		7 (12.3)	0 (0.0)	0 (0.0)	0 (0.0)	7 (22.6)
Exhaustion							
I felt that everything I did was an effort	Total	Raw score	1.4 ± 1.2	1.1 ± 1.1 *	0.4 ± 0.7 **	1.3 ± 1.3	2.0 ± 1.1
	M		1.0 ± 1.1 †	0.7 ± 0.9	0.2 ± 0.5	1.2 ± 1.4	1.6 ± 1.1 †
	F		1.8 ± 1.1	1.5 ± 1.1	0.7 ± 0.8	1.5 ± 0.7	2.4 ± 0.9
I could not get going	Total	Raw score	1.4 ± 1.3	0.8 ± 1.1 *	0.6 ± 0.9 *	1.6 ± 1.4	2.0 ± 1.2
	M		1.1 ± 1.2 †	0.6 ± 0.9	0.5 ± 0.8	1.5 ± 1.4	1.6 ± 1.2 †
	F		1.7 ± 1.3	1.0 ± 1.3	0.8 ± 1.1	2.0 ± 1.4	2.4 ± 1.0
Total	M	Frail n (%)	21 (27.6)	1 (7.1)	1 (5.3)	5 (35.7)	14 (48.3)
	F		30 (52.6)	4 (30.8)	1 (9.1)	0 (0.0)	25 (80.6)
Gait speed (m/s)	Total	Raw score	0.87 ± 0.48	1.03 ± 0.44 *	1.27 ± 0.36 **	0.92 ± 0.48 ***	0.59 ± 0.36
	M	Raw score	0.98 ± 0.52 †	1.21 ± 0.47 †	1.34 ± 0.40	0.98 ± 0.48	0.63 ± 0.40
	M	Frail n (%)	27 (35.5)	2 (14.3)	0 (0.0)	5 (35.7)	20 (69.0)
	F	Raw score	0.73 ± 0.38	0.85 ± 0.31	1.15 ± 0.24	0.51 ± 0.24	0.55 ± 0.33
	F	Frail n (%)	33 (57.9)	6 (46.2)	1 (9.1)	1 (50.0)	25 (80.6)
Level of physical activity (Katz independence in ADL)	Total	Raw score	5.2 ± 1.3	5.5 ± 1.1 *	6.0 ± 0.0 **	5.4 ± 1.1	4.7 ± 1.5
	M	Raw score	5.3 ± 1.3	5.6 ± 1.1	6.0 ± 0.0	5.3 ± 1.1	4.7 ± 1.5
	M	Frail n (%)	24 (31.6)	2 (14.3)	0 (0.0)	5 (35.7)	17 (58.6)
	F	Raw score	5.1 ± 1.3	5.5 ± 1.1	6.0 ± 0.0	6.0 ± 0.0	4.6 ± 1.5
	F	Frail n (%)	20 (35.1)	3 (23.1)	0 (0.0)	0 (0.0)	17 (54.8)
Handgrip strength (kg)	Total	Raw score	26.7 ± 11.8	30.7 ± 13.2 *	33.1 ± 11.1 **	31.1 ± 9.0 ***	20.5 ± 9.1
	M	Raw score	33.3 ± 10.7 †	38.8 ± 13.3 †	39.0 ± 9.3 †	33.0 ± 7.7	27.1 ± 7.9 †
	M	Frail n (%)	31 (40.8)	3 (21.4)	5 (26.3)	3 (21.4)	20 (69.0)
	F	Raw score	17.9 ± 6.2	22.0 ± 4.9	22.9 ± 4.7	17.9 ± 6.2	14.4 ± 4.9
	F	Frail n (%)	35 (61.4)	4 (30.8)	3 (27.3)	1 (50.0)	27 (87.1)
Total frailty score	Total	Raw score	1.8 ± 1.6	1.0 ± 1.2 *	0.5 ± 0.8 **	1.5 ± 1.5 ***	3.0 ± 1.4
	M		1.5 ± 1.6 †	0.6 ± 1.2	0.5 ± 0.8	1.6 ± 1.6	2.6 ± 1.4
	F		2.2 ± 1.6	1.3 ± 1.3	0.5 ± 0.7	1.0 ± 1.4	3.3 ± 1.2

ADL, activities of daily living; CABG, coronary artery bypass grafting; CORO, coronarography; F females; HF, heart failure; kg, kilogram; M, males; n, number; PCI, percutaneous coronary intervention; s, seconds; SD, standard deviation; $p < 0.05$ * CORO vs. HF; ** PCI vs. HF; *** CABG vs. HF; † $p < 0.05$ between sexes. Results are expressed as mean ± SD.

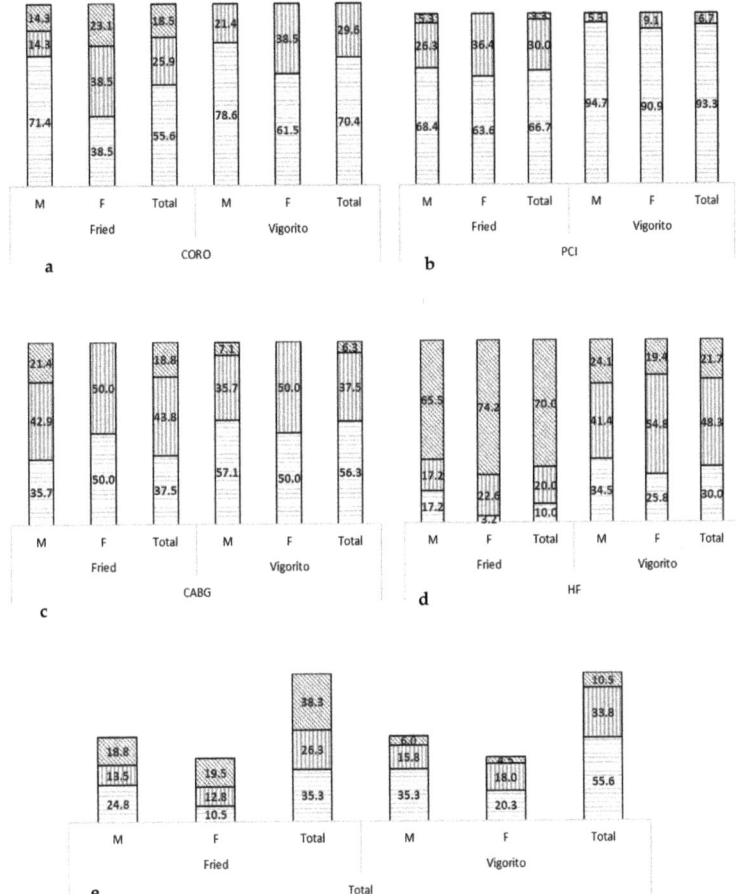

Figure 1. Distribution of the different levels of frailty (%) according to Fried and Vigorito for male and female CORO (**a**), PCI (**b**), CABG (**c**) and HF (**d**) patients. The different levels of frailty are represented as no frailty (horizontal lines), pre-frailty (Fried) or mild frailty (Vigorito) (vertical lines) and frailty (Fried) or moderate frailty (Vigorito) (diagonal lines). Note: Severe frailty (Vigorito) was not detected in the subjects and, thus, are not represented in the figure. Results are expressed as % within males and within females per CVD for each subcategory of frailty (in CORO, PCI, CABG and HF patients) or as % within CVD for total results (in CORO, PCI, CABG and HF patients) or as % within total population (for total results in last graph) (**e**). CABG, coronary artery bypass grafting; CORO, coronarography; F, females; HF, heart failure; M, males; PCI, percutaneous coronary intervention.

3.3. Frailty Characteristics Based on Vigorito et al.'s Frailty Assessment Tool

Based on the comprehensive multi-perspective frailty assessment tool developed by Vigorito et al. [26], 44% of the patients were categorised as having minor to severe frailty, of which significantly more CVD patients suffered from minor vs. moderate frailty (34% vs. 10%, $p < 0.001$), while severe frailty was not detected. The highest prevalence of frailty was detected in HF patients (70%) and CABG patients (44%), while the frailty prevalence rates were lower in CORO (30%) and PCI (7%) patients. Major differences between HF patients and other patient populations were identified for nearly all outcomes ($p < 0.05$). Moreover, frailty was more prevalent in females than in males (53% vs. 38%, respectively) in the total population and within each CVD individually because of significant differences in gait speed, handgrip strength and TUG ($p < 0.05$) (see Tables 3 and 4 and Figure 1).

Table 3. Frailty assessment using Vigorito et al.'s tool.

			CORO		PCI		CABG		HF	
			M (n = 14)	F (n = 13)	M (n = 19)	F (n = 11)	M (n = 14)	F (n = 2)	M (n = 29)	F (n = 31)
MNA	NF/MiF/ModF/SF	n	10/3/1/0	9/3/1/0	16/3/0/0	8/2/1/0	7/5/2/0	0/2/0/0	9/15/5/0	4/16/7/4
		%	71.4/21.4/7.1/0.0	69.2/23.1/7.7/0.0	84.2/15.8/0.0/0.0	72.7/18.2/9.1/0.0	50.0/35.7/14.3	0.0/100/0.0/0.0	31.0/51.7/17.2/0.0	12.9/51.6/22.6/12.9
Katz independence in ADL	NF/MiF/ModF/SF	n	12/2/0/0	10/3/0/0	19/0/0/0	11/0/0/0	11/3/0/0	2/0/0/0	19/6/4/0	17/12/2/0
		%	85.7/14.3/0.0/0.0	76.9/23.1/0.0/0.0	100/0.0/0.0/0.0	100/0.0/0.0/0.0	78.6/21.4/0.0/0.0	100/0.0/0.0/0.0	65.5/20.7/13.8/0.0	54.8/38.7/6.5/0.0
Gait speed	NF/MiF/ModF/SF	n	11/2/0/1	6/3/4/0	17/2/0/0	10/1/0/0	8/1/4/1	0/1/0/1	7/5/7/10	5/2/14/10
		%	78.6/14.3/0.0/7.1	46.2/23.1/30.8/0.0	89.5/10.5/0.0/0.0	90.9/9.1/0.0/0.0	57.1/7.1/28.6/7.1 *	0.0/50.0/0.0/50.0	24.1/17.2/24.1/34.5	16.1/6.5/45.2/32.3
TUG	NF/MiF/ModF/SF	n	11/2/0/1	6/2/4/1	17/2/0/0	8/2/1/0	8/2/3/1	1/0/1/0	6/5/8/10	6/6/10/9
		%	78.6/14.3/0.0/7.1	46.2/15.4/30.8/7.7	89.5/10.5/0.0/0.0	72.7/18.2/9.1/0.0	57.1/14.3/21.4/7.1	50.0/0.0/0.0/50.0	20.7/17.2/27.6/34.5	19.4/19.4/32.3/29.0
Handgrip strength	NF/MiF/ModF/SF	n	11/1/1/1	13/0/0/0	14/3/2/0	10/1/0/0	10/2/1/1	1/1/0/0	9/8/10/2	14/7/9/1
		%	78.6/7.1/7.1/7.1	100/0.0/0.0/0.0	73.7/15.8/10.5/0.0	90.9/9.1/0.0/0.0	71.4/14.3/7.1/7.1	50.0/50.0/0.0/0.0	31.0/27.6/34.5/6.9	45.2/22.6/29.0/3.2
MMSE	NF/MiF/ModF/SF	n	13/1/0/0	10/2/1/0	19/0/0/0	11/0/0/0	13/0/0/1	2/0/0/0	16/11/2/0	22/5/3/1
		%	92.9/7.1/0.0/0.0	76.9/15.4/7.7/0.0	100/0.0/0.0/0.0	100/0.0/0.0/0.0	92.9/0.0/0.0/7.1	100/0.0/0.0/0.0	55.2/37.9/6.9/0.0	71.0/16.1/9.7/3.2
GDS	NF/MiF/ModF/SF	n	7/5/2/0	8/2/3/0	14/4/1/0	6/4/1/0	8/4/2/0	0/2/0/0	8/16/5/0	9/15/7/0
		%	50.0/35.7/14.3/0.0	61.5/15.4/23.1/0.0	73.7/21.1/5.3/0.0	54.5/36.4/9.1/0.0	57.1/28.6/14.3/0.0	0.0/100/0.0/0.0	27.6/55.2/17.2/0.0	29.0/48.4/22.6/0.0
Number of medications	NF/MiF/ModF/SF	n	5/6/3/0	4/5/3/1	3/11/5/0	2/4/5/0	0/8/5/1	0/1/1/0	1/12/8/8	0/16/7/8
		%	35.7/42.9/21.4/0.0	30.8/38.5/23.1/7.7	15.8/57.9/26.3/0.0	18.2/36.4/45.5/0.0	0.0/57.1/35.7/7.1	0.0/50.0/50.0/0.0	3.4/41.4/27.6/27.6	0.0/51.6/22.6/25.8

CABG, coronary artery bypass grafting; CORO, coronarography; F, females; HF, heart failure; M, males; MiF, mild frailty; ModF, moderate frailty; n, number; NF, not frail; PCI, percutaneous coronary intervention; SF, severe frailty; TUG, timed up-and-go test. Results are expressed as n or % (% within males or within females per CVD); * $p < 0.05$ association between level (severity) of frailty and sex per CVD.

Table 4. Analysis of the frailty component scores, according to CVD and sex, based on Vigorito et al.'s frailty assessment tool.

		Total (n = 133)	CORO (n = 27)	PCI (n = 30)	CABG (n = 16)	HF (n = 60)
MNA (/30)	Total	23.6 ± 3.6	25.8 ± 3.2 *	25.3 ± 2.2 **	23.8 ± 3.2	21.8 ± 3.4
	M	24.2 ± 3.1	25.8 ± 3.3	25.5 ± 1.7	23.8 ± 3.4	22.9 ± 2.9 †
	F	22.8 ± 4.0	25.8 ± 3.2	25.0 ± 2.9	23.8 ± 0.4	20.8 ± 3.7
Katz independence in ADL (n)	Total	5.2 ± 1.3	5.5 ± 1.1 *	6.0 ± 0.0 **	5.4 ± 1.1	4.7 ± 1.5
	M	5.3 ± 1.3	5.6 ± 1.1	6.0 ± 0.0	5.3 ± 1.1	4.7 ± 1.5
	F	5.1 ± 1.3	5.5 ± 1.1	6.0 ± 0.0	6.0 ± 0.0	4.6 ± 1.5
Gait speed (m/s)	Total	0.87 ± 0.48	1.03 ± 0.44 *	1.27 ± 0.36 **	0.92 ± 0.48 ***	0.59 ± 0.36
	M	0.98 ± 0.52 †	1.21 ± 0.47 †	1.34 ± 0.40	0.98 ± 0.48	0.63 ± 0.40
	F	0.73 ± 0.38	0.85 ± 0.31	1.15 ± 0.24	0.51 ± 0.24	0.55 ± 0.33
TUG (s)	Total	14.4 ± 9.0	11.5 ± 6.9 *	8.3 ± 2.5 **	12.9 ± 7.7	19.1 ± 9.8
	M	13.5 ± 9.3 †	10.3 ± 8.4 †	7.8 ± 2.1	11.8 ± 6.3	19.5 ± 10.5
	F	15.6 ± 8.5	12.9 ± 4.8	9.2 ± 2.9	20.6 ± 14.9	18.7 ± 9.3
Handgrip strength (kg)	Total	26.7 ± 11.8	30.7 ± 13.2 *	33.1 ± 11.1 **	31.1 ± 9.0 ***	20.5 ± 9.1
	M	33.3 ± 10.7 †	38.8 ± 13.3 †	39.0 ± 9.3 †	33.0 ± 7.7	27.1 ± 7.9 †
	F	17.9 ± 6.2	22.0 ± 4.9	22.9 ± 4.7	17.9 ± 6.2	14.4 ± 4.9
MMSE (/30)	Total	26.2 ± 3.2	27.3 ± 2.5 *	27.6 ± 1.7 **	26.8 ± 4.1 ***	24.9 ± 3.4
	M	26.3 ± 3.3	27.7 ± 2.2	27.7 ± 1.7	26.6 ± 4.3	24.6 ± 3.3
	F	26.1 ± 3.2	26.9 ± 2.9	27.5 ± 1.8	28.0 ± 1.4	25.1 ± 3.4
GDS-15 (/15)	Total	3.2 ± 2.3	3.3 ± 3.0	2.2 ± 1.8 **	2.8 ± 1.9	3.9 ± 2.0
	M	3.0 ± 2.2	3.3 ± 2.7	2.0 ± 1.6	2.5 ± 2.0	3.9 ± 2.1
	F	3.5 ± 2.4	3.4 ± 3.4	2.6 ± 2.0	4.5 ± 0.7	3.8 ± 2.0
Number of medications (n)	Total	8.3 ± 3.4	6.6 ± 3.2 *	7.2 ± 2.4 **	7.8 ± 2.5	9.9 ± 3.4
	M	8.2 ± 3.6	6.2 ± 3.4	6.8 ± 2.3	7.8 ± 2.6	10.0 ± 3.8
	F	8.6 ± 3.1	6.9 ± 3.0	7.7 ± 2.4	7.5 ± 2.1	9.7 ± 3.2
Total frailty score	Total	6.2 ± 4.8	3.8 ± 3.8 *	2.4 ± 2.1 **	5.6 ± 4.2	9.4 ± 4.2
	M	5.6 ± 4.7	3.2 ± 3.7	2.2 ± 2.0	5.3 ± 4.4	9.2 ± 4.2
	F	7.0 ± 4.8	4.5 ± 4.0	2.7 ± 2.5	7.5 ± 3.5	9.6 ± 4.3

ADL, activities of daily living; CABG, coronary artery bypass grafting; cm, centimetre; CORO, coronarography; F, females; GDS, Geriatric Depression Scale; HF, heart failure; kg, kilogram; M, males; m, metre; MNA, Mini Nutritional Assessment; MMSE, Mini-Mental State Examination; n, number; PCI, percutaneous coronary intervention; s, seconds; SD, standard deviation; TUG, timed up-and-go test; $p < 0.05$ * CORO vs. HF; ** PCI vs. HF; *** CABG vs. HF; † $p < 0.05$ between sexes. Results are expressed as mean ± SD.

3.4. Comparison between Vigorito and Fried Frailty Criteria

Some level of frailty was detected in 44% of the patients according to Vigorito et al.'s frailty assessment tool (from mild to severe frailty) and in 65% of the patients according to the Fried phenotype (from pre-frail to frail) ($x^2 = 57.95$, $p < 0.001$) (see Figure 1). However, according to Vigorito et al.'s tool, significantly more CVD patients suffered from minor vs. moderate frailty (34% vs. 10%, $p < 0.001$), while the Fried phenotype did not succeed in detecting any significant difference in the number of pre-frail vs. frail patients (26% vs. 38%, $p = 0.11$).

Moreover, 51 patients were detected as being frail according to Fried. However, of these patients, Vigorito criteria classified 25% as having moderate frailty, 69% as having minor frailty and 6% as being non-frail. Similarly, of the 35 patients classified as pre-frail according to Fried, only 3% of the patients were classified as having moderate frailty, and 29% had minor frailty, while 69% of them were not frail according to Vigorito. As the largest proportion of pre-frail patients based on Fried seem to not be frail according to Vigorito and frail patients based on Fried seem to mainly have minor frailty according to Vigorito, we suggest that, based on these data, the Fried criteria may overestimate frailty and its severity. The same findings emerged when a comparison was made between older and younger CVD patients. Moreover, based on this analysis, a significant association was found between age and frailty status (see Appendix A Table A4).

3.5. Creation of New Frailty Test Battery

To examine which frailty measurements could contribute to the prediction of frailty in CVD patients and should thus be executed in clinical settings, multivariate correlations between all frailty assessments (in particular, the components of the Fried and Vigorito frailty assessments and all additional frailty measurements) and the total frailty score according to Vigorito et al. were determined. From these analyses, the following parameters correlated significantly ($p < 0.05$) with the total Vigorito frailty score: walking time (r = 0.854), TUG (r = 0.845), gait speed (r = −0.823), TCST (r = 0.740), MNA (r = −0.727), Katz scale (r = −0.694), number of medications (r = 0.641), handgrip strength (r = −0.607), MMSE (r = −0.559), knee extension strength (right leg) (r = −0.549), hip flexion strength (right leg) (r = −0.548), hip flexion strength (left leg) (r = −0.539), GDS−15 (r = 0.531) and knee extension strength (left leg) (−0.526).

Finally, a multivariate regression model was built to decide which test should be maintained so that it has as few measurements as possible but optimal predictive power. In this model, the total frailty score of Vigorito et al.'s frailty assessment tool was considered the dependent variable, while all frailty assessments/parameters were considered independent variables. To detect frailty ($R^2 = 0.95$), sex, MNA, Katz scale, TUG, handgrip strength, MMSE, GDS-15, total number of medications and the interaction of Katz scale and TUG should be assessed.

Based on these parameters, which are components of Vigorito et al.'s frailty assessment tool, a new formula was developed (r = 0.98 with Vigorito score, $p < 0.001$):

Total frailty score = [(18.221173 + (1.1454217 × sex] + (−0.267283 × MNA score)] + (−0.947011 × Katz scale score) + (0.2157993 × TUG score) + (−0.081659 × handgrip strength score) + [−0.18281 × MMSE score) + (0.2700342 × GDS-15 score) + (0.2264091 × total number of medications) + [0.0453303 × (Katz scale score − 5.21805) × (TUG score − 14.3608)]]

In order to avoid false-negative frailty diagnoses, a sensitivity of 1.0 was determined with a corresponding specificity of 0.54, resulting in a cut-off score of ≥5.56 pointing towards frailty according to this newly proposed frailty score (see Table 5 and Figure 2).

Table 5. Cut-off scores and corresponding sensitivity and specificity analyses of the newly developed frailty assessment battery.

Cut-Off Score	Sensitivity	Specificity
−1.71	1.00	0.00
−0.34	1.00	0.03
0.09	1.00	0.06
0.42	1.00	0.08
0.65	1.00	0.10
0.85	1.00	0.13
1.09	1.00	0.17

Table 5. Cont.

Cut-Off Score	Sensitivity	Specificity
3.04	1.00	0.35
5.56	**1.00**	**0.54**
7.02	0.63	0.60
7.17	0.50	0.60
7.27	0.38	0.60
7.46	0.25	0.61
7.92	0.13	0.64
9.09	0.00	0.67
11.2	0.00	0.83
13.3	0.00	0.91
15.07	0.00	0.96
17.32	0.00	0.98
18.90	0.00	1.00

Note: The bold format indicates the preferred cut-off score which should be used when implementing the newly proposed frailty assessment tool to detect frailty.

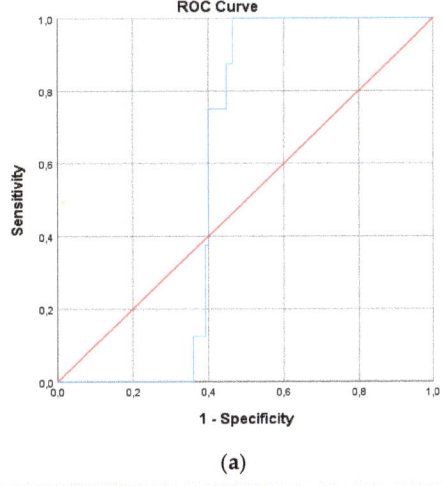

(a)

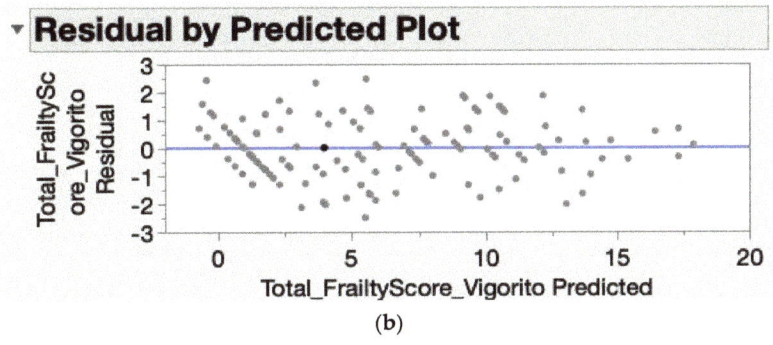

(b)

Figure 2. ROC curve (**a**) and plot (**b**) of the new regression formula vs. the total frailty score of Vigorito et al.

3.6. Association of Frailty with 6-Month Clinical Outcomes

To examine the association of frailty with clinical outcomes, hospitalisations and mortality up to six months after the initial hospital admission were examined. During this period, 39% of the patients were readmitted to the hospital, and 56% of these hospitalisations were attributed to HF patients. The hospital admissions were mainly of cardiovascular, pulmonary or metabolic origin (65%), followed by orthopaedic (e.g., falls, fractures, amputations) (13%) and neurological events (e.g., stroke) (3%), while 20% were classified as another event (e.g., epistaxis, wound problems, hematomas, etc.). Six months after the initial hospital admission, 7% of the subjects died, of which 89% were HF patients (OR 11.1).

Significant associations between (markers of) frailty and 6-month clinical outcomes can be found in Table 6. Frailty and specific markers of frailty (e.g., handgrip strength) were significantly associated with mortality and 6-month general, urgent, orthopaedic and cardiovascular hospitalisations. Especially orthopaedic hospital admissions were associated with frailty and several frailty components. Furthermore, specific Vigorito components are more feasible for predicting mortality, while specific Fried components can better predict 6-month (urgent) hospitalisations.

Table 6. Significant associations between markers of frailty and 6-month clinical outcomes.

6-Month Clinical Outcomes	Frailty Marker	*p*-Value
Mortality	Frailty status according to Fried	$p = 0.002$
	Frailty status according to Vigorito	$p = 0.011$
	MNA	$p = 0.003$
	Gait speed	$p = 0.023$
	TUG	$p = 0.001$
	MMSE	$p = 0.042$
	Handgrip strength	$p = 0.006$
	Frailty status according to the newly developed frailty assessment battery	$p = 0.017$
6-month hospitalisations	Frailty status according to Fried	$p = 0.030$
	Handgrip strength	$p = 0.004$
	Exhaustion	$p = 0.011$
6-month urgent hospitalisations	Frailty status according to Fried	$p = 0.032$
	Handgrip strength	$p = 0.013$ (Fried) $p = 0.019$ (Vigorito)
	Exhaustion	$p = 0.032$
	Physical activity	$p = 0.03$
	Frailty status according to the newly developed frailty assessment battery	$p = 0.04$
Orthopaedic hospitalisations	Frailty status according to Fried	$p = 0.005$
	Handgrip strength	$p = 0.033$
	Gait speed	$p = 0.023$
	Frailty status according to Vigorito	$p = 0.022$
	Gait speed	$p = 0.025$
	MNA	$p = 0.018$
	GDS-15	$p = 0.003$
Cardiovascular hospitalisations	Handgrip strength (Fried)	$p = 0.028$

GDS-15, Geriatric Depression Scale; MMSE, Mini-Mental State Examination; MNA, Mini Nutritional Assessment; TUG, timed up-and-go test.

Moreover, subgroup analysis (HF vs. CAD) did not reveal any significant associations with the newly proposed frailty assessment battery.

4. Discussion

This was the first study that aimed to analyse the prevalence of frailty in hospitalised CVD patients using the Fried vs. Vigorito criteria. Moreover, we were able to define which tests should be included in such an assessment to generate a time- and cost-efficient frailty assessment tool for CVD patients, allowing the development of a multi-component and sex-specific frailty assessment tool.

In this study, 70% of HF patients and 44% of CABG patients were frail, compared with only 30% of CORO patients and 7% of PCI patients. These data confirm that the more severe CVD patients (HF and CABG) more often suffer from (more severe) frailty. Indeed, while moderate frailty was mostly detected in CABG and HF patients, CORO and PCI patients mostly suffered from minor frailty. These higher prevalence rates and more severe levels of frailty in HF patients could be mainly explained by the more severe disease characteristics, such as dyspnoea, exhaustion or peripheral oedema. This is further confirmed by the high prevalence rates of frailty in older ($\geq$80 years) as well as in younger (<80 years) HF patients (82.4% vs. 53.8% according to Vigorito and 85.3% vs. 50.0% according to Fried). However, severe frailty was not detected even in the most severe CVDs such as HF. This could be explained by the fact that most HF patients were classified as New York Heart Association (NYHA) class II or III. Frailty was more prevalent in females than in males in the total population (53% vs. 38%) as well as within each CVD individually. This was mainly due to significantly lower/worse outcomes in gait speed, handgrip strength and TUG and a trend for a lower MNA score, although lower results can be expected in females than in males. We thus can conclude that, despite the finding that most of the participants were not frail or mildly frail, CABG and HF patients are especially at risk for developing or experiencing frailty, particularly females, which is supported by previous evidence [12]. Frailty is related to several adverse health outcomes, such as functional decline with an increased risk of dependency (because of falls, difficulties with mobility, impairment of basic and instrumental ADL), poor cognition (with an increased incidence of dementia and delirium) and a decreased quality of life (subjective health, mood, engagement and social relations), resulting in increased healthcare consumption with more frequent hospitalisations (such as emergency room visits and surgical complications), institutionalisation and, finally, premature death [11]. Therefore, it might be advisable to execute frailty screenings more often in clinical practice in these patients and initiate preventive measures accordingly. In this regard, exercise training, in combination with nutritional support, is highly recommended [37–41].

Along with the potential of the Vigorito frailty assessment tool to detect frailty in several domains (physical, psychosocial, cognitive) in CVD patients (in contrast to the Fried phenotype), Vigorito et al.'s frailty assessment tool reported a lower prevalence of frailty (44%) and of minor (34%) compared to moderate (10%) frailty. The Fried phenotype reported a larger percentage of frailty (64%) and of frail compared to pre-frail patients. By examining frailty in several domains, Vigorito et al.'s tool has the capacity to only consider a patient frail when several domains are affected and could be more sensitive in detecting small differences in frailty severity, while the Fried tool may have a smaller latitude and be limited by a ceiling effect. Moreover, the Fried phenotype can be somewhat subjective, as, for example, the two questions regarding exhaustion are often difficult for patients to answer correctly. Furthermore, registration of involuntary weight loss only does not always fully capture the nutritional status of the patients.

However, the Vigorito frailty assessment tool is not yet validated in CVD patients. Therefore, based on all frailty measurements that we performed in this study, we tried to analyse which measurements could contribute to the prediction of frailty and related hospitalisations and mortality in CVD patients based on the model proposed by Vigorito et al. Based on multivariate regression analysis, sex, MNA, Katz scale, TUG, handgrip strength,

MMSE, GDS-15 and total number of medications are collectively the best predictors of frailty (model $R^2 = 0.95$). Based on this specific frailty assessment tool, which comprises components of Vigorito et al.'s frailty assessment tool, the presence of frailty in CVD patients can be feasibly detected in a time- and cost-efficient way, as is it takes only 10–15 min, while, except for a handgrip dynamometer, no expensive equipment is required. Thus, this score calculator can be implemented in clinical practice and/or validated in subsequent studies:

$$[(18.221173 + (1.1454217 \times sex] + (-0.267283 \times \text{MNA score})] + (-0.947011 \times \text{Katz scale score}) + (0.2157993 \times \text{TUG score}) + (-0.081659 \times \text{handgrip strength score}) + [-0.18281 \times \text{MMSE score}) + (0.2700342 \times \text{GDS-15 score}) + (0.2264091 \times \text{total number of medications}) + [0.0453303 \times (\text{Katz scale score} - 5.21805) \times (\text{TUG score} - 14.3608)]]$$

Moreover, given the importance of avoiding false-negative frailty diagnoses in clinical practice, a cut-off score corresponding to a sensitivity of 1.00 was determined. According to this model, a frailty diagnosis is thus made with a score of 5.56 or higher, which corresponds to a 100% probability of correctly detecting frailty with a false-positive probability of 46%.

Finally, we examined whether frailty is related to 6-month clinical outcomes. As all three frailty assessment batteries (Fried $\chi^2 = 10.431$, $p = 0.002$; Vigorito $\chi^2 = 7.755$, $p = 0.011$; and the newly developed battery $\chi^2 = 5.953$, $p = 0.017$) found significant associations between frailty and mortality, we can conclude that frailty indeed increases the mortality risk. These increased mortality rates in frail CVD patients were previously confirmed in a recent systematic review [12]. Moreover, given the significant association between hospitalisations and frailty according to Fried, there are indications that frailty also increases the risk for (urgent) hospital admissions. Based on a logistic regression model, the stronger association of frailty with mortality, in comparison with hospitalisations, was further confirmed, given the significant associations between several frailty assessment components (MNA, Katz scale, walking time, gait speed, TUG, MMSE and number of medications) and mortality in comparison with hospitalisations (only walking time, handgrip strength and GDS). It thus seems possible that frailty in CVD patients is more related to increased mortality instead of increased risk for hospitalisation. Moreover, when we examine the specific frailty components of Fried vs. Vigorito, it seems that mainly specific Vigorito components are more able to predict mortality, while specific Fried components can better predict 6-month (urgent) hospitalisations. Furthermore, as especially orthopaedic hospital admissions were associated with frailty and several frailty components, there are indications that especially a low handgrip strength and gait speed, a worse nutritional status and a depressed state can result in hospital admissions due to fall incidents and related fractures. These findings again confirm the importance of the early detection and multidisciplinary treatment of frailty in order to prevent hospitalisations and mortality.

Based on the multivariate regression model, we were able to select specific frailty measurements that were highly qualified to predict frailty. Based on this newly proposed frailty assessment tool, it will now be possible to examine frailty in a sex-specific and multidimensional way. Moreover, by using the proposed formula, the exact score of each frailty measurement can be input, which will then result in an automatic and therefore simple and time-efficient calculation of the frailty score. As this easy-to-use tool does not necessitate extensive education, it will therefore be accessible for all members of the healthcare professional, which will further encourage a multidisciplinary frailty approach. Usage of this exact score is an important advantage over the Vigorito tool, in which it is unclear how raw data of MNA and TUG should be rounded to interpret the frailty severity. Moreover, the Vigorito tool only takes into account specific criteria for men vs. women for the handgrip strength criteria, in contrast to other sex-influenced criteria such as TUG and gait speed. Furthermore, based on the sensitivity and specificity curves (Table 5), it will be possible to check the sensitivity and accompanying specificity of the preferred cut-off scores. We thus can conclude that this newly developed frailty assessment battery provides several advantages over the Fried and Vigorito tools to more objectively examine frailty in CVD patients.

Some study limitations should be taken into account. First, the sample sizes were not equal across all of the different CVDs, and especially CABG patients were underrepresented in this study. Second, the frailty assessment battery was not performed on the same day of hospitalisation for all patients, which could have caused differences in the physical status of the patients. Moreover, a modified version of the Fried criteria was used by implementing the Katz scale to examine the level of physical activity instead of the original Minnesota Leisure Time Activity questionnaire. Although this Katz scale was more in accordance with the study population, the use of a modified version of the Fried criteria has to be acknowledged. Moreover, as no severely frail patients were detected in this study, it may be worthwhile to further evaluate the diagnostic power of the Vigorito frailty assessment tool in a larger population of CVD patients. Furthermore, we aimed to develop a new frailty assessment battery based on a multivariate regression model with the total Vigorito frailty score as a dependent variable. However, it remains important to acknowledge that this Vigorito frailty assessment tool has not yet been validated and thus requires further research.

Finally, there are indications that certain biomarkers (such as NT-proBNP) may be associated with the presence of frailty in older HF patients. To further optimize frailty diagnosis, it may thus be promising to explore the potential role of biomarkers in future research [42].

5. Conclusions

To detect frailty, including at an early stage, in patients with CVD, sex, MNA, Katz scale, TUG, handgrip strength, MMSE, GDS-15 and total number of medications play a key role. A new simple, time- and cost-efficient test battery for frailty with sufficient sensitivity and specificity, accessible for all healthcare professionals, is proposed in this study.

Author Contributions: Investigation, K.B., L.H., T.J. and Y.V.; Writing—original draft, N.M.; Writing—review & editing, C.V., F.G., P.D., R.M., M.S., J.S. and D.H. All authors have read and agreed to the published version of the manuscript.

Funding: This research received no external funding. Internal faculty funding was received.

Institutional Review Board Statement: The study was conducted in accordance with the Declaration of Helsinki and approved by the Institutional Review Board (or Ethics Committee) of JESSA HOSPITAL (protocol code 19.81-REVA19.05, date of approval 7 November 2019).

Informed Consent Statement: Informed consent was obtained from all subjects involved in the study.

Data Availability Statement: All data tables are included in this manuscript.

Conflicts of Interest: The authors declare no conflict of interest.

Appendix A

Table A1. Frailty phenotype according to Fried et al. [13].

Weight loss	"In the last year, have you lost more than 10 pounds unintentionally (i.e., not due to dieting or exercise)?" If yes, then frail for weight loss criterion. At follow-up, weight loss was calculated as: (Weight in previous year–current measured weight)/(weight in previous year) = K. If $K \geq 0.05$ and the subject does not report that he/she was trying to lose weight (i.e., unintentional weight loss of at least 5% of previous year's body weight), then frail for weight loss = Yes.
Exhaustion	Using the CES–D Depression Scale, the following two statements are read. (a) I felt that everything I did was an effort; (b) I could not get going. The question is asked: "How often in the last week did you feel this way?" 0 = rarely or none of the time (<1 day) 1 = some or a little of the time (1–2 days) 2 = a moderate amount of the time (3–4 days) 3 = most of the time. Subjects answering "2" or "3" to either of these questions are categorized as frail for the exhaustion criterion.

Table A1. *Cont.*

Physical activity	Based on the short version of the Minnesota Leisure Time Activity questionnaire, asking about walking, chores (moderately strenuous), mowing the lawn, raking, gardening, hiking, jogging, biking, exercise cycling, dancing, aerobics, bowling, golf, singles tennis, doubles tennis, racquetball, calisthenics and swimming, kcals per week expended are calculated using standardised algorithm. This variable is stratified by gender. Men: Those with kcals of physical activity per week < 383 are frail. Women: Those with kcals per week < 270 are frail.

	Cut-off for time to walk 15 feet criterion for frailty (Stratified by gender and height)	
	Men	
	Height ≤ 173 cm	≥7 s
Walk time	Height > 173 cm	≥6 s
	Women	
	Height ≤ 159 cm	≥7 s
	Height > 159 cm	≥6 s

	Cut-off for grip strength (kg) criterion for frailty (stratified by gender and BMI quartiles)	
	Men	
	BMI ≤ 24	≤29
	BMI 24.1–26	≤30
	BMI 26.1–28	≤30
Grip strength	BMI > 28	≤32
	Women	
	BMI ≤ 23	≤17
	BMI 23.1–26	≤17.3
	BMI 26.1–29	≤18
	BMI > 29	≤21

BMI, body mass index; kcals, kilocalories; CES-D, Center of Epidemiologic Studies—depression subscale; kg, kilogram.

Table A2. Vigorito et al.'s frailty assessment tool.

	No Frailty	Minor Frailty	Moderate Frailty	Severe Frailty
	Score 0	Score 1	Score 2	Score 3
MNA (/30)	A validated screening and assessment tool to identify persons of 65 years or older who are malnourished or at risk of malnutrition based on 6 screening questions and 12 assessment questions. A lower score indicates a higher risk of malnutrition.			
	≥25	21–24	17–20	<17
Katz independence in ADL (6 activities)	A screening tool to examine the level of (in)dependence in activities of daily living (ADL) (bathing, dressing, transfers, toileting, continence and eating). Complete independence in performing these activities results in a score of 1, while any dependence (from partial to full help required) is scored as 0. This results in a total score from 0 to 6 (i.e., number of independent activities), in which the highest score is associated with complete independence in 6 ADLs.			
	5–6 activities	3–4 activities	1–2 activities	0 activities
Gait speed (m/s)	Evaluation of the gait speed (expressed in metres per second (m/s) based on a 4.6 m walking test (use of walking aids is permitted).			
	≥0.80	0.61–0.79	0.40–0.60	<0.40

Table A2. *Cont.*

	No Frailty	Minor Frailty	Moderate Frailty	Severe Frailty
	Score 0	Score 1	Score 2	Score 3
TUG (s)	A test that evaluates a combination of mobility, balance and lower-extremity strength. The subject has to stand up from a chair (use of armrests permitted), walk 3 m, return and sit down in the chair again as quickly but safely as possible (use of walking aids is permitted). The walking time is registered in seconds.			
	≤10	11–14	15–20	>20
Handgrip strength (kg)	Evaluation of the handgrip strength (kg) of the dominant hand with a handheld dynamometer. The subject has to squeeze three times, and the highest value is taken into account for the evaluation of frailty severity.			
	F >15.6	11.4–15.6	7.3–11.3	≤7.2
	M ≥30.6	25.7–30.5	19.0–25.6	≤18.9
MMSE (/30)	A valid and reliable screening tool to detect cognitive disabilities in older adults in the domains of orientation in time and space, registration, attention and calculation, recall, language and copying. A lower score indicates a lower level of cognitive abilities.			
	>24	21–24	16–20	≤15
GDS-15 (/15)	A screening tool for older adults consisting of 15 questions to detect the presence of a depressive mood. A higher score indicates a more depressed state.			
	<3	3–5	6–10	11–15
Number of medications (*n*)	Registration of the use of medications. Vitamins, minerals and food supplements are not included.			
	1–4	5–8	9–12	>12
TOTAL SCORE	0–6	7–12	13–18	19–24

ADL, activities of daily living; GDS. Geriatric Depression Scale; m, metre; MMSE, Mini-Mental State Examination; MNA, Mini Nutritional Assessment; s, seconds; TUG, timed up-and-go test.

Table A3. Additional frailty measures.

IPAQ (long version) (METS/min/week)	An evaluation tool that examines the level of physical activity spent in the previous seven days in the domains of work, transportation, domestic/garden and recreation/sport/leisure time as well as the time spent sitting. A higher score indicates a higher level of physical activity.
Muscle strength (kg)	Evaluation of the muscle strength of the knee extensors (sitting position with hip and knee flexed 90°) and hip flexors (supine position with hip flexed 90°) of both legs, measured with the MicroFET® dynamometer (Hoggan Health Industries Inc., West Jordan, UT, USA). Each measurement is repeated three times, and the highest value is used in the data analysis.
Timed chair stand test (s)	A test that evaluates the functional muscle strength of the lower limbs. The subject has to stand up five times from a chair, without using armrests (arms crossed at the chest), and has to return to the sitting position as fast and as safely as possible. The time is registered in seconds.
FES-I (/64)	A questionnaire that examines the level of concern about falling during 16 social and physical activities. A higher score indicates a higher level of concern about falling.

FES-I, Falls Efficacy Scale International; IPAQ, International Physical Activity Questionnaire; kg, kilograms; METS, metabolic equivalents; min, minutes; s, seconds.

Table A4. (1) Frailty analysis (in %) according to the Fried phenotype per age group ($p < 0.001$). (2) Frailty analysis (in %) according to the Vigorito frailty assessment tool per age group ($p = 0.022$). (3) Frailty analysis (in %) according to the newly developed frailty assessment tool per age group ($p < 0.001$).

	(1)	
	65–75 years	>75 years
Not frail	49.0	26.8
Pre-frail	33.3	22.0
Frail	17.6	51.2
	(2)	
	65–75 years	>75 years
Not frail	70.6	46.3
Mild frail	21.6	41.5
Moderate frail	7.8	12.2
	(3)	
	65–75 years	>75 years
Not frail	70.6	37.8
Frail	29.4	62.2

References

1. Townsend, N.; Wilson, L.; Bhatnagar, P.; Wickramasinghe, K.; Rayner, M.; Nichols, M. Cardiovascular disease in Europe: Epidemiological update 2016. *Eur. Heart J.* **2016**, *37*, 3232–3245. [CrossRef] [PubMed]
2. Carneiro, J.A.; Cardoso, R.R.; Durães, M.S.; Guedes, M.C.; Santos, F.L.; Costa, F.M.; Caldeira, A.P. Frailty in the elderly: Prevalence and associated factors. *Rev. Bras. Enferm.* **2017**, *70*, 747–752. [CrossRef]
3. Ferrucci, L.; Giallauria, F.; Guralnik, J.M. Epidemiology of aging. *Radiol. Clin. N. Am.* **2008**, *46*, 643–652. [CrossRef]
4. Heidenreich, P.A.; Trogdon, J.G.; Khavjou, O.A.; Butler, J.; Dracup, K.; Ezekowitz, M.D.; Finkelstein, E.A.; Hong, Y.; Johnston, S.C.; Khera, A.; et al. Forecasting the future of cardiovascular disease in the United States: A policy statement from the American Heart Association. *Circulation* **2011**, *123*, 933–944. [CrossRef]
5. Easterwood, R.M.; Bostock, I.C.; Nammalwar, S.; McCullough, J.N.; Iribarne, A. The evolution of minimally invasive cardiac surgery: From minimal access to transcatheter approaches. *Future Cardiol.* **2018**, *14*, 75–87. [CrossRef] [PubMed]
6. Prescott, E.; Eser, P.; Mikkelsen, N.; Holdgaard, A.; Marcin, T.; Wilhelm, M.; Gil, C.P.; González-Juanatey, J.R.; Moatemri, F.; Iliou, M.C.; et al. Cardiac rehabilitation of elderly patients in eight rehabilitation units in western Europe: Outcome data from the EU-CaRE multi-centre observational study. *Eur. J. Prev. Cardiol.* **2020**, *27*, 1716–1729. [CrossRef]
7. Peersen, K.; Munkhaugen, J.; Gullestad, L.; Liodden, T.; Moum, T.; Dammen, T.; Perk, J.; Otterstad, J.E. The role of cardiac rehabilitation in secondary prevention after coronary events. *Eur. J. Prev. Cardiol.* **2017**, *24*, 1360–1368. [CrossRef] [PubMed]
8. Eichler, S.; Völler, H.; Reibis, R.; Wegscheider, K.; Butter, C.; Harnath, A.; Salzwedel, A. Geriatric or cardiac rehabilitation? Predictors of treatment pathways in advanced age patients after transcatheter aortic valve implantation. *BMC Cardiovasc. Disord.* **2020**, *20*, 158.
9. Okwuosa, I.S.; Lewsey, S.C.; Adesiyun, T.; Blumenthal, R.S.; Yancy, C.W. Worldwide disparities in cardiovascular disease: Challenges and solutions. *Int. J. Cardiol.* **2016**, *202*, 433–440. [CrossRef]
10. World Report on Ageing and Health. Available online: https://apps.who.int/iris/bitstream/handle/10665/186463/97892406948 11_eng.pdf;jsessionid=96E25B91F60EBDEF561148FC471C5D78?sequence=1 (accessed on 20 September 2019).
11. Junius-Walker, U.; Onder, G.; Soleymani, D.; Wiese, B.; Albaina, O.; Bernabei, R.; Marzetti, E. The essence of frailty: A systematic review and qualitative synthesis on frailty concepts and definitions. *Eur. J. Intern. Med.* **2018**, *56*, 3–10. [CrossRef] [PubMed]
12. Marinus, N.; Vigorito, C.; Giallauria, F.; Haenen, L.; Jansegers, T.; Dendale, P.; Feys, P.; Meesen, R.; Timmermans, A.; Spildooren, J. Frailty is highly prevalent in specific cardiovascular diseases and females, but significantly worsens prognosis in all affected patients: A systematic review. *Ageing Res. Rev.* **2020**, *66*, 101233. [CrossRef] [PubMed]
13. Fried, L.P.; Tangen, C.M.; Walston, J.; Newman, A.B.; Hirsch, C.; Gottdiener, J.; Seeman, T.; Tracy, R.; Kop, W.J.; Burke, G. Frailty in older adults: Evidence for a phenotype. *J. Gerontol. A Biol. Sci. Med. Sci.* **2001**, *56*, M146–M156. [CrossRef]
14. Evans, S.J.; Sayers, M.; Mitnitski, A.; Rockwood, K. The risk of adverse outcomes in hospitalized older patients in relation to a frailty index based on a comprehensive geriatric assessment. *Age Ageing* **2014**, *43*, 127–132. [CrossRef] [PubMed]

15. Pilotto, A.; Veronese, N.; Daragjati, J.; Cruz-Jentoft, A.J.; Polidori, M.C.; Mattace-Raso, F.; Paccalin, M.; Topinkova, E.; Siri, G.; Greco, A. Using the multidimensional prognostic index to predict clinical outcomes of hospitalized older persons: A prospective, multicenter, international study. *J. Gerontol. A Biol. Sci. Med. Sci.* **2019**, *74*, 1643–1649. [CrossRef] [PubMed]
16. Schoenenberger, A.W.; Stortecky, S.; Neumann, S.; Moser, A.; Jüni, P.; Carrel, T.; Huber, C.; Gandon, M.; Bischoff, S.; Schoenenberger, C.M. Predictors of functional decline in elderly patients undergoing transcatheter aortic valve implantation (TAVI). *Eur. Heart J.* **2013**, *34*, 684–692. [CrossRef] [PubMed]
17. Needham, M.J.; Webb, C.E.; Bryden, D.C. Postoperative cognitive dysfunction and dementia: What we need to know and do. *Br. J. Anaesth.* **2017**, *119* (Suppl. 1), i115–i125. [CrossRef]
18. Evered, L.; Scott, D.A.; Silbert, B.; Maruff, P. Postoperative cognitive dysfunction is independent of type of surgery and anesthetic. *Anesth Analg.* **2011**, *112*, 1179–1185. [CrossRef] [PubMed]
19. Itagaki, A.; Sakurada, K.; Matsuhama, M.; Yajima, J.; Yamashita, T.; Kohzuki, M. Impact of frailty and mild cognitive impairment on delirium after cardiac surgery in older patients. *J. Cardiol.* **2020**, *76*, 147–153. [CrossRef] [PubMed]
20. Li, H.C.; Wei, Y.C.; Hsu, R.B.; Chi, N.H.; Wang, S.S.; Chen, Y.S.; Chen, S.Y.; Chen, C.C.; Inouye, S.K. Surviving and thriving 1 year after cardiac surgery: Frailty and delirium matter. *Ann. Thorac. Surg.* **2020**, *111*, 1578–1584. [CrossRef] [PubMed]
21. Gao, L.; Taha, R.; Gauvin, D.; Othmen, L.B.; Wang, Y.; Blaise, G. Postoperative cognitive dysfunction after cardiac surgery. *Chest* **2005**, *128*, 3664–3670. [CrossRef]
22. Tachibana, H.; Hiraoka, A.; Saito, K.; Naito, Y.; Chikazawa, G.; Tamura, K.; Totsugawa, T.; Yoshitaka, H.; Sakaguchi, T. Incidence and impact of silent brain lesions after coronary artery bypass grafting. *J. Thorac. Cardiovasc. Surg.* **2019**, *161*, 636–644. [CrossRef] [PubMed]
23. Havranek, E.P.; Mujahid, M.S.; Barr, D.A.; Blair, I.V.; Cohen, M.S.; Cruz-Flores, S.; Davey-Smith, G.; Dennison-Himmelfarb, C.R.; Lauer, M.S.; Lockwood, D.W.; et al. Social determinants of risk and outcomes for cardiovascular disease: A scientific statement from the american heart association. *Circulation* **2015**, *132*, 873–898. [CrossRef] [PubMed]
24. Vigorito, C.; Abreu, A.; Ambrosetti, M.; Belardinelli, R.; Corra, U.; Cupples, M.; Davos, C.H.; Hoefer, S.; Iliou, M.C.; Schmid, J.P.; et al. Frailty and cardiac rehabilitation: A call to action from the EAPC Cardiac Rehabilitation Section. *Eur. J. Prev. Cardiol.* **2017**, *24*, 577–590. [CrossRef] [PubMed]
25. Richter, D.; Guasti, L.; Walker, D.; Lambrinou, E.; Lionis, C.; Abreu, A.; Savelieva, I.; Fumagalli, S.; Bo, M.; Rocca, B.; et al. Frailty in cardiology: Definition, assessment and clinical implications for general cardiology. A consensus document of the Council for Cardiology Practice (CCP), Acute Cardiovascular Care Association (ACCA), Association of Cardiovascular Nursing and Allied Professions (ACNAP), European Association of Preventive Cardiology (EAPC), European Heart Rhythm Association (EHRA), Council on Valvular Heart Diseases (VHD), Council on Hypertension (CHT), Council of Cardio-Oncology (CCO), Working Group (WG) Aorta and Peripheral Vascular Diseases, WG e-Cardiology, WG Thrombosis, of the European Society of Cardiology, European Primary Care Cardiology Society (EPCCS). *Eur. J. Prev. Cardiol.* **2022**, *29*, 216–227.
26. Vigorito, C.; Abreu, A. Cardiac rehabilitation for geriatric and frail patients. In *The ESC Handbook of Cardiovascular Rehabilitation*; Abreu, A., Schmid, J.P., Piepoli, M., Eds.; O.U. Press: Oxford, UK, 2020.
27. Green, P.; Woglom, A.E.; Genereux, P.; Daneault, B.; Paradis, J.M.; Schnell, S.; Hawkey, M.; Maurer, M.S.; Kirtane, A.J.; Kodali, S.; et al. The impact of frailty status on survival after transcatheter aortic valve replacement in older adults with severe aortic stenosis: A single-center experience. *JACC Cardiovasc. Interv.* **2012**, *5*, 974–981. [CrossRef]
28. Tanaka, S.; Kamiya, K.; Hamazaki, N.; Matsuzawa, R.; Nozaki, K.; Maekawa, E.; Noda, C.; Yamaoka-Tojo, M.; Matsunaga, A.; Masuda, T.; et al. Incremental value of objective frailty assessment to predict mortality in elderly patients hospitalized for heart failure. *J. Card. Fail.* **2018**, *24*, 723–732. [CrossRef]
29. Green, P.; Arnold, S.V.; Cohen, D.J.; Kirtane, A.J.; Kodali, S.K.; Brown, D.L.; Rihal, C.S.; Xu, K.; Lei, Y.; Hawkey, M.C.; et al. Relation of frailty to outcomes after transcatheter aortic valve replacement (from the PARTNER trial). *Am. J. Cardiol.* **2015**, *116*, 264–269. [CrossRef]
30. Boujemaa, H.; Yilmaz, A.; Robic, B.; Koppo, K.; Claessen, G.; Frederix, I.; Dendale, P.; Völler, H.; van Loon, L.J.; Hansen, D. The effect of minimally invasive surgical aortic valve replacement on postoperative pulmonary and skeletal muscle function. *Exp. Physiol.* **2019**, *104*, 855–865. [CrossRef]
31. Mathiowetz, V.; Kashman, N.; Volland, G.; Weber, K.; Dowe, M.; Rogers, S. Grip and pinch strength: Normative data for adults. *Arch. Phys. Med. Rehabil.* **1985**, *66*, 69–74.
32. Folstein, M.F.; Folstein, S.E.; McHugh, P.R. "Mini-mental state". A practical method for grading the cognitive state of patients for the clinician. *J. Psychiatr. Res.* **1975**, *12*, 189–198. [CrossRef]
33. Sheikh, J.I.; Yesavage, J.A. Geriatric Depression Scale (GDS): Recent evidence and development of a shorter version. *Clin. Gerontol.* **1986**, *5*, 165–173.
34. International Physical Activity Questionnaire. Available online: https://sites.google.com/site/theipaq/ (accessed on 8 April 2020).
35. Hsieh, C.Y.; Phillips, R.B. Reliability of manual muscle testing with a computerized dynamometer. *J. Manipulative Physiol. Ther.* **1990**, *13*, 72–82. [PubMed]
36. Yardley, L.; Beyer, N.; Hauer, K.; Kempen, G.; Piot-Ziegler, C.; Todd, C. Development and initial validation of the Falls Efficacy Scale-International (FES-I). *Age Ageing* **2005**, *34*, 614–619. [CrossRef]

37. Billot, M.; Calvani, R.; Urtamo, A.; Sánchez-Sánchez, J.L.; Ciccolari-Micaldi, C.; Chang, M.; Roller-Wirnsberger, R.; Wirnsberger, G.; Sinclair, A.; Vaquero-Pinto, N.; et al. Preserving mobility in older adults with physical frailty and sarcopenia: Opportunities, challenges, and recommendations for physical activity interventions. *Clin. Interv. Aging* **2020**, *15*, 1675–1690. [CrossRef] [PubMed]
38. Flint, K.M.; Stevens-Lapsley, J.; Forman, D.E. Cardiac rehabilitation in frail older adults with cardiovascular disease: A new diagnostic and treatment paradigm. *J. Cardiopulm. Rehabil. Prev.* **2020**, *40*, 72–78. [CrossRef] [PubMed]
39. Goldfarb, M.; Afilalo, J. Cardiac rehabilitation: Are we missing an important means to defrail and reverse adverse consequences of aging? *Can. J. Cardiol.* **2020**, *36*, 457–458. [CrossRef]
40. Kamiya, K.; Sato, Y.; Takahashi, T. Multidisciplinary cardiac rehabilitation and long-term prognosis in patients with heart failure. *Circ. Heart Fail.* **2020**, *13*, e006798. [CrossRef]
41. Lutz, A.H.; Delligatti, A.; Allsup, K.; Afilalo, J.; Forman, D.E. Cardiac rehabilitation is associated with improved physical function in frail older adults with cardiovascular disease. *J. Cardiopulm. Rehabil. Prev.* **2020**, *40*, 310–318. [CrossRef]
42. Aguilar-Iglesias, L.; Merino-Merino, A.; Sanchez-Corral, E.; Garcia-Sanchez, M.J.; Santos-Sanchez, I.; Saez-Maleta, R.; Perez-Rivera, J.A. Differences according to age in the diagnostic performance of cardiac biomarkers to predict frailty in patients with acute heart failure. *Biomolecules* **2022**, *12*, 245. [CrossRef]

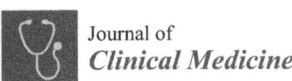

Article

Implementation of EHMRG Risk Model in an Italian Population of Elderly Patients with Acute Heart Failure

Lorenzo Falsetti [1,*], Vincenzo Zaccone [1,*], Emanuele Guerrieri [2], Giulio Perrotta [3], Ilaria Diblasi [2], Luca Giuliani [2], Linda Elena Gialluca Palma [4], Giovanna Viticchi [5], Agnese Fioranelli [6], Gianluca Moroncini [7], Adolfo Pansoni [8], Marinella Luccarini [8], Marianna Martino [6], Caterina Scalpelli [6], Maurizio Burattini [6] and Nicola Tarquinio [6]

1. Internal and Subintensive Medicine Department, Azienda Ospedaliero-Universitaria "Ospedali Riuniti" di Ancona, 60100 Ancona, Italy
2. Emergency Medicine Residency Program, Marche Polytechnic University, 60100 Ancona, Italy; e.guerrieri93@gmail.com (E.G.); ilariadiblasi@gmail.com (I.D.); luca.giuliani33@gmail.com (L.G.)
3. General and Emergency Surgical Clinic, Azienda Ospedaliero-Universitaria "Ospedali Riuniti", 60126 Ancona, Italy; info@giulioperrotta.com
4. Internal Medicine Residency Program, Marche Polytechnic University, 60126 Ancona, Italy; elena.giallucapalma@gmail.com
5. Neurologic Clinic, Marche Polytechnic University, 60126 Ancona, Italy; viticchi.g@gmail.com
6. Internal Medicine Department, INRCA-IRCCS di Osimo, 60027 Ancona, Italy; agnese.fioranelli@gmail.com (A.F.); mariannamartino88@gmail.com (M.M.); caterina.scalpelli@gmail.com (C.S.); m.burattini@inrca.it (M.B.); n.tarquinio@inrca.it (N.T.)
7. Clinica Medica, Marche Polytechnic University, 60124 Ancona, Italy; g.moroncini@univpm.it
8. Emergency Department, INRCA-IRCCS di Osimo, 60027 Ancona, Italy; a.pansoni@inrca.it (A.P.); m.luccarini@inrca.it (M.L.)
* Correspondence: lorenzo.falsetti@ospedaliriuniti.marche.it (L.F.); vincenzozaccone@libero.it (V.Z.); Tel.: +39-071-596-5269 (L.F.); +39-071-596-3565 (V.Z.)

Abstract: Acute heart failure (AHF) is a cardiac emergency with an increasing incidence, especially among elderly patients. The Emergency Heart failure Mortality Risk Grade (EHMRG) has been validated to assess the 7-days AHF mortality risk, suggesting the management of patients admitted to an emergency department (ED). EHMRG has never been implemented in Italian ED nor among elderly patients. We aimed to assess EHMRG score accuracy in predicting in-hospital death in a retrospective cohort of elderly subjects admitted for AHF from the ED to an Internal Medicine Department. We enrolled, in a 24-months timeframe, all the patients admitted to an Internal Medicine Department from ED for AHF. We calculated the EHMRG score, subdividing patients into six categories, and assessing in-hospital mortality and length of stay. We evaluated EHMRG accuracy with ROC curve analysis and survival with Kaplan–Meier and Cox models. We collected 439 subjects, with 45 in-hospital deaths (10.3%), observing a significant increase of in-hospital death along with EHMRG class, from 0% (class 1) to 7.7% (class 5b; $p < 0.0001$). EHMRG was fairly accurate in the whole cohort (AUC: 0.75; 95%CI: 0.68–0.83; $p < 0.0001$), with the best cutoff observed at >103 (Se: 71.1%; Sp: 72.8%; LR+: 2.62; LR-: 0.40; PPV: 23.0%; NPV: 95.7%), but performed better considering the events in the first seven days of admission (AUC: 0.83; 95%; CI: 0.75–0.91; $p < 0.0001$). In light of our observations, EHMRG can be useful also for the Italian emergency system to predict the risk of short-term mortality for AHF among elderly patients. EHMRG performance was better in the first seven days but remained acceptable when considering the whole period of hospitalization.

Keywords: EHMRG; acute heart failure; prognosis; emergency department

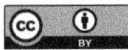

1. Introduction

Acute heart failure (AHF) represents a cardiac emergency that is often managed in the emergency departments (ED) and then treated, according to its severity and prognosis, in

ED short stay areas, internal medicine or cardiology wards, or—in the most severe cases—in subintensive or intensive care units [1]. Both de novo AHF and acutely decompensated heart failure (ADHF) are characterized by high mortality and increased hospitalization and re-hospitalization rates, which result in increased healthcare costs and significant mortality and morbidity [2,3].

Therefore, physicians involved in the decision-making process of AHF/ADHF are required to decide whether to admit, place them in short-stay or observation or directly discharge patients with AHF/ADHF. A relevant proportion of these subjects are directly discharged from ED, and this subpopulation is at the highest risk of short-term adverse events, including early re-hospitalization and death [4,5]. Physician's clinical gestalt is often adopted to assess patients' prognosis and decide the disposition, although it is widely recognized as a non-accurate method [6,7] that can lead to unnecessary hospitalizations or, on the other side, to serious adverse events related to an early discharge. Of note, there is a substantial overlap in the prognostic profiles of ED patients who are subsequently discharged or hospitalized. This phenomenon can be explained by the fact that diagnostic approaches are often not clear and linear, with the risk of admitting low-risk patients and discharging subjects with only an apparent low risk, thus increasing the risk of serious events. Therefore, several prognostic algorithms have been studied to improve AHF prognostic evaluation in the ED [8].

Several factors have been considered in AHF prognosis, and several authors suggested evaluating six fundamental dimensions in these patients: blood pressure, heart rate, heart rhythm, precipitating factors, comorbid conditions, and clinical severity [9]. Previous prognostic studies have focused on AHF/ADHF patients who have been hospitalized but have resoundingly excluded those discharged from the ED [10–13], although it should be pointed out that those discharged from the ED may be a substantial proportion of all patients with HF and may also be at significant risk of acute mortality [7]. This observation limits the use of previous hospitalization-based risk algorithms in the broader context of ED. Thus, there is no guarantee that AHF risk algorithms developed in patients already admitted will identify those who can be safely discharged from ED [14].

Most of the risk stratification tools for AHF were designed in cohorts of cardiology inpatients [10,12], therefore, not being applicable to other populations, like ED patients [15,16]. Among the others, the most adopted tools to stratify AHF prognosis in clinical practice are the OPTIMIZE-HF and the ADHERE risk scales, which were specifically designed to improve in-hospital management of patients with AHF/ADHF [17,18]. However, since the derivation and validation cohorts were used in specific clinical settings, the possibilities to extend these clinical prediction rulers (CPRs) in other clinical settings, such as in ED or Internal Medicine, and in the short-term prognosis are limited [19]. Recently, several authors proposed specific risk scores for the ED to fill this gap: among the others, the Ottawa Heart Failure Risk Scale (OHFRS), the MEESSI risk score, and the Emergency Heart Failure Mortality Risk Grade (EHMRG) are the most studied and validated scores in this setting [20–22]. EHMRG is based on commonly adopted parameters but is very complex to calculate without a smartphone app and can only predict mortality, while the other CPRs are usually simpler to calculate but adopt some parameters that are more difficult to collect during the primary assessment of a critical patient [20,22].

EHMRG was originally engineered and validated in Canada, then validated in other countries, such as Spain, showing similar performances [23]. Italian patients are often older and less burdened by atherosclerosis than American populations, while they are more clinically and socially similar to Spanish subjects. However, a study on the implementation of this score in the Italian sanitary system and in the Italian geriatric population is missing. With this paper, we aimed to assess the efficacy of EHMRG score in predicting in-hospital death in a cohort of elderly Italian subjects admitted for AHF in the ED.

2. Materials and Methods

Background: Methods of this study have already been described elsewhere [24]. The INRCA-IRCSS (National Institute for Care and Research in Aging, Ancona, Italy) Hospital of Osimo (Ancona, Italy) is a primary hospital specializing in the acute care of elderly subjects. Regarding AHF/ADHF, patients admitted to the ED can directly access the Internal Medicine department. However, AHF associated with other acute conditions (STE/NSTE myocardial infarction requiring revascularization, brady- or tachyarrhythmias requiring pacing or other device therapy, acute valvular and cardiac diseases requiring cardiac surgery, or severe associated critical illnesses, such as pulmonary embolism, septic or cardiogenic shock that require admission to intensive care unit) are directly sent or to the cardiac care unit of the same institute or to a tertiary-care hospital after pre-hospital or ED evaluation. As such, very-high risk patients are not present in this sample, which mainly includes subjects affected by ADHF or de novo AHF due to medical conditions, such as arrhythmias, hypertensive crises, and other causes. ADHF/AHF was diagnosed by the attending physician according to the ESC 2016 guidelines that were current at the moment of the study [25].

Ethical Issues: This study was authorized on 6 May 2021 by the INRCA-IRCSS Ethical Committee (CE INRCA, protocol n° 21011/21-CE) and then approved by INRCA Hospital (protocol n° 193, 26 May 2021). All patients gave their informed consent and were treated according to the guidelines current at the time of the study. We followed the Declaration of Helsinki Ethical Principles for Medical Research Involving Human Subjects.

Enrolment, Inclusion, and Exclusion Criteria: In a 24-months timeframe (1 January 2018–30 December 2019), we retrospectively enrolled all the patients aged 60 or more years and assessed in the ED, and then admitted to the Internal Medicine Department with ADHF/AHF diagnosis. We adopted the same exclusion criteria of the original EHMRG study [22]: (i) transfer from another department (ICU, Cardiology, Pneumology) or direct admission from the heart failure ward, (ii) patients in end-of-life care due to active cancer or other terminal comorbidities, (iii) dialysis-dependent subjects. We also excluded patients with incomplete data that did not allow us to correctly calculate the EHMRG score.

Data Collection: We gathered history and vital signs at the ED arrival. For each patient, we collected: age, modality of ED transport, systolic blood pressure (SBP), heart rate (HR), oxygen saturation (SpO2), serum creatinine, serum potassium, serum troponin, presence of active cancer, and metolazone use at home. From these items, we calculated the absolute EHMRG score according to its original definition, as shown in Table 1, and then recategorized the subjects into the six EHMRG categories (Class 1: −49.1; Class 2: from −49.0 to −15.9; Class 3: from −15.8 to 17.9; Class 4: from 18.0 to 56.5; Class 5a: from 56.6 to 89.3; Class 5b: 89.4). Last, we evaluated the length of admission and in-hospital mortality.

Statistical Analysis: We presented continuous variables with normal distribution as mean and standard deviation (SD) and compared them with a t-test for independent variables. We synthesized non-normally distributed variables with median and interquartile range [IQR], adopting the Mann–Whitney U test. We presented categorical variables as absolute number and percent, comparing them with the chi-squared test. We evaluated the EHMRG accuracy for in-hospital death with ROC curve analysis, considering both the events (discharge or in-hospital mortality) during the whole time of observation and the events observed in the first seven days. We identified the best cutoff point with a critical ROC curve assessment and adopted the Youden Index. We performed a univariate test to select covariates, choosing the ones associated with the outcome of interest at a level of $p < 0.10$ and excluding the items already considered in the EHMRG score to avoid multi-collinearity. Last, we performed a Cox multivariate model considering days of admission as the time variable, in-hospital death as the event variable, EHMRG category as the main predictor, and the covariates selected by univariate test, both in the full sample and in the seven days sample. We considered as significant all the differences at a level of $p < 0.05$. We performed the analysis with SPSS 13.0 for Windows Systems (SPSS Inc., Chicago, IL, USA).

Table 1. EHMRG Score.

Variable	Units	Factor
Age	Years	2 × age
ED arrival by ambulance	If "yes"	+60
SBP	mmHg	−1 × SBP
Heart rate	beats/min	1 × HR
Oxygen saturation	%	−2 × Oxygen Saturation
Creatinine	mg/dL	20 × Creatinine
Serum potassium	• 4.0–4.5 mmol/L • ≥4.6 mmol/L • ≤3.9 mmol/L	• 0 • +30 • +5
Serum troponin	>ULN	+60
Active cancer	If "yes"	+45
Metolazone at home	If "yes"	+60
Adjustment factor		+12
Total		

Legend: EHMRG = Emergency Heart Failure Mortality Risk Grade; ED = emergency department; SBP = systolic blood pressure; ULN = upper limit of normal.

3. Results

We obtained a cohort of 439 subjects with 45 (10.3%) deaths. Baseline characteristics of the full cohort and of the events observed at seven days are synthesized in Table 2, while differences between surviving and non-surviving subjects are shown in the Supplementary Materials (Table S1).

Table 2. Baseline characteristics of the sample.

Clinical Variables	Full Cohort (n = 439)	7 Days (n = 138)
Age, years, (±SD)	84.6 (±7.7)	84.1 (± 8.3)
Males (n, %)	180 (41.0%)	64 (46.4%)
In-hospital death (n, %)	45 (10.3%)	22 (15.9%)
NYHA class, [IQR]	4 [1]	3 [1]
Length of hospitalization, days, [IQR]	10 [7]	-
BNP on admission, pg/mL, [IQR]	600.5 [805]	560.5 [846]
SBP, mmHg, (±SD)	127.5 (±28.1)	128.0 (±28.2)
HR, bpm, (±SD)	89.4 (±24.6)	90.4 (±23.9)
SpO2, %, (±SD)	91.8 (±7.3)	92.0 (±7.07)
Creatinine, mg/dl, (±SD)	1.6 (±1.0)	1.45 (±0.99)
Potassium, mmol/l, (±SD)	4.00 (±0.69)	4.04 (±0.65)
Out of range Potassium, (n, %)	180 (41.1%)	74 (53.6%)
Troponin, ng/mL, [IQR]	0.05 [0.10]	0.05 [0.11]
Increased troponin, (n, %)	204 (46.5%)	63 (45.7%)
ED arrival by ambulance, (n, %)	284 (64.7%)	83 (60.1%)
Active cancer, (n, %)	77 (17.9%)	16 (11.6%)
Metolazone use, (n, %)	11 (2.6%)	1 (0.72%)

Table 2. Cont.

Clinical Variables	Full Cohort (n = 439)	7 Days (n = 138)
EHMRG, [IQR]	69 [98.4]	60,8 [99.3]
EHMRG Class, [IQR]	5 [2]	5 [3]
AHF characteristics		
ADHF (n, %)	370 (84.2%)	109 (78.9%)
AHF de novo (n, %)		
• Arrhythmia	• 36 (8.20%)	• 11 (7.97%)
• Hypertensive crisis	• 21 (4.78%)	• 12 (8.69%)
• Other	• 12 (2.73%)	• 6 (4.34%)

Legend: AHF = acute heart failure; ADHF = acutely decompensated heart failure; BNP = brain-derived natriuretic peptide; EHMRG = Emergency Heart Failure Mortality Risk Grade; HR = heart rate; IQR = interquartile range; SBP = systolic blood pressure; NYHA = New York Heart Academy; SD = standard deviation; SpO2 = oxygen saturation.

EHMRG predicted with fair accuracy in-hospital death in the whole cohort when treated as continuous (AUC: 0.754; 95%CI: 0.68–0.83; $p < 0.0001$) and categorial (AUC: 0.727; 95%CI: 0.66–0.80; $p < 0.0001$), as shown in Figure 1A.

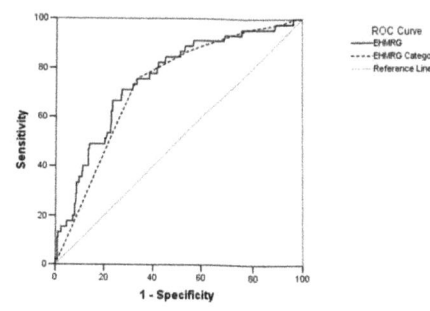
(A) Whole sample (n = 439)

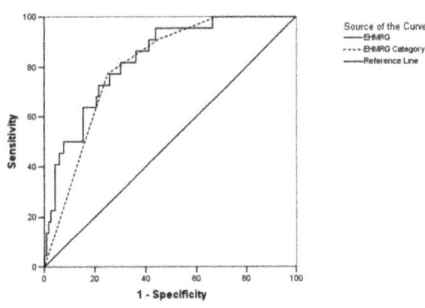
(B) 7-days (n = 138)

Figure 1. ROC curve analysis of continuous and categorial EHMRG for in-hospital death (panel (A): whole sample; panel (B): first 7 days of admission).

Analyzing the ROC curve drawn from the continuous EHMRG variable, we observed, at the optimal cutoff of 103, a sensitivity of 71.1% (95%CI: 55.7–83.6%), a specificity of 72.8% (95%CI: 68.2–77.2%), a positive likelihood ratio of 2.62 (95%CI: 2.0–3.4), a negative likelihood ratio of 0.40 (95%CI: 0.2–0.6), a positive predictive value of 23.0% (95%CI: 16.3–30.9%), a negative predictive value of 95.7% (92.7–97.7%). On the other hand, analyzing the ROC curve drawn from the categorial EHMRG variable, we observed, at the optimal cutoff of 3, a sensitivity of 95.6% (95%CI: 84.9–99.5%), a specificity of 22.1% (95%CI: 18.1–26.5%), a positive likelihood ratio of 1.23 (95%CI: 1.1–1.3), a negative likelihood ratio of 0.20 (95%CI: 0.05–0.8), a positive predictive value of 12.3% (95%CI: 9.0–16.2%), a negative predictive value of 97.8% (95%CI: 92.1–99.7%), which was comparable to the one observed in the original cohort. Prevalence of in-hospital death increased significantly across EHMRG categories, ranging from 0% in the first to 7.7% in the last category, as shown in Table 3 and in the Supplementary Materials (Figure S1, Panel A).

Table 3. Distribution of in-hospital death according to EHMRG score ($p < 0.0001$).

EHMRG Category In-Hospital Death	Full Sample ($n = 439$)	7-Days Observation ($n = 138$)
EHMRG Category 1 (n, %)	0 (0.0%)	0 (0.0%)
EHMRG Category 2 (n, %)	1 (0.2%)	0 (0.0%)
EHMRG Category 3 (n, %)	1 (0.2%)	0 (0.0%)
EHMRG Category 4 (n, %)	4 (4.1%)	2 (1.4%)
EHMRG Category 5a (n, %)	5 (1.1%)	3 (2.2%)
EHMRG Category 5b (n, %)	34 (7.7%)	17 (12.3%)
Total	45 (10.3%)	22 (15.9%)

Legend: EHMRG = Emergency Heart Failure Mortality Risk Grade.

When reducing the observation period to the events of the first seven days (138 patients, 22 in-hospital deaths), EHMRG accuracy significantly increased for both continuous (AUC: 0.83; 95%CI: 0.75–0.91; $p < 0.0001$) and categorial (AUC: 0.80; 95%CI: 0.72–0.89; $p < 0.0001$) variables, as shown in Figure 1B. According to these results, the optimal cut-off was 4, holding a sensitivity of 90.9% (70.8–98.9%), a specificity of 55.2% (45.7–64.4%), a positive likelihood ratio of 2.03 (95%CI: 1.6–2.6), a negative likelihood ratio of 0.16 (95%CI: 0.04–0.6), a positive predictive value of 27.8% (95%CI: 17.8–39.7%) and a negative predictive value of 97.0% (95%CI: 89.5–99.6%), which was comparable to the one observed in the original cohort. Prevalence of in-hospital death increased significantly across EHMRG categories, ranging from 0% in the first to 12.3% in the last category: in this subgroup, the distribution of deaths was even more shifted towards higher EHMRG categories, with a significant difference in the distribution ($p < 0.0001$), as synthesized in Table 3 and in the Supplementary Materials (Figure S1, Panel B).

We observed in the univariate analysis that EHMRG class, NYHA category, BNP at the admission, and sex were associated with in-hospital death, thus, we maintained these variables in the final multivariate model. We did not include the other collected variables from the multivariate model since they were already considered in the EHMRG score: adding these features could have increased the risk of multicollinearity and the overinflation of the model. Cox regression analysis underlined that both in the whole cohort and in the seven-day events cohort, a one-unit increase in EHMRG category was associated with an increased hazard ratio (HR) of in-hospital death (HR: 2.85; 95%CI: 1.64–4.98; $p < 0.0001$). Furthermore, NYHA class was associated with an increased HR (HR: 2.84; 95%CI: 1.78–4.54; $p < 0.0001$), while BNP at the admission and sex became non-significant in the multivariate analysis. The full model is shown in the Supplementary Materials (Table S2, Panel A). Considering the events in the first seven days, we observed similar results, as shown in the Supplementary Materials (Table S2, Panel B).

4. Discussion

The EHMRG score has among its main strengths, the ease of use and the limited number of items required for the calculation that makes this CPR ideal for use in an Emergency Department. Particularly, EHMRG can be calculated only by vital parameters and data retrieved from the first contact between the patient and the triage nurse, and laboratory exams that are measured virtually in all the ED patients. However, despite its usability, its accuracy should be assessed, especially when translated to populations or emergency systems that differ from the original cohort, like all the clinical scores [24,26,27].

Our population varied from the original one [22] for a significantly older age (75.4 ± 11.4 years in the original cohort versus 84.6 ± 7.7 years in our cohort), a different pattern of comorbidities, and a different sanitary system. Despite these differences, EHMRG maintained a similar accuracy in predicting in-hospital death in the first seven days (original cohort AUC: 0.81; 95%CI: 0.77–0.85; this cohort AUC: 0.83; 95%CI: 0.75–0.91). Our sample had characteristics similar to a recently published Spanish cohort [23], however, the accuracy was probably different for the different populations considered (ED patients in the Spanish cohort, ED subjects admitted to Internal Medicine in this sample), and the inclusion in that cohort of palliative patients.

When we extended the observation to the whole observation period, which was longer than the original one, we observed that EHMRG maintained a fair accuracy (AUC: 0.75; 95%CI: 0.68–0.83), suggesting the potential use of this score both for the ED and the Internal Medicine specialist.

However, at its best cutoffs (>103 in the continuous variable and >3 in the categorical variable), EHMRG showed a remarkable capacity to identify subjects at low risk of short-term events. According to our data, EHMRG accuracy in predicting death peaked when considering the events observed in the first seven days, which is the original timeframe for which EHMRG was designed to predict mortality. In this short period, EHMRG accuracy improved, as underlined by a significant AUC increase, from 75 to 83%, which is similar to the accuracy observed in the original and in the validation cohorts [22,23]. However, the most important datum in all the ROC curve analyses performed is the negative likelihood ratio, which was 0.20 when considering the whole cohort and 0.16 in the first seven days, underlining an important capacity of this score in excluding the events, best if in the very short-term. Moreover, the negative predictive values observed in this cohort are similar to the ones observed in the original derivation and validation cohort. The capacity of EHMRG in identifying very low-risk subjects seems to be especially useful in the ED, where the physician needs to accurately identify patients that will not undergo complications after an early discharge. On the other side, the capability of identifying low-risk subjects even after the strict seven days can be useful both for the ED physician to choose the best care setting, thus optimizing economic resources, and for the Internal Medicine specialist, who could be able to assess the short-term prognosis even during the admission to choose the most appropriate follow-up.

This study has its strengths: the population under exam comprises most of the patients admitted in our ED since the internal protocols, in the presence of a very small, short-stay area, did not allow to directly discharge the AHF patients. All the patients were followed up during the admission to Internal Medicine, and this is another important point since there were no patients lost after the ED disposition.

Limitations: the current study's main limitation is related to its retrospective nature and the relatively small sample size. Multicentric, prospective studies with larger samples are necessary to obtain more reliable results in the same population. Moreover, to further reduce the risk of bias, it would be important to perform these studies by enrolling the subjects directly in the ED and following them up independently of their destination (discharge, short-stay, regular or subintensive ward), which could be, however, very difficult for the actual organization of the regional sanitary system, which allocates patients with different degrees of severity in different hospitals and departments. Another point is related to the lack of follow-up after discharge, which could be useful for assessing the early readmission rates. This point could represent a potential implementation for future studies assessing not only in-hospital mortality but also early readmissions rates: in fact, this composite outcome could be a more reliable marker of therapeutic failure in these patients. Last, this score does not suggest different therapeutic management during the in-hospital stay: a potential implementation for future studies could be to assess whether a different treatment according to this stratification could translate into better clinical outcomes.

5. Conclusions

The implementation of the EHMRG score can be useful to assess short-term prognosis in elderly patients with AHF evaluated in the ED and then managed in Internal Medicine in the Italian geriatric population. This score, however, seems to be more important to rule-out short-term mortality than to rule-in events, especially in lower-risk classes.

Supplementary Materials: The following supporting information can be downloaded at: https://www.mdpi.com/article/10.3390/jcm11112982/s1, Table S1: Differences between surviving and non-surviving patients; Table S2: Cox regression analysis; Figure S1: Cumulative percentage of in-hospital deaths according to EHMRG categories ($p < 0.0001$).

Author Contributions: Conceptualization, L.F., V.Z. and N.T.; methodology: L.F., V.Z., E.G., G.M., M.B. and N.T.; software: L.F.; validation: L.F., V.Z., A.F., G.V., M.B. and N.T.; formal analysis: L.F., V.Z. and N.T.; investigation: L.F., V.Z., E.G., G.P., I.D., L.G., L.E.G.P., G.V., A.P., M.L., M.M., C.S., M.B. and N.T.; resources: A.P., M.L., M.M., C.S., M.B. and N.T.; data curation: L.F., N.T., M.M., C.S. and E.G.; writing–original draft preparation: L.F., E.G., G.P., I.D., L.G., L.E.G.P., G.V., A.F., G.M., A.P., M.L., M.M., C.S., M.B. and N.T.; writing—review and editing: L.F., E.G., G.P., I.D., L.G., L.E.G.P., G.V., A.F., G.M., A.P., M.L., M.M., C.S., M.B. and N.T.; supervision: G.M., A.P. and M.B. All authors have read and agreed to the published version of the manuscript.

Funding: This research received no external funding.

Institutional Review Board Statement: This study was authorized on 6 May 2021 by the INRCA-IRCSS Ethical Committee (CE INRCA, protocol n° 21011/21-CE) and then approved by INRCA Hospital (protocol n° 193, 26 May 2021).

Informed Consent Statement: All patients gave their informed consent and were treated according to the guidelines current at the time of the study. We followed the Declaration of Helsinki Ethical Principles for Medical Research Involving Human Subjects.

Data Availability Statement: The data presented in this study are available on request from the corresponding author. The data are not publicly available due to privacy issues.

Conflicts of Interest: The authors declare no conflict of interest.

References

1. McDonagh, T.A.; Metra, M.; Adamo, M.; Gardner, R.S.; Baumbach, A.; Böhm, M.; Burri, H.; Butler, J.; Čelutkienė, J.; Chioncel, O.; et al. 2021 ESC Guidelines for the diagnosis and treatment of acute and chronic heart failure. *Eur. Heart J.* **2021**, *42*, 3599–3726. [CrossRef] [PubMed]
2. Jencks, S.F.; Williams, M.V.; Coleman, E.A. Rehospitalizations among Patients in the Medicare Fee-for-Service Program. *N. Engl. J. Med.* **2009**, *360*, 1418–1428. [CrossRef] [PubMed]
3. Sanderson, J.E.; Tse, T. Heart failure: A global disease requiring a global response. *Heart* **2003**, *89*, 585–586. [CrossRef] [PubMed]
4. Collins, S.P.; Schauer, D.P.; Gupta, A.; Brunner, H.; Storrow, A.B.; Eckman, M.H. Cost-effectiveness analysis of ED decision making in patients with non-high-risk heart failure. *Am. J. Emerg. Med.* **2009**, *27*, 293–302. [CrossRef] [PubMed]
5. Ezekowitz, J.A.; Bakal, J.A.; Kaul, P.; Westerhout, C.M.; Armstrong, P.W. Acute heart failure in the emergency department: Short and long-term outcomes of elderly patients with heart failure. *Eur. J. Heart Fail.* **2008**, *10*, 308–314. [CrossRef]
6. Butler, J.; Hanumanthu, S.; Chomsky, D.; Wilson, J.R. Frequency of low-risk hospital admissions for heart failure. *Am. J. Cardiol.* **1998**, *81*, 41–44. [CrossRef]
7. Lee, D.S.; Schull, M.J.; Alter, D.A.; Austin, P.C.; Laupacis, A.; Chong, A.; Tu, J.V.; Stukel, T.A. Early deaths in patients with heart failure discharged from the emergency department: A population-based analysis. *Circ. Heart Fail.* **2010**, *3*, 228–235. [CrossRef]
8. Peacock, W.F.; Braunwald, E.; Abraham, W.; Albert, N.; Burnett, J.; Christenson, R.; Collins, S.; Diercks, D.; Fonarow, G.; Hollander, J.; et al. National Heart, Lung, and Blood Institute working group on emergency department management of acute heart failure: Research challenges and opportunities. *J. Am. Coll. Cardiol.* **2010**, *56*, 343–351. [CrossRef]
9. Gheorghiade, M.; Braunwald, E. A proposed model for initial assessment and management of acute heart failure syndromes. *JAMA* **2011**, *305*, 1702–1703. [CrossRef]
10. Fonarow, G.C.; Adams, K.F.; Abraham, W.T.; Yancy, C.W.; Boscardin, W.J.; ADHERE Scientific Advisory Committee, Study Group and Investigators. Risk stratification for in-hospital mortality in acutely decompensated heart failure: Classification and regression tree analysis. *JAMA* **2005**, *293*, 572–580. [CrossRef]
11. Chin, M.H.; Goldman, L. Correlates of major complications or death in patients admitted to the hospital with congestive heart failure. *Arch. Intern. Med.* **1996**, *156*, 1814–1820. [CrossRef] [PubMed]
12. Auble, T.E.; Hsieh, M.; Gardner, W.; Cooper, G.F.; Stone, R.A.; McCausland, J.B.; Yealy, D.M. A prediction rule to identify low-risk patients with heart failure. *Acad. Emerg. Med.* **2005**, *12*, 514–521. [CrossRef] [PubMed]
13. Lee, D.S.; Austin, P.C.; Rouleau, J.L.; Liu, P.P.; Naimark, D.; Tu, J.V. Predicting mortality among patients hospitalized for heart failure: Derivation and validation of a clinical model. *JAMA* **2003**, *290*, 2581–2587. [CrossRef] [PubMed]
14. Justice, A.C.; Covinsky, K.E.; Berlin, J.A. Assessing the generalizability of prognostic information. *Ann. Intern. Med.* **1999**, *130*, 515–524. [CrossRef]

15. Furlan, L.; Gianni, F.; Costantino, G. Prediction tools in clinical practice: Carefully read instructions before use. *Eur. J. Intern. Med.* **2022**, *98*, 37–38. [CrossRef]
16. Adams, S.T.; Leveson, S.H. Clinical prediction rules. *Bmj* **2012**, *344*, d8312. [CrossRef]
17. Fonarow, G.C.; Abraham, W.T.; Albert, N.M.; Gattis, W.A.; Gheorghiade, M.; Greenberg, B.; O'Connor, C.M.; Yancy, C.W.; Young, J. Organized Program to Initiate Lifesaving Treatment in Hospitalized Patients with Heart Failure (OPTIMIZE-HF): Rationale and design. *Am. Heart J.* **2004**, *148*, 43–51. [CrossRef]
18. Fonarow, G.C.; ADHERE Scientific Advisory Committee. The Acute Decompensated Heart Failure National Registry (ADHERE): Opportunities to improve care of patients hospitalized with acute decompensated heart failure. *Rev. Cardiovasc. Med.* **2003**, *4* (Suppl. S7), S21–S30. [PubMed]
19. Win, S.; Hussain, I.; Hebl, V.B.; Dunlay, S.M.; Redfield, M.M. Inpatient Mortality Risk Scores and Postdischarge Events in Hospitalized Heart Failure Patients. *Circ. Heart Fail.* **2017**, *10*, e003926. [CrossRef]
20. Stiell, I.G.; Clement, C.M.; Brison, R.J.; Rowe, B.H.; Borgundvaag, B.; Aaron, S.D.; Lang, E.; Calder, L.A.; Perry, J.J.; Forster, A.J.; et al. A risk scoring system to identify emergency department patients with heart failure at high risk for serious adverse events. *Acad. Emerg. Med.* **2013**, *20*, 17–26. [CrossRef]
21. Miró, Ò.; Rosselló, X.; Gil, V.; Martín-Sánchez, F.J.; Llorens, P.; Herrero, P.; Jacob, J.; López-Grima, M.L.; Gil, C.; Lucas Imbernón, F.J.; et al. The Usefulness of the MEESSI Score for Risk Stratification of Patients With Acute Heart Failure at the Emergency Department. *Rev. Española Cardiol. (Engl. Ed.)* **2019**, *72*, 198–207. [CrossRef]
22. Lee, D.S.; Stitt, A.; Austin, P.C.; Stukel, T.A.; Schull, M.J.; Chong, A.; Newton, G.E.; Lee, J.S.; Tu, J.V. Prediction of heart failure mortality in emergent care: A cohort study. *Ann. Intern. Med.* **2012**, *156*, 767–775. [CrossRef] [PubMed]
23. Gil, V.; Miró, Ò.; Schull, M.J.; Llorens, P.; Herrero-Puente, P.; Jacob, J.; Ríos, J.; Lee, D.S.; Martín-Sánchez, F.J. Emergency Heart Failure Mortality Risk Grade score performance for 7-day mortality prediction in patients with heart failure attended at the emergency department: Validation in a Spanish cohort. *Eur. J. Emerg. Med.* **2018**, *25*, 169–177. [CrossRef]
24. Falsetti, L.; Zaccone, V.; Viticchi, G.; Fioranelli, A.; Diblasi, I.; Guerrieri, E.; Ferrini, C.; Scarponi, M.; Giuliani, L.; Scalpelli, C.; et al. Improving the EHMRG Prognostic Evaluation of Acute Heart Failure with TAPSE/PASp: A Sequential Approach. *Diagnostics* **2022**, *12*, 478. [CrossRef]
25. Ponikowski, P.; Voors, A.A.; Anker, S.D.; Bueno, H.; Cleland, J.G.F.; Coats, A.J.S.; Falk, V.; González-Juanatey, J.R.; Harjola, V.-P.; Jankowska, E.A.; et al. 2016 ESC Guidelines for the diagnosis and treatment of acute and chronic heart failure. *Eur. Heart J.* **2016**, *37*, 2129–2200. [CrossRef] [PubMed]
26. Falsetti, L.; Proietti, M.; Zaccone, V.; Guerra, F.; Nitti, C.; Salvi, A.; Viticchi, G.; Riccomi, F.; Sampaolesi, M.; Silvestrini, M.; et al. Impact of atrial fibrillation in critically-ill patients admitted to a stepdown unit. *Eur. J. Clin. Investig.* **2020**, *50*, e13317. [CrossRef]
27. Falsetti, L.; Rucco, M.; Proietti, M.; Viticchi, G.; Zaccone, V.; Scarponi, M.; Giovenali, L.; Moroncini, G.; Nitti, C.; Salvi, A. Risk prediction of clinical adverse outcomes with machine learning in a cohort of critically ill patients with atrial fibrillation. *Sci. Rep.* **2021**, *11*, 18925. [CrossRef]

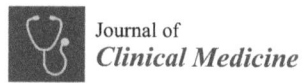

Article

Quality of Life in Older Patients after a Heart Failure Hospitalization: Results from the SENECOR Study

Daniele Luiso [1,2], Marta Herrero-Torrus [3], Neus Badosa [1,4], Cristina Roqueta [2,3], Sonia Ruiz-Bustillo [1,4,5], Laia C. Belarte-Tornero [1,4], Sandra Valdivielso-Moré [1,4], Ronald O. Morales [1], Olga Vázquez [3] and Núria Farré [1,2,4,*]

[1] Heart Failure Unit, Cardiology Department, Hospital del Mar, 08003 Barcelona, Spain; d.luiso@gmail.com (D.L.); nbadosa@psmar.cat (N.B.); sruiz@psmar.cat (S.R.-B.); lbelarte@psmar.cat (L.C.B.-T.); svaldivielso@psmar.cat (S.V.-M.); romoralesmurillo@psmar.cat (R.O.M.)
[2] Department of Medicine, Universitat Autónoma de Barcelona, 08193 Barcelona, Spain; croqueta@psmar.cat
[3] Geriatrics Department, Hospital del Mar, 08003 Barcelona, Spain; mherrero@psmar.cat (M.H.-T.); ovazquez@psmar.cat (O.V.)
[4] Biomedical Research Group on Heart Disease, Hospital del Mar Medical Research Group (IMIM), 08003 Barcelona, Spain
[5] Department of Medicine, Universidad Pompeu Fabra, 08002 Barcelona, Spain
* Correspondence: nfarrelopez@psmar.cat

Citation: Luiso, D.; Herrero-Torrus, M.; Badosa, N.; Roqueta, C.; Ruiz-Bustillo, S.; Belarte-Tornero, L.C.; Valdivielso-Moré, S.; Morales, R.O.; Vázquez, O.; Farré, N. Quality of Life in Older Patients after a Heart Failure Hospitalization: Results from the SENECOR Study. *J. Clin. Med.* **2022**, *11*, 3035. https://doi.org/10.3390/jcm11113035

Academic Editors: Claudio Montalto, Nuccia Morici, Aung Myat and Alberto Domínguez-Rodríguez

Received: 25 April 2022
Accepted: 26 May 2022
Published: 27 May 2022

Publisher's Note: MDPI stays neutral with regard to jurisdictional claims in published maps and institutional affiliations.

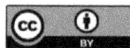

Copyright: © 2022 by the authors. Licensee MDPI, Basel, Switzerland. This article is an open access article distributed under the terms and conditions of the Creative Commons Attribution (CC BY) license (https://creativecommons.org/licenses/by/4.0/).

Abstract: Background: Information about health-related quality of life (HRQoL) in heart failure (HF) in older adults is scarce. Methods: We aimed to describe the HRQoL of the SENECOR study cohort, a single-center, randomized trial comparing the effects of multidisciplinary intervention by a geriatrician and a cardiologist (intervention group) to that of a cardiologist alone (control group) in older patients with a recent HF hospitalization. Results: HRQoL was assessed by the short version of the disease-specific Kansas Cardiomyopathy Questionnaire (KCCQ-12) in 141 patients at baseline and was impaired (KCCQ-12 < 75) in almost half of the cohort. Women comprised 50% of the population, the mean age was 82.2 years, and two-thirds of patients had preserved ejection fraction. Comorbidities were highly prevalent. Patients with impaired HRQoL had a worse NYHA functional class, a lower NT-proBNP, a lower Barthel index, and a higher Clinical Frailty Scale. One-year all-cause mortality was 22.7%, significantly lower in the group with good-to-excellent HRQoL (14.5% vs. 30.6%; hazard ratio 0.28; 95% confidence interval 0.10–0.78; $p = 0.014$). In the group with better HRQoL, all-cause hospitalization was lower, and there was a trend towards lower HF hospitalization. Conclusions: The KCCQ-12 questionnaire can provide inexpensive prognostic information even in older patients with HF. (Funded by grant Primitivo de la Vega, Fundación MAPFRE. ClinicalTrials number, NCT03555318).

Keywords: quality of life; heart failure; older patients; prognosis

1. Introduction

Heart failure (HF) is one of Western society's major public health problems. The epidemiological dimension of HF, its clinical complexity, the impact on patients' quality of life, and the burden it represents for a health system with finite resources [1] make this syndrome one of the greatest health, organizational, and economic challenges of the present day.

The clinical practice guidelines of the European Society of Cardiology [2] establish that the main goals of the treatment of patients with HF are to improve quality of life, reduce mortality, and reduce hospitalizations. Classically, the efficacy endpoint used to evaluate new therapies in HF is to reduce mortality. On the one hand, mortality has the advantage that it is a strong and an easy-to-measure event. On the other hand, it has an important disadvantage: being the final manifestation of the disease, it does not represent the clinical course until the fatal outcome, or the evolution of those patients who do not die [3]. Thus, considering that HF is a chronic and progressive disease with florid symptoms and significant repercussions on functionalism, an ideal efficacy endpoint should reflect both the symptoms and the patient's subjective perception of their health status [3–6]. In this way, assessing health-related quality of life (HRQoL) as an efficacy endpoint in HF is crucial. It provides precious information on both the patients who survive and those who die. It has been shown that HRQoL in HF correlates well with both disease severity and mortality and allows cost-effectiveness evaluations when implementing new therapeutic options [7,8]. The measurement of HRQoL is easy and inexpensive since it is carried out through questionnaires that can be generic or specific to the disease. HRQoL is a multidimensional concept that includes four fundamental aspects: physical, psychological, social, and functional status. The multidimensional nature of HRQoL allows for capturing a complete perspective of the patient. The impairment of HRQoL in HF is reflected, above all, in the functional dimension, with particular repercussions in the domains that inform about mobility and activities of daily living [9].

Information on HRQoL in HF in older adults is scarce. Most of the data reported in the literature on HRQoL in HF come from studies that include non-older patients and patients with reduced left ventricular ejection fraction (LVEF) [8,10–15]. Describing HRQoL and its correlation with prognosis in older people with HF could provide valuable clinical information, since the improvement in HRQoL in this population could have an even higher value than a reduction in mortality, both for patients and health professionals [16].

2. Materials and Methods

2.1. Study Design

The SENECOR study was a single-center, randomized trial comparing the effects of multidisciplinary intervention by a geriatrician and a cardiologist (intervention group) to that of a cardiologist alone (control group) in older patients with a recent HF hospitalization. The primary endpoint for the trial was all-cause hospitalization. Quality-of-life assessment was a pre-specified secondary endpoint of the SENECOR study. The Ethics Committee approved the study (number 2017/7653/I) and all patients signed written informed consent forms. The details of the study design and results have been published [17] and the trial is registered with ClinicalTrials.gov (NCT03555318). Briefly, patients 75 years or older and hospitalized due to HF were randomized to a follow-up performed by a cardiologist (usual care) or by a cardiologist and a geriatrician. All patients were assessed with the Canadian Study of Health and Aging (CSHA) Clinical Frailty Scale during hospitalization [18]. Frailty was defined as a CSHA equal to or higher than 4. Functional status was assessed with the Lawton [19] and Barthel index [20] and cognitive status with the Spanish version of the Pfeiffer Questionnaire (Short Portable Mental Status Questionnaire (SPMSQ)) [21]. The 12-item Kansas City Cardiomyopathy Questionnaire (KCCQ-12) was used to assess HRQoL specifically related to HF [22]. The functional class was evaluated by the New York Heart Association (NYHA) classification. In patients randomized to the intervention group, the geriatrician assessed the social sphere with the Gijón socio-family assessment scale (abbreviated and modified) (Barcelona version) [23], the emotional sphere with the Geriatric Depression Scale Short Form (GDS-SF) Yesavage [24], nutritional status with the Mini Nutritional Assessment Short Form (MNA-SF) [25] and plasma albumin, and the presence of geriatric syndromes. After the geriatrician assessment and depending on the patient's needs, up to eighteen interdisciplinary interventions were carried out in each area evaluated. The study showed that the multidisciplinary intervention by the cardiologist and geriatrician was associated with a decrease in all-cause hospitalization at one-year follow-up (62.7% in the intervention group and 77.3% in the control group) (hazard ratio 0.67; 95% confidence interval 0.46–0.99; $p = 0.046$) [17].

In the SENECOR study, the calculated sample size to detect a statistically significant difference between the two groups was 114 patients in the intervention group and 114 patients in the control group for 1 year [17]. However, patients with exclusion criteria or who refused to participate were higher than expected, and the estimated patient goal was not reached. On the other hand, the number of events was much higher than anticipated. Of the 150 patients who were finally included in the SENECOR study, we only included in the present study patients who had answered the KCCQ-12 at baseline, leaving a sample size of 141 patients (Figure 1).

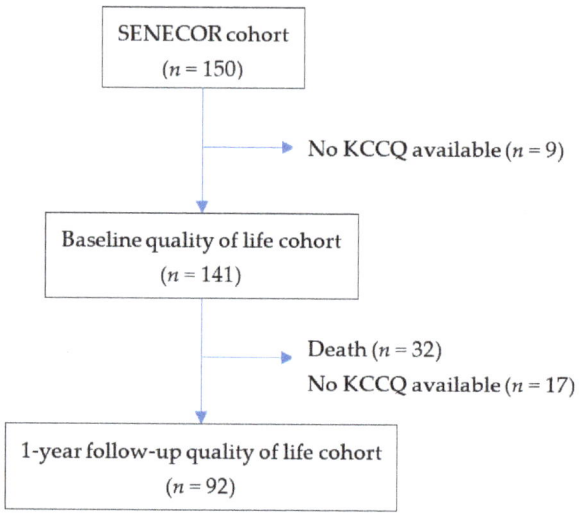

Figure 1. Flow diagram of the study.

2.2. Quality-of-Life Assessment

The KCCQ-12 is the short version (12-item) of the Kansas City Cardiomyopathy Questionnaire (KCCQ) (23-item). This self-administered test measures symptoms, physical and social limitations, and quality of life in patients with HF. It has been validated in HF both with reduced and preserved ejection fractions [8,26]. Moreover, it has proven to be both reproducible and sensitive to important changes in HF health status [26–29]. The shorter version has shown to be more feasible to implement while preserving the psychometric properties of the full instrument [22]. Scores for each domain are summarized by the KCCQ summary score, which has values between 0 and 100, with higher scores indicating better HF-specific health status. An increase of fewer than 5 points is considered a small clinical change [28]. Several studies have established a KCCQ-12 cut-off point of 75 or higher to identify patients with good-to-excellent HRQoL [30]. Therefore, we considered HRQoL impaired if KCCQ-12 was below 75. In the SENECOR study, KCCQ-12 was measured during the baseline visit. At one-year follow-up, all the baseline assessments including KCCQ-12 were repeated in those who survived.

2.3. Study Outcome

The main aim was to evaluate whether a good-to-excellent HRQoL was associated with lower all-cause mortality at one-year follow-up.

The secondary objectives were to evaluate whether a good-to-excellent HRQoL was associated with lower all-cause hospitalization and HF hospitalization at one-year follow-up and evaluate the extent of change in the KCCQ-12 scores at one-year follow-up.

2.4. Statistical Analysis

Mean and standard deviation were used to describe continuous variables, and numbers and proportions to describe the categorical variables. The chi-square test or Fisher's exact test for categorical variables and the Student's t-test for continuous variables were used to assess the baseline differences between patients with KCCQ-12 below and over 75.

Time-to-event data were evaluated using Kaplan–Meier estimates and Cox proportional-hazards models. The adjusted hazard ratio (HR) of HF hospitalization for HRQoL measured by the KCCQ-12 was analyzed using Cox proportional hazard models. The models were adjusted for potential confounders selected among patient characteristics that were significantly associated with a better HRQoL status. We included all variables with $p < 0.05$. We decided to include age and gender due to their known prognostic value.

Study data were collected and managed using REDCap electronic data capture tools hosted at Parc de Salut Mar [31,32]. REDCap (Research Electronic Data Capture) is a secure, web-based software platform designed to support data capture for research studies, providing (1) an intuitive interface for validated data capture; (2) audit trails for tracking data manipulation and export procedures; (3) automated export procedures for seamless data downloads to common statistical packages; and (4) procedures for data integration and interoperability with external sources.

3. Results

One hundred and fifty patients were randomized between 2 July 2018 and 15 November 2019. A total of 141 patients answered the KCCQ-12 at baseline and were included in the analysis. Figure 1 shows the flow diagram of the study.

HRQoL was impaired in almost half of the cohort. Only 2 patients (1.4%) had very-poor-to-poor HRQoL (KCCQ-12 0–24), 30 patients (21.3%) had poor-to-fair HRQoL (KCCQ-12 25–49), and 40 patients (28.4%) a fair-to-good HRQoL (KCCQ-12 50–74). A good-to-excellent HRQoL (KCCQ 75–100) was present in 48.9% of patients at the baseline visit. Women comprised 50% of the population, the mean age was 82.2 years, and two-thirds of patients had HF with a preserved ejection fraction. Comorbidities were highly prevalent. Baseline characteristics were not different between patients with impaired and non-impaired HRQoL (Table 1).

Table 1. Baseline clinical and demographic characteristics of the patients included in the study.

	KCCQ < 75 (n = 72)	KCCQ 75–100 (n = 69)	p-Value
Age (years)	81.7 ± 4.8	82.3 ± 4.7	0.43
Female	37 (51.4)	34 (49.3)	0.80
Hypertension	63 (90)	62 (89.9)	0.98
Diabetes mellitus	31 (44.3)	28 (41.2)	0.71
Dyslipidemia	47 (66.2)	41 (59.4)	0.41
Stroke/TIA	9 (13.4)	10 (15.4)	0.75
Chronic kidney disease	54 (75)	44 (63.8)	0.15
Anemia	42 (58.3)	39 (56.5)	0.83
Peripheral vascular disease	9 (12.7)	14 (20.6)	0.21
Chronic lung disease	28 (38.9)	18 (26.1)	0.11
Cancer	16 (22.5)	19 (27.9)	0.43
Myocardial infarction	18 (25)	11 (15.9)	0.18
Coronary percutaneous intervention	14 (19.4)	10 (14.5)	0.43
TAVI or Mitraclip	1 (1.4)	2 (2.9)	0.48
Cardiac surgery:			
CABG	2 (2.8)	3 (4.3)	
Valve replacement	4 (5.6)	6 (8.7)	0.60
CABG and valve replacement	3 (4.2)	2 (2.8)	
Atrial fibrillation or flutter	54 (75)	43 (62.3)	0.10
Moderate-to-severe valve disease	22 (31.4)	22 (32.8)	0.86
Device therapy:			
Pacemaker	12 (16.7)	10 (14.5)	0.52
CRT or ICD	1 (1.4)	4 (5.7)	

Table 1. Cont.

	KCCQ < 75 (n = 72)	KCCQ 75–100 (n = 69)	p-Value
Previous history of HF	43 (59.7)	38 (55.1)	0.58
Duration of HF *:			
<3 months	12 (27.9)	3 (7.9)	
3–6 months	1 (2.3)	3 (7.9)	
6–12 months	4 (9.3)	5 (13.2)	0.18
1–5 years	17 (39.5)	15 (39.5)	
>5 years	9 (20.9)	11 (28.9)	
HF hospitalization the previous year *	19 (45.2)	12 (32.4)	0.25
HF categories:			
HFpEF (LVEF $\geq$ 50%)	48 (66.7)	46 (66.7)	
HFmrEF (LVEF 40–49%)	9 (12.5)	6 (8.7)	0.70
HFrEF (LVEF < 40%)	15 (20.8)	17 (24.6)	
Ecocardiographic parameters:			
LVEF (%)	52.1 ± 13.6	52.7 ± 15.2	0.79
Left ventricular mass index (g/m^2), n = 134	120.2 ± 30.7	134.2 ± 36.7	0.018
TAPSE (mm), n = 126	17.5 ± 4.3	17.3 ± 3.6	0.72
Right ventricle (mm), n = 88	28.9 ± 6.7	29.7 ± 7.3	0.56
Heart failure etiology			
Ischaemic	10 (14.1)	12 (17.4)	
Hypertensive	11 (15.5)	12 (17.4)	
Dilated cardiomyopathy	4 (5.6)	6 (8.7)	0.16
Valve heart disease	21 (29.6)	17 (24.6)	
Other/unknown	25 (35.2)	22 (31.9)	
Medications at discharge:			
ACEI/ARB-II/ARNI	35 (49.3)	39 (57.4)	0.34
MRA	9 (12.7)	12 (17.6)	0.41
Betablockers	52 (73.2)	49 (72.1)	0.87
Diuretics	68 (95.8)	67 (98.5)	0.62
Anticoagulation	53 (74.6)	46 (67.6)	0.36
Antiplatelet therapy	12 (16.9)	14 (20.6)	0.58
Oral antidiabetic drugs	24 (34.3)	20 (29.4)	0.54
Insulin	14 (19.7)	10 (14.7)	0.43
Proton-pump inhibitors	48 (67.6)	46 (67.6)	1.00
Statin	50 (70.4)	37 (54.4)	0.051
Calcium channel antagonists	25 (36.2)	17 (25.0)	0.15
Nitrates	16 (22.5)	10 (14.7)	0.24
Hydralazine	10 (14.1)	7 (10.3)	0.50
Amiodarone	16 (22.9)	8 (11.8)	0.09
Digoxin	3 (4.3)	1 (1.5)	0.62
Vitamin D supplements	25 (35.2)	20 (29.4)	0.47
Oral iron supplements	19 (26.8)	19 (27.9)	0.88
Benzodiazepines	16 (22.5)	14 (20.6)	0.78
Antidepressant drugs	20 (28.2)	16 (23.5)	0.53
Bronchodilators	27 (38.0)	20 (29.4)	0.28

Data are numbers (percentage) or mean ± standard deviation. ACEI: angiotensin-converting enzyme inhibitors; ARB-II: angiotensin II receptor blockers; ARNI: angiotensin receptor and neprilysin inhibition; CABG: coronary artery bypass grafting; CRT: cardiac resynchronization therapy; HF: heart failure; HFrEF: heart failure with reduced ejection fraction. HFmrEF: heart failure with mildly reduced ejection fraction; HFpEF: heart failure with preserved ejection fraction; ICD: implantable cardioverter defibrillator; LVEF: left ventricular ejection fraction; MRA: mineralocorticoid receptor antagonists; TIA: transient ischemic attack; TAPSE: tricuspid annular plane systolic excursion; TAVI: transcatheter aortic valve implantation. * Only for patients with a previous history of HF.

The only statistically significant differences were a lower NYHA functional class and a surprisingly higher NT-proBNP and left ventricular mass index in the group with better HRQoL. These patients also had a higher Barthel index and a lower Clinical Frailty Scale (Table 2).

Table 2. Hospitalization and first appointment characteristics.

	KCCQ < 75 (n = 72)	KCCQ 75–100 (n = 69)	p-Value
NT-proBNP at discharge, pg/mL	1977.5 (950.5–3917.0)	2774.5 (1767.0–6191.5)	0.018
High-sensitivity T troponin (Hs-TnT) at discharge, ng/L	37.5 (26.6–65.1)	43.7 (30.5–70.2)	0.26
eGFR (mL/min) at discharge	46.4 ± 19.9	47.3 ± 20.4	0.81
Frailty (Clinical Frailty Scale) ≥ 4	44 (61.1)	27 (40.3)	0.014
Clinical Frailty Scale	4.2 ± 1.4	3.7 ± 1.1	0.02
Barthel index	81.8 ± 19.7	90.4 ± 12.3	0.002
Basic activities of daily living (Barthel index):			
Independent (100)	17 (23.6)	25 (36.2)	
Minimally dependent (61–99)	45 (62.5)	41 (59.4)	0.07
Partially to totally dependent (0–60)	10 (13.9)	3 (4.3)	
Instrumental activities of daily living (Lawton index)	4.6 ± 2.3	5.3 ± 1.9	0.054
Pfeiffer Short Portable Mental Status Questionnaire (SPMSQ)	1 (1–3)	1 (0–2)	0.08
NYHA functional class	2.5 ± 0.6	2 ± 0.4	<0.001
Intervention geriatrician and cardiologist	31 (43.1)	40 (58)	0.08
KCCQ-12 at baseline	53 ± 15.9	88.3 ± 7.8	<0.001

Data are number (percentage), mean ± standard deviation, or median (interquartile range). eGFR: estimated glomerular filtration rate; NT-proBNP: N-terminal prohormone of brain natriuretic peptide; NYHA: New York Heart Association; KCCQ-12: Kansas City Cardiomyopathy Questionnaire-12.

One-year all-cause mortality was 22.7% and was significantly lower in the group with good HRQoL (14.5% vs. 30.6%; hazard ratio 0.28; 95% confidence interval 0.10–0.78; $p = 0.014$). In the group with better HRQoL, all-cause hospitalization was lower, and there was a trend towards lower HF hospitalization (Figure 2) (Table 3).

Table 3. Primary and secondary outcomes during follow-up.

	KCCQ < 75 (n = 72)	KCCQ 75–100 (n = 69)	p-Value
All-cause mortality	22 (30.6)	10 (14.5)	0.014
All-cause hospitalization	55 (76.4)	43 (62.3)	0.017
HF hospitalization	30 (41.7)	19 (27.5)	0.051

Data are numbers (percentage). HF: heart failure. The model is adjusted for age, female sex, Barthel index, Clinical Frailty Scale, NT-proBNP value at discharge, New York Heart Association functional class, and Kansas City Cardiomyopathy Questionnaire 75–100.

In patients with a KCCQ-12 measured at one year, there was a statistically significant increase in KCCQ-12. KCCQ-12 went from 71.5 ± 21.5 to 83.1 ± 20.8, $p < 0.001$, and 69.6% of patients had good-to-excellent HRQoL (Figure 3).

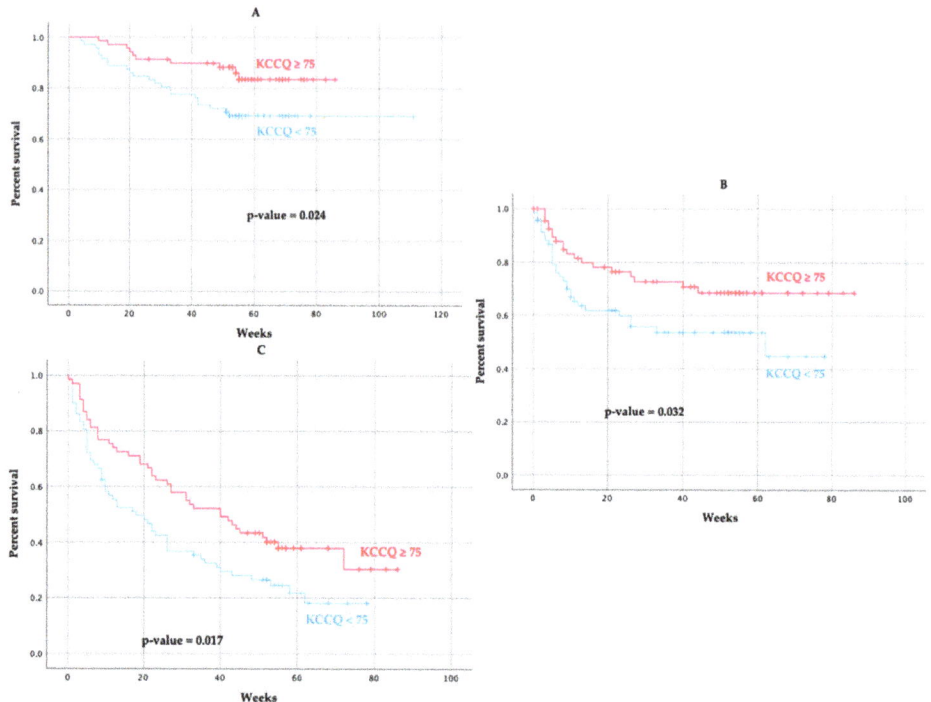

Figure 2. Unadjusted Kaplan–Meier for (**A**) all-cause death, (**B**) heart failure hospitalization, and (**C**) all-cause hospitalization.

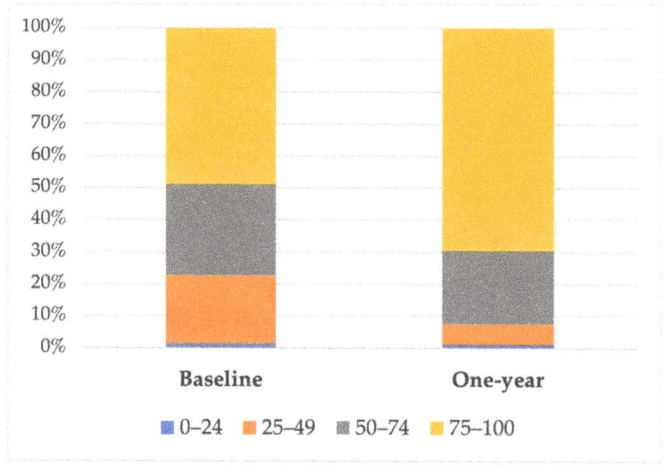

Figure 3. Change in KCCQ-12 at one-year follow-up.

Of the 72 patients with impaired HRQoL at baseline, 44 repeated the KCCQ-12 assessment at 12 months. Of those, 15 patients did not improve HRQoL (KCCQ-12 < 75) and 29 patients improved (KCCQ-12 > 75). Baseline characteristics of patients with impaired HRQoL at baseline who did not improve and who improved to a good-to-excellent HRQoL at one-year follow-up are summarized in Tables 4 and 5. A lower proportion of all-cause hospitalization was found in the group with HRQoL improvement, although statistical significance was not reached (62.1% vs. 86.7%, $p = 0.09$).

Table 4. Baseline clinical and demographic characteristics of the patients included in the study according to the improvement of KCCQ-12 at one-year follow-up.

	No KCCQ Improvement (n = 15)	KCCQ Improvement (n = 29)	p-Value
Age (years)	80.0 ± 4.4	81.9 ± 5.08	0.23
Female	11 (73.3)	12 (41.4)	0.04
Hypertension	14 (93.3)	25 (89.3)	1.00
Diabetes mellitus	8 (53.3)	14 (50)	0.84
Dyslipidemia	11 (73.3)	19 (65.5)	0.74
Stroke/TIA	2 (13.3)	4 (14.8)	1.00
Chronic kidney disease	11 (73.3)	22 (75.9)	1.00
Anemia	9 (60)	14 (48.3)	0.46
Peripheral vascular disease	2 (14.3)	4 (13.8)	1.00
Chronic lung disease	6 (40)	9 (31)	0.55
Cancer	2 (13.3)	10 (34.5)	0.17
Myocardial infarction	2 (13.3)	4 (13.8)	1.00
Coronary percutaneous intervention	2 (13.3)	7 (24.1)	0.69
TAVI or Mitraclip	1 (7.1)	0 (0)	0.33
Cardiac surgery:	2 (13.3)	4 (13.8)	0.69
Atrial fibrillation or flutter	10 (66.7)	23 (79.3)	0.47
Moderate to severe valve disease	4 (28.6)	8 (27.6)	1.00
Device therapy:			
Pacemaker	12 (16.7)	10 (14.5)	0.52
CRT or ICD	1 (1.4)	4 (5.7)	
Previous history of HF	7 (46.7)	18 (62.1)	0.33
HF hospitalization the previous year *	2 (28.6)	5 (29.4)	1.00
LVEF (%)	62.3 ± 3.9	49.3 ± 13.2	<0.001

Data are number (percentage) or mean ± standard deviation. HF: heart failure; LVEF: left ventricular ejection fraction; TIA: transient ischemic attack; TAVI: transcatheter aortic valve implantation. * Only for patients with a previous history of HF.

Table 5. Hospitalization and first appointment characteristics according to the improvement of KCCQ-12 at one-year follow-up.

	No KCCQ Improvement (n = 15)	KCCQ Improvement (n = 29)	p-Value
NT-proBNP at discharge, pg/mL	1162 (606.6–3579.0)	1799.5 (801.9–3562.5)	0.44
High-sensitivity T troponin (Hs-TnT) at discharge, ng/L	31.6 (22.9–44.5)	46.9 (22.4–73.0)	0.21
eGFR (mL/min) at discharge	52.9 ± 23.2	46.0 ± 22.1	0.36
Frailty (Clinical Frailty Scale) ≥ 4	12 (80.0)	16 (55.2)	0.11
Clinical Frailty Scale	4.5 ± 1.4	3.9 ± 1.1	0.14
Barthel index	76.2 ± 22.0	86.1 ± 15.3	0.09
Instrumental activities of daily living (Lawton index)	4.5 ± 2.3	4.6 ± 2.0	0.82
Pfeiffer Short Portable Mental Status Questionnaire (SPMSQ)	1 (1–2)	1 (1–3)	0.62
NYHA functional class	2.7 ± 0.7	2.2 ± 0.6	0.053
Intervention geriatrician and cardiologist	8 (53.3)	15 (51.7)	0.92
KCCQ-12 at baseline	55.1 ± 15.3	52.6 ± 17.5	0.64

Data are number (percentage), mean ± standard deviation, or median (interquartile range). eGFR: estimated glomerular filtration rate; NT-proBNP: N-terminal prohormone of brain natriuretic peptide; NYHA: New York Heart Association; KCCQ-12: Kansas City Cardiomyopathy Questionnaire-12.

4. Discussion

In our study involving older patients with a recent HF hospitalization, almost half of the patients had impaired HRQoL measured by the KCCQ-12 questionnaire. Surprisingly, baseline characteristics did not allow the identification of patients with worse HRQoL, except for parameters usually associated with aging, such as frailty and functional status measured by Barthel index, NYHA functional class, NT-proBNP, and left ventricular mass index. A good-to-excellent HRQoL was significantly associated with lower one-year all-cause mortality and hospitalization. In patients with HRQoL measured at one year, there was a significant improvement in the KCCQ-12 score.

This study extends prior works describing the association between HRQoL and clinical outcomes. It has already been shown that KCCQ provides prognostic information independent of other clinical data in patients with HF [8,10–15]. However, none of these studies examined the prognostic significance of KCCQ-12 in a prospective elderly cohort with a recent admission for HF. Indeed, our series differs from those previously published in two relevant aspects that should be noted. First, with a mean age of 82.2 years, our population was more than 10 years older than the oldest cohort published to date [33]. Second, the patients' profiles were rather different from what has been published so far. In fact, the prevalence of HF with a preserved ejection fraction was higher than in previous studies (66.7%), probably concerning the age of the population. Finally, the presence of comorbidities was substantial.

It has been reported that, among a cohort of stable patients with HF, no significant changes were detected by the KCCQ questionnaire at mid-term follow-up. In contrast, large changes were observed among a cohort of patients recovering from admission for decompensated HF [27]. Since the HRQoL assessment in the SENECOR study had a median (interquartile range) of 6 (5–9) after discharge from decompensated HF, our results are in line with previous evidence. Interestingly, patients with impaired HRQoL at baseline who did not have HRQoL improvement at one-year follow-up were more likely to be women. This is consistent with the previous finding that, in a cohort of patients with HF and reduced ejection fraction, women reported significantly worse HRQoL than men, although HRQoL was independently associated with outcome similarly in men and women [34]. On the other hand, patients who did not improve HRQoL also had a higher baseline LVEF than patients who improved. This could be explained by a potential improvement in LVEF over time in the group with a lower baseline LVEF, which could be associated with improvements in HRQoL. However, it could also reflect the several pitfalls that the actual classification of HF based on LVEF values has [35]. Moreover, in our study, a trend towards a lower proportion of all-cause hospitalization was found in the group with HRQoL improvement. Anyway, we must consider a possible selection bias in this analysis due to patients who died or did not repeat the HRQoL assessment at a one-year follow-up.

Better strategies are needed to help physicians efficiently target healthcare resources to HF patients at the highest risk. Our findings suggest that noninvasive risk stratification based on HRQoL measurement by the KCCQ-12 questionnaire can provide prognostic information even in older patients with HF, which could be an essential reference for subsequent treatment decisions when identifying candidates for disease management for whom increased care may reduce hospitalization and prevent death. Future studies are needed to establish whether the assessment of HRQoL in older HF patients with questionnaires such as KCCQ-12 can improve outcomes. It is worth noting that the baseline characteristics did not allow us to identify patients with worse HRQoL. Hence, HRQoL should be assessed in all patients to identify high-risk patients.

Limitations

Since this was a single-center study with a relatively small sample size, our data must be interpreted with caution. Moreover, HRQoL measurements in our study were administered as a part of routine outpatient follow-up visits within a clinical trial. In the setting of a clinical trial, the self-perception of HRQoL may increase regardless of the intervention due to multiple factors (extra care, more intensive management, optimism, etc.) [36,37]. Whether HRQoL assessments will have similar prognostic value outside this setting remains to be established. Finally, although our results were adjusted for multiple demographic and clinical patient factors, a possibility of residual unmeasured confounding factors cannot be definitively excluded, and our findings need to be validated in a larger-cohort multicenter study.

5. Conclusions

In older patients with a recent hospital admission for HF, good-to-excellent HRQoL was significantly associated with lower one-year all-cause mortality and hospitalization. These data support the assessment of HRQoL in relation to HF in the older population.

Author Contributions: Conceptualization, N.F. and C.R.; methodology, D.L., N.F. and C.R.; validation, D.L., N.F. and C.R.; formal analysis, N.F. and D.L.; investigation, D.L., M.H.-T., N.F., S.R.-B., L.C.B.-T., S.V.-M. and R.O.M.; resources, N.F. and O.V.; data curation, D.L., M.H.-T., N.F., C.R. and N.B.; writing—original draft preparation, D.L.; writing—review and editing, D.L., N.F. and C.R.; supervision, N.F. and C.R.; project administration, N.B.; funding acquisition, N.F. All authors have read and agreed to the published version of the manuscript.

Funding: This research was funded by Fundación MAPFRE, grant Primitivo de la Vega.

Institutional Review Board Statement: The study was conducted in accordance with the Declaration of Helsinki, and approved by the Ethics Committee of Parc de Salut Mar (protocol code number 2017/7653/I, approved on 8 February 2018).

Informed Consent Statement: Informed consent was obtained from all subjects involved in the study.

Data Availability Statement: The data presented in this study are available on request from the corresponding author. The data are not publicly available due to ethical restrictions.

Acknowledgments: We are indebted to all patients and families who agreed to participate in the study, especially those who decided to continue in the middle of the pandemic.

Conflicts of Interest: The authors declare no conflict of interest. The funders had no role in the design of the study; in the collection, analyses, or interpretation of data; in the writing of the manuscript, or in the decision to publish the results.

References

1. Farré, N.; Vela, E.; Clèries, M.; Bustins, M.; Cainzos-Achirica, M.; Enjuanes, C.; Moliner, P.; Ruiz, S.; Verdú-Rotellar, J.M.; Comín-Colet, J. Medical Resource Use and Expenditure in Patients with Chronic Heart Failure: A Population-Based Analysis of 88 195 Patients. *Eur. J. Heart Fail.* **2016**, *18*, 1132–1140. [CrossRef]
2. McDonagh, T.A.; Metra, M.; Adamo, M.; Gardner, R.S.; Baumbach, A.; Böhm, M.; Burri, H.; Butler, J.; Čelutkienė, J.; Chioncel, O.; et al. 2021 ESC Guidelines for the Diagnosis and Treatment of Acute and Chronic Heart Failure. *Eur. Heart J.* **2021**, *42*, 3599–3726. [CrossRef]
3. Anand, I.S.; Florea, V.G.; Fisher, L. Surrogate End Points in Heart Failure. *J. Am. Coll. Cardiol.* **2002**, *39*, 1414–1421. [CrossRef]
4. McMurray, J. Heart Failure: We Need More Trials in Typical Patients. *Eur. Heart J.* **2000**, *21*, 699–700. [CrossRef]
5. Cohn, J.; Cleland, J.G.F.; Lubsen, J.; Borer, J.S.; Steg, P.G.; Perelman, M.; Zannad, F. Unconventional End Points in Cardiovascular Clinical Trials: Should We Be Moving Away from Morbidity and Mortality? *J. Card. Fail.* **2009**, *15*, 199–205. [CrossRef]
6. Al-Kaade, S.; Hauptman, P.J. Health-Related Quality of Life Measurement in Heart Failure: Challenges for the New Millennium. *J. Card. Fail.* **2001**, *7*, 194–201. [CrossRef]
7. Sullivan, M.D.; Levy, W.C.; Russo, J.E.; Crane, B.; Spertus, J.A. Summary Health Status Measures in Advanced Heart Failure: Relationship to Clinical Variables and Outcome. *J. Card. Fail.* **2007**, *13*, 560–568. [CrossRef]
8. Heidenreich, P.A.; Spertus, J.A.; Jones, P.G.; Weintraub, W.S.; Rumsfeld, J.S.; Rathore, S.S.; Peterson, E.D.; Masoudi, F.A.; Krumholz, H.M.; Havranek, E.P.; et al. Health Status Identifies Heart Failure Outpatients at Risk for Hospitalization or Death. *J. Am. Coll. Cardiol.* **2006**, *47*, 752–756. [CrossRef]
9. Comín-Colet, J.; Garin, O.; Lupón, J.; Manito, N.; Crespo-Leiro, M.G.; Gómez-Bueno, M.; Ferrer, M.; Artigas, R.; Zapata, A.; Elosua, R.; et al. Validation of the Spanish Version of the Kansas City Cardiomyopathy Questionnaire. *Rev. Esp. Cardiol.* **2011**, *64*, 51–58. [CrossRef]
10. Kosiborod, M.N.; Jhund, P.S.; Docherty, K.F.; Diez, M.; Petrie, M.C.; Verma, S.; Nicolau, J.C.; Merkely, B.; Kitakaze, M.; DeMets, D.L.; et al. Effects of Dapagliflozin on Symptoms, Function, and Quality of Life in Patients With Heart Failure and Reduced Ejection Fraction: Results From the DAPA-HF Trial. *Circulation* **2020**, *141*, 90–99. [CrossRef]

11. Kosiborod, M.; Soto, G.E.; Jones, P.G.; Krumholz, H.M.; Weintraub, W.S.; Deedwania, P.; Spertus, J.A. Identifying Heart Failure Patients at High Risk for Near-Term Cardiovascular Events with Serial Health Status Assessments. *Circulation* **2007**, *115*, 1975–1981. [CrossRef]
12. Luo, N.; Teng, T.-H.K.; Tay, W.T.; Anand, I.S.; Kraus, W.E.; Liew, H.B.; Ling, L.H.; O'Connor, C.M.; Piña, I.L.; Richards, A.M.; et al. Multinational and Multiethnic Variations in Health-Related Quality of Life in Patients with Chronic Heart Failure. *Am. Heart J.* **2017**, *191*, 75–81. [CrossRef]
13. Ambrosy, A.P.; Hernandez, A.F.; Armstrong, P.W.; Butler, J.; Dunning, A.; Ezekowitz, J.A.; Felker, G.M.; Greene, S.J.; Kaul, P.; McMurray, J.J.; et al. The Clinical Course of Health Status and Association with Outcomes in Patients Hospitalized for Heart Failure: Insights from ASCEND-HF. *Eur. J. Heart Fail.* **2016**, *18*, 306–313. [CrossRef]
14. Dunlay, S.M.; Gheorghiade, M.; Reid, K.J.; Allen, L.A.; Chan, P.S.; Hauptman, P.J.; Zannad, F.; Maggioni, A.P.; Swedberg, K.; Konstam, M.A.; et al. Critical Elements of Clinical Follow-up after Hospital Discharge for Heart Failure: Insights from the EVEREST Trial. *Eur. J. Heart Fail.* **2010**, *12*, 367–374. [CrossRef]
15. Ekman, I.; Chassany, O.; Komajda, M.; Böhm, M.; Borer, J.S.; Ford, I.; Tavazzi, L.; Swedberg, K. Heart Rate Reduction with Ivabradine and Health Related Quality of Life in Patients with Chronic Heart Failure: Results from the SHIFT Study. *Eur. Heart J.* **2011**, *32*, 2395–2404. [CrossRef]
16. Lewis, E.F.; Johnson, P.A.; Johnson, W.; Collins, C.; Griffin, L.; Stevenson, L.W. Preferences for Quality of Life or Survival Expressed by Patients with Heart Failure. *J. Heart Lung Transplant.* **2001**, *20*, 1016–1024. [CrossRef]
17. Herrero-Torrus, M.; Badosa, N.; Roqueta, C.; Ruiz-Bustillo, S.; Solé-González, E.; Belarte-Tornero, L.C.; Valdivielso-Moré, S.; Vázquez, O.; Farré, N. Randomized Controlled Trial Comparing a Multidisciplinary Intervention by a Geriatrician and a Cardiologist to Usual Care after a Heart Failure Hospitalization in Older Patients: The SENECOR Study. *J. Clin. Med.* **2022**, *11*, 1932. [CrossRef]
18. Rockwood, K. A Global Clinical Measure of Fitness and Frailty in Elderly People. *Can. Med. Assoc. J.* **2005**, *173*, 489–495. [CrossRef]
19. Lawton, M.P.; Brody, E.M. Assessment of Older People: Self-Maintaining and Instrumental Activities of Daily Living. *Gerontologist* **1969**, *9*, 179–186. [CrossRef]
20. Mahoney, F.I.; Barthel, D.W. Functional Evaluation: The Barthel Index. *Md. State Med. J.* **1965**, *14*, 61–65.
21. Pfeiffer, E. A Short Portable Mental Status Questionnaire for the Assessment of Organic Brain Deficit in Elderly Patients. *J. Am. Geriatr. Soc.* **1975**, *23*, 433–441. [CrossRef]
22. Spertus, J.A.; Jones, P.G. Development and Validation of a Short Version of the Kansas City Cardiomyopathy Questionnaire. *Circ. Cardiovasc. Qual. Outcomes* **2015**, *8*, 469–476. [CrossRef]
23. Garcia-Caselles, P.; Miralles, R.; Arellano, M.; Torres, R.M.; Aguilera, A.; Pi-Figueras, M.; Cervera, A.M. Validation of A Modified Version of the Gijon's Social-Familial Evaluation Scale (Sfes): The "Barcelona Sfes Version", for Patients with Cognitive Impairment. *Arch. Gerontol. Geriatr.* **2004**, *38*, 201–206. [CrossRef]
24. Martí, D.; Miralles, R.; Llorach, I.; García Palleiro, P.; Esperanza, A.; Guillem, J.; Cervera, A.M. Depressive Mood Disorders in an Inpatient Convalescence Unit: Experience and Validation of a 15-Items Spanish Version of the Yesavage Geriatric Depression Scale. *Rev. Esp. Geriatr. Gerontol.* **2000**, *35*, 7–14.
25. Rubenstein, L.Z.; Harker, J.O.; Salva, A.; Guigoz, Y.; Vellas, B. Screening for Undernutrition in Geriatric Practice: Developing the Short-Form Mini-Nutritional Assessment (MNA-SF). *J. Gerontol. Ser. A Biol. Sci. Med. Sci.* **2001**, *56*, M366–M372. [CrossRef]
26. Joseph, S.M.; Novak, E.; Arnold, S.V.; Jones, P.G.; Khattak, H.; Platts, A.E.; Dávila-Román, V.G.; Mann, D.L.; Spertus, J.A. Comparable Performance of the Kansas City Cardiomyopathy Questionnaire in Patients With Heart Failure With Preserved and Reduced Ejection Fraction. *Circ. Heart Fail.* **2013**, *6*, 1139–1146. [CrossRef]
27. Green, C.P.; Porter, C.B.; Bresnahan, D.R.; Spertus, J.A. Development and Evaluation of the Kansas City Cardiomyopathy Questionnaire: A New Health Status Measure for Heart Failure. *J. Am. Coll. Cardiol.* **2000**, *35*, 1245–1255. [CrossRef]
28. Spertus, J.; Peterson, E.; Conard, M.W.; Heidenreich, P.A.; Krumholz, H.M.; Jones, P.; McCullough, P.A.; Pina, I.; Tooley, J.; Weintraub, W.S.; et al. Monitoring Clinical Changes in Patients with Heart Failure: A Comparison of Methods. *Am. Heart J.* **2005**, *150*, 707–715. [CrossRef]
29. Hauptman, P.J.; Masoudi, F.A.; Weintraub, W.S.; Pina, I.; Jones, P.G.; Spertus, J.A. Variability in the Clinical Status of Patients with Advanced Heart Failure. *J. Card. Fail.* **2004**, *10*, 397–402. [CrossRef]
30. Spertus, J.A.; Jones, P.G.; Sandhu, A.T.; Arnold, S.V. Interpreting the Kansas City Cardiomyopathy Questionnaire in Clinical Trials and Clinical Care. *J. Am. Coll. Cardiol.* **2020**, *76*, 2379–2390. [CrossRef]
31. Harris, P.A.; Taylor, R.; Minor, B.L.; Elliott, V.; Fernandez, M.; O'Neal, L.; McLeod, L.; Delacqua, G.; Delacqua, F.; Kirby, J.; et al. The REDCap Consortium: Building an International Community of Software Platform Partners. *J. Biomed. Inform.* **2019**, *95*, 103208. [CrossRef]
32. Harris, P.A.; Taylor, R.; Thielke, R.; Payne, J.; Gonzalez, N.; Conde, J.G. Research Electronic Data Capture (REDCap)—A Metadata-Driven Methodology and Workflow Process for Providing Translational Research Informatics Support. *J. Biomed. Inform.* **2009**, *42*, 377–381. [CrossRef]
33. Pokharel, Y.; Khariton, Y.; Tang, Y.; Nassif, M.E.; Chan, P.S.; Arnold, S.V.; Jones, P.G.; Spertus, J.A. Association of Serial Kansas City Cardiomyopathy Questionnaire Assessments with Death and Hospitalization in Patients With Heart Failure With Preserved and Reduced Ejection Fraction. *JAMA Cardiol.* **2017**, *2*, 1315. [CrossRef]

34. Ravera, A.; Santema, B.T.; Sama, I.E.; Meyer, S.; Lombardi, C.M.; Carubelli, V.; Ferreira, J.P.; Lang, C.C.; Dickstein, K.; Anker, S.D.; et al. Quality of Life in Men and Women with Heart Failure: Association with Outcome, and Comparison between the Kansas City Cardiomyopathy Questionnaire and the EuroQol 5 Dimensions Questionnaire. *Eur. J. Heart Fail.* **2021**, *23*, 567–577. [CrossRef]
35. Severino, P.; D'Amato, A.; Prosperi, S.; Dei Cas, A.; Mattioli, A.V.; Cevese, A.; Novo, G.; Prat, M.; Pedrinelli, R.; Raddino, R.; et al. Do the Current Guidelines for Heart Failure Diagnosis and Treatment Fit with Clinical Complexity? *J. Clin. Med.* **2022**, *11*, 857. [CrossRef]
36. Bekelman, D.B.; Plomondon, M.E.; Carey, E.P.; Sullivan, M.D.; Nelson, K.M.; Hattler, B.; McBryde, C.F.; Lehmann, K.G.; Gianola, K.; Heidenreich, P.A.; et al. Primary Results of the Patient-Centered Disease Management (PCDM) for Heart Failure Study. *JAMA Intern. Med.* **2015**, *175*, 725. [CrossRef]
37. Lewis, E.F. Are Hospitalizations for Heart Failure the Great Equalizer? *JACC Heart Fail.* **2015**, *3*, 539–541. [CrossRef]

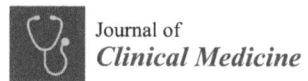
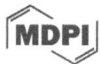

Article

Clinical Characteristics and Prognostic Relevance of Different Types of Caregivers for Elderly Patients with Acute Heart Failure—Analysis from the RICA Registry

Manuel Méndez-Bailon [1], Noel Lorenzo-Villalba [2,*], Jorge Rubio-Garcia [3], María Carmen Moreno-García [4], Guillermo Ropero-Luis [5], Eduardo Martínez-Litago [6], Raúl Quirós-López [7], Sara Carrascosa-García [8], Alvaro González-Franco [9], Emmanuel Andrès [2], Jesús Casado-Cerrada [10] and Manuel Montero-Pérez-Barquero [11]

1. Internal Medicine Department, Hospital Clínico San Carlos, Instituto de Investigación Sanitaria (IdISSC), Universidad Complutense, 28040 Madrid, Spain; manuelmenba@hotmail.com
2. Service de Médecine Interne, Diabète et Maladies Métaboliques, Hôpitaux Universitaires de Strasbourg, 67000 Strasbourg, France; emmanuel.andres@chru-strasbourg.fr
3. Internal Medicine Department, Hospital Clínico Universitario Lozano Blesa, 50009 Zaragoza, Spain; jorgerubiogracia@gmail.com
4. Internal Medicine Department, Hospital de Manises, 46940 Valencia, Spain; mcmorenogarcia@gmail.com
5. Internal Medicine Department, Hospital de la Serranía de Ronda, 29400 Malaga, Spain; guillermo.ropero.sspa@juntadeandalucia.es
6. Internal Medicine Department, Hospital Santa Bárbara, 13500 Ciudad Real, Spain; emartinezl@sescam.jccm.es
7. Internal Medicine Department, Hospital Costa del Sol, 29603 Málaga, Spain; quiroslopez77@gmail.com
8. Internal Medicine Department, Consorcio Hospital General Universitario de Valencia, 46014 Valencia, Spain; saracarrascosagarcia@gmail.com
9. Internal Medicine Department, Hospital Universitario Central de Asturias, 33011 Oviedo, Spain; alvarogfranco@yahoo.com
10. Internal Medicine Department, Hospital Universitario de Getafe, 28905 Madrid, Spain; casadocerrada@telefonica.net
11. Internal Medicine Department, IMIBIC, Hospital Universitario Reina Sofía, 14004 Córdoba, Spain; montero.manolo@gmail.com
* Correspondence: noellorenzo@gmail.com

Abstract: Background: Patients with heart failure encompass a heterogeneous group, but they are mostly elderly patients with a large burden of comorbid conditions. Objective: The aim of this study was to compare the clinical characteristics and the prognostic impact on hospital admissions and mortality in a population of patients with HF with different types of caregivers (family members, professionals, and the patient himself). Methods: We conducted an observational study from a prospective registry. Patients from the National Registry of Heart Failure (RICA), which belongs to the Working Group on Heart Failure and Atrial Fibrillation of the Spanish Society of Internal Medicine (SEMI), were included. Patients with heart failure were classified, according to the type of main caregiver, into four groups: the patient himself/herself, a partner, children, or a professional caregiver. A bivariable analysis was performed between the clinical, analytical, therapeutic, and prognostic characteristics of the different groups. The endpoints of the study were all-cause mortality at 1 year; mortality at 120 days; and the readmission rate for HF at 30 days, 120 days, and 1 year of follow-up. In all cases, the level of statistical significance was set at $p < 0.05$. Results: A total of 2147 patients were enrolled in this study; women represented 52.4%, and the mean age was 81 years. The partner was the caregiver for 703 patients, children were caregivers for 1097 patients, 199 patients had a professional caregiver, and only 148 patients were their own caregivers. Women were more frequently cared for by their children (65.8%) or a professional caregiver (61.8%); men were more frequently cared for by their spouses (68.7%) and more frequently served as their own caregivers (59.5%) ($p < 0.001$). No statistically significant differences were observed in relation to readmissions or mortality at one year of follow-up between the different groups. A lower probability of readmission and death was observed for patients who received care from a partner or children/relative, with log-rank scores of 11.2 with $p = 0.010$ and 10.8 with $p = 0.013$. Conclusions: Our study showed that the presence of a family caregiver for elderly patients with heart failure was associated with a lower

Citation: Méndez-Bailon, M.; Lorenzo-Villalba, N.; Rubio-Garcia, J.; Moreno-García, M.C.; Ropero-Luis, G.; Martínez-Litago, E.; Quirós-López, R.; Carrascosa-García, S.; González-Franco, A.; Andrès, E.; et al. Clinical Characteristics and Prognostic Relevance of Different Types of Caregivers for Elderly Patients with Acute Heart Failure—Analysis from the RICA Registry. *J. Clin. Med.* 2022, 11, 3516. https://doi.org/10.3390/jcm11123516

Academic Editor: Filippos Triposkiadis

Received: 10 April 2022
Accepted: 16 June 2022
Published: 18 June 2022

Publisher's Note: MDPI stays neutral with regard to jurisdictional claims in published maps and institutional affiliations.

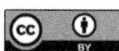

Copyright: © 2022 by the authors. Licensee MDPI, Basel, Switzerland. This article is an open access article distributed under the terms and conditions of the Creative Commons Attribution (CC BY) license (https://creativecommons.org/licenses/by/4.0/).

readmission rate and a lower mortality rate at 120 days of follow-up. Our study also demonstrated that elderly patients with good cognitive and functional status can be their own caregivers, as they obtained good health outcomes in terms of readmission and mortality. More prospective studies and clinical trials are needed to evaluate the impact of different types of caregivers on the outcomes of patients with heart failure.

Keywords: heart failure; caregivers; mortality; hospital readmission

1. Introduction

Heart failure (HF) is a chronic disease that is increasing worldwide. Patients with heart failure encompass a heterogeneous group, but they are mostly elderly patients with a large burden of comorbid conditions [1].

To reduce hospitalizations and mortality rates, it is recommended that patients with HF practice self-care, which also includes adherence to treatment. Self-care for HF is defined as the naturalistic decision-making process used by patients to maintain the stability of their disease (self-care maintenance), monitor signs and symptoms of HF (symptom awareness), and manage HF exacerbation (self-care). Evidence shows that HF self-care improves patient outcomes, such as the use of health care services and mortality. A recently published article demonstrated that worse self-care is an independent predictor of long-term mortality (both all-cause and cardiovascular), HF hospitalization, and the combination of these endpoints in patients with chronic HF [2]. Despite its positive effects, patients with HF have difficulty performing self-care.

In the self-care, management, and treatment of HF, the role of the caregiver is key, especially in patients with a profile of greater vulnerability due to their cognitive, functional, and social status, among other aspects. In this setting, most patients depend on support from relatives, friends, or some other external help in order to comply with medication and self-care. Thus, caregivers represent an important tool in the management of this group of patients. Both patients and caregivers must engage in medication management, adherence to diet and physical activity regimens, and symptom recognition [3–5]. Community nurses and other health care professionals also play important roles in HF care by optimizing the management, assessment, and evaluation of the patient's clinical condition and care during transitions from the hospital to the home [6].

Some studies have demonstrated the effects of education of family caregivers at discharge on reducing hospital readmission in these patients [7]. However, the prognostic impact of different types of caregivers on the care of HF patients has not been evaluated [7]. The aim of this study was to compare the clinical characteristics and the prognostic impact on hospital admissions and mortality in a population of patients with HF with different types of caregivers (family members, professionals, and the patient himself/herself).

2. Methods

2.1. Design—Type of Study

We conducted an observational study from a prospective registry. Patients from the National Registry of Heart Failure (RICA), which belongs to the Working Group on Heart Failure and Atrial Fibrillation of the Spanish Society of Internal Medicine (SEMI), were included. The latter is a prospective, multicenter registry that has been active since 2008. It includes consecutive individual patients over 50 years of age with a diagnosis of HF at hospital discharge (acute decompensated or new-onset HF), according to European cardiology guidelines published in 2008.

2.2. Inclusion and Exclusion Criteria

Inclusion criteria: Subjects were included in the registry after hospital discharge and followed for at least one year. A total of 2147 patients were included. In the present analysis, we included patients older than 65 years who were registered from March 2008 to December 2020. Exclusion criteria: Patients who did not sign the informed consent to participate in the study were excluded.

2.3. Variables

We used personal history, physical examination, and clinical analysis records. Left ventricular ejection fraction (LVEF) as assessed by 2D echocardiography was included. The Charlson comorbidity index and Pfeiffer test were also collected. The Charlson comorbidity index predicts the one-year mortality for a patient who may have a range of comorbid conditions, such as heart disease, AIDS, or cancer (a total of 22 conditions are included). Each condition is assigned a score of 1, 2, 3, or 6, depending on the risk of dying associated with each one. Scores are summed to provide a total score to predict mortality. The Pfeiffer test is a short, reliable instrument used to detect the presence of intellectual impairment and determine its degree, if any.

Patients were classified, according to the type of main caregiver, into four groups: the patient himself/herself, partner, children, or a paid professional caregiver.

2.4. Statistical Analysis

Quantitative variables are expressed as means (standard deviation) and qualitative variables are expressed as absolute values (percentages). Quantitative variables were compared using ANOVA, and qualitative variables were compared using the Chi-square test. The post hoc Tukey method was used. Kaplan–Meier curves were constructed, comparing the groups using the log-rank test. A bivariable analysis was performed between the clinical, analytical, therapeutic, and prognostic characteristics of the different groups. The endpoints of the study were all-cause mortality at 1 year; mortality at 120 days; and the readmission rate for HF at 30 days, 120 days, and 1 year of follow-up. We performed a survival analysis for patients with HF at 120 days of follow-up with Kaplan–Meier curves. In all cases, the level of statistical significance was set at $p < 0.05$. Statistical analysis was performed using the IBM Statistical Package for Social Sciences (version 22.0, SPSS Inc., Chicago, IL, USA).

2.5. Ethical Aspects

The registry protocol was initially approved by the Ethics Committee of the Hospital Universitario Reina Sofía de Córdoba and was subsequently approved by each of the committees of the participating hospitals, code 18/349-E, with the last update approved by the CEIC on 9 August 2018. All patients signed an informed consent form prior to inclusion in the registry. The data were collected from a web page (www.registrorica.org, accessed on 1 March 2008) containing the anonymous database and accessed by each investigator through a personalized password. The registry's design was previously published [8].

3. Results

A total of 2147 patients were enrolled in this study. Women represented 52.4% of patients, and the mean age was 81 years. The partner was the caregiver for 703 patients, children were the caregivers for 1097 patients, 199 patients had professional caregivers, and only 148 patients were their own caregivers. Hypertension and atrial fibrillation were seen in 88% and 54% of patients, respectively. The mean Barthel index was 81.2, and the mean Charlson score was 3.05. The mean left ventricular ejection fraction was 51.8% and was more frequently reduced for patients without a caregiver (44.7) ($p < 0.001$). Women were more frequently cared for by their children (65.8%) or a professional caregiver (61.8%); men were more frequently cared for by their wives (68.7) and more frequently served as their own caregivers (59.5%) ($p < 0.001$). (Table 1) In the latter case, the patients had a better functional status (Barthel index of 95) and cognitive situation (Pfeiffer of 0.5) than patients with other types of caregivers ($p < 0.001$). In relation to self-care, 1814 and 1555 patients followed low-sodium intake and weight monitoring regimens, respectively. Statistically significant differences were seen in relation to water restriction, which was lower for patients without an external caregiver (Table 1). The majority of patients were on beta blockers and ACE/ARA-2 inhibitors or anti-aldosterone agents. Statistically significant differences were observed in relation to the prescription of beta blockers (85.1%) and sacubitril valsartan (25.4%) in the group of patients without external caregivers ($p < 0.01$).

Table 1. Baseline characteristics and outcomes of patients with HF according to caregiver.

Variable	All (n= 2147)	Partner Caregiver (n = 703)	Children Caregiver (n = 1097)	Professional Caregiver (n = 199)	No Caregiver (n = 148)	p-Value
Age, median (SD)	81.06 (8.7)	77.28 (9.05)	83.63 (7.02)	83.53 (8.2)	76.6 * (10.7)	<0.001
Sex: male, n (%)	1022 (47.6)	483 (68.7) *	375 (34.2)	76 (38.2)	88 (59.5)	<0.001
Sex: female, n (%)	1125 (52.4)	220 (31.3)	722 (65.8) *	123 (61.8)	60 (40.5)	<0.001
Comorbidities						
Hypertension, n (%)	1889 (88)	604 (85.9)	989 (90.2)	176 (88.4)	120 (81.1) *	<0.001
T2DM, n (%)	993 (46.3)	367 (52.2)	467 (42.6)	82 (41.2) *	77 (52)	<0.001
COPD, n (%)	448 (20.9)	182 (25.9) *	203 (18.5)	34 (17.1)	29 (19.6)	0.001
Atrial fibrillation, n (%)	1172 (54.6)	361 (51.4)	629 (57.3)	119 (59.8)	63 (42.6) *	<0.001
Ischemic heart disease, n (%)	481 (22.4)	190 (27)	213 (19)	167 (16)	102 (31) *	<0.001
Pfeiffer index, median (SD)	1.5 (1.9)	1.08 (1.6)	1.31 (1.7)	2.02 (2.3)	0.5 * (1.09)	<0.001
Barthel index, median (SD)	81.2 (24.09)	89.2 (18.02)	75.3 (25.9)	73.8 (26.6)	95.9 * (9.7)	<0.001
Charlson score, median (SD)	3.05 (2.5)	3.2 (2.6)	3.02 (2.4)	2.9 (2.4)	2.6 * (3.2)	0.035
LVEF, median (SD)	51.8 (15.7)	50.3 (15.4)	53.3 (15.7)	54.5 (15.3)	44.7 * (15.3)	<0.001
Laboratory, n (%)						
Hemoglobin, (g/dL) median (SD)	12.09 (2.04)	12.3 (2.09)	11.9 (1.9)	11.8 * (1.9)	12.5 (2.2)	<0.001
Creatinine (ml/min/m^3), median (SD)	1.3 (2.6)	1.2 (0.5)	1.4 (3.6)	1.2 (0.7)	1.2 (0.5)	0.692
proBNP (pg/mL), median	6654.6	5697.2	7108.06	7296.9	7555.1	0.058
Non-pharmacological treatment	19(0.88)					
Fluid restriction, n (%)	1365 (70.5)	417 (66.3)	741 (73.7)	124 (68.5)	83 (65.9)	0.008
Weight monitoring, n (%)	1555 (80)	497 (79.1)	803 (41.3)	153 (84.1)	102 (81)	0.510
Low-sodium diet, n (%)	1814 (93)	583 (92.4)	949 (93.9)	172 (94.5)	110 (88)	0.072

Table 1. Cont.

Variable	All (n= 2147)	Partner Caregiver (n = 703)	Children Caregiver (n = 1097)	Professional Caregiver (n = 199)	No Caregiver (n = 148)	p-Value
Pharmacological treatment, n (%)						
Beta blockers, n (%)	1522 (70.9)	516 (73.4)	753 (68.6)	127 (63.8)	126 (85.1) *	<0.001
ACE inhibitors/ARA-2, n (%)	1266 (59)	404 (57.5)	654 (59.6%)	131 (65.8) *	77 (52)	0.054
Sacubitril valsartan, n (%)	138 (6.4)	42 (6)	55 (5)	6 (3)	35 (25.4) *	<0.001
Anti-aldosterone agents	486 (22.6)	180 (37) *	233 (21.2)	38 (19.1)	35 (23.6)	0.099
Endpoints n (%)						
Mortality at 30 days, n (%)	546 (27.9)	155 (29.2)	299 (35.3)	67 (35.3)	25 (22.9) *	0.011
30-day readmission, n (%)	383 (19.7)	109 (17.3) *	201 (19.7)	49 (26.1)	24 (22.4)	0.053
Mortality at 120 days, n (%)	630 (32.1)	177 (27.8) *	341 (33.3)	76 (40)	336 (33)	0.010
120-day readmission, n (%)	691 (35.5)	207 (32.8) *	355 (34.8)	87 (46.3)	42 (39.3)	0.006
One-year readmission, n (%)	1365 (70.1)	430 (68.1)	718 (70.4)	142 (75.5)	75 (70.1)	0.279
One-year mortality, n (%)	1208 (61.6)	380 (59.7)	635 (62)	121 (63.7)	72 (66.1)	0.524

Legend: * adjusted residuals are outside the ranges +2 −2. T2DM: type 2 diabetes mellitus; COPD: chronic obstructive pulmonary disease; LVEF: left ventricular ejection fraction; ACE inhibitors: angiotensin-converting enzyme inhibitors; ARA-2: angiotensin II receptor antagonists.

In relation to the endpoints analyzed, no statistically significant differences were observed in terms of readmission and mortality at 1 year of follow-up between the different types of caregivers. We did observe statistically significant differences in terms of readmission and mortality at 120 days, with lower rates of these events in patients with HF who had family members (child or partner) as their main caregivers (Table 1).

Figures 1 and 2 show the tendency to present fewer admission and death events in these types of caregivers, with log-rank scores of 11.2 with $p = 0.010$ and 10.8 with $p = 0.013.4$.

In Table S1 and Figure S1, we include the bivariate and Kaplan–Meier analysis for patients with heart failure, only considering the presence or absence of caregivers.

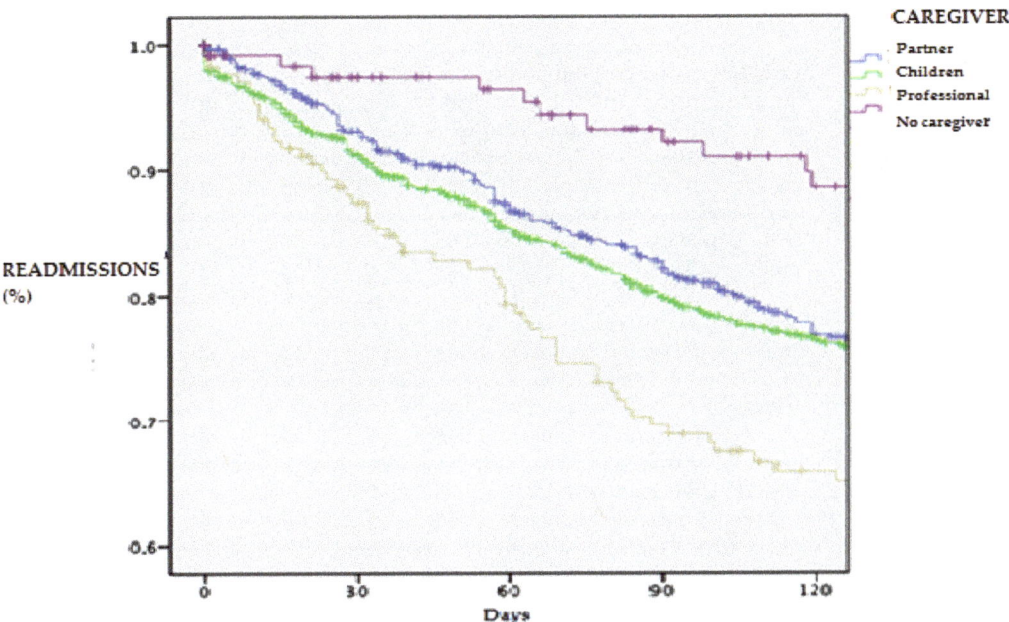

Figure 1. Survival analysis for readmissions in patients with HF according to caregiver type at 120-day follow-up.

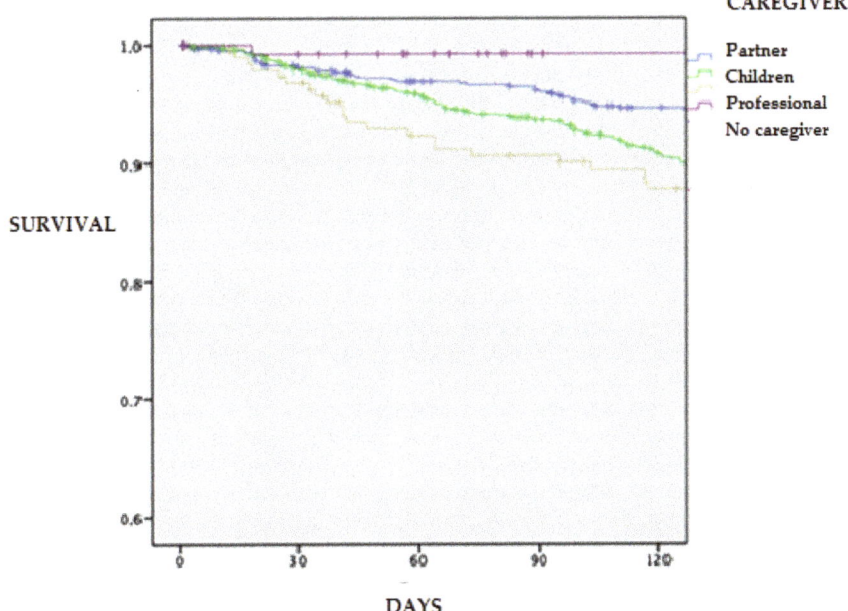

Figure 2. Survival analysis for mortality in patients with HF according to caregiver type at 120-day follow-up.

4. Discussion

The results of our investigation highlight that in our sample, HF patients who were admitted to the hospital and had a family caregiver had a more favorable prognosis regarding readmission and survival at 120 days of follow-up after hospitalization than patients with heart failure who were their own main caregiver or had a professional caregiver. This study is the largest of its kind in our country to evaluate the prognostic impact of the different types of caregivers on patients with HF admitted to hospitals. Our study demonstrates that elderly patients with good cognitive and functional status can also be their own caregivers, as they obtained good health outcomes in terms of readmission and mortality.

In relation to the characteristics of our series, we should highlight the important role played by family caregivers, initially the partners and later the children. This may be due to the characteristics of our aging population and the cultural aspects of our Spanish society; family values in the care of the elderly are deeply rooted in our country [9]. A low proportion of patients do not have caregivers, and this may be due to the fact that the great majority of elderly patients admitted to internal medicine services have a low capacity for self-care due to their high levels of dependency and cognitive deterioration [10]. In this sense, we emphasize that patients with HF who were their own main caregivers were younger and presented better cognitive and functional situations than the rest. Patients with HF for whom the caregiver was the patient had the smallest sample size, and it may be difficult to obtain solid conclusions in this regard. In relation to self-care, the patients in this group presented poorer adherence to measures such as control of water intake [11].

In relation to family caregivers, more than 60% of men received care from their wives, and more than 60% of women received care from their children or professional caregivers [12]. This may be due to the longer life expectancy of women in our country [13], which means that the main caregiver is less frequently the husband. The presence of a family caregiver in our study was accompanied by a favorable trend in terms of readmission and mortality in the short- and medium-term and attenuated at one year of follow-up. These findings may be due to the fact that the effects of family self-care have a higher impact in short- and medium-term follow-up than in long-term follow-up, in which the progressive evolution of the disease and the clinical situation of comorbidity and functional deterioration of the patient may lead to a higher risk of readmission and death [10]. In another study, the education levels of HF patients and caregivers were not correlated with readmission or mortality rates [14]. In the self-care measures evaluated, we only observed differences in relation to water restriction, which were in favor of patients with HF with caregivers, but we did not evaluate other measures recommended by clinical practice guidelines, such as self-adjustment of diuretics and monitoring of alarm signs [15].

The degree of clinical follow-up in heart failure programs carried out by each of the groups evaluated is also unknown. This study is limited by its retrospective nature and the fact that the RICA registry was not designed to evaluate the hypothesis of our investigation; the variables of self-care and the main caregiver were collected by the medical researchers, but no structured analysis of the patient's self-care capacity—such as the European self-care scale—was carried out, and no evaluation of the degree of caregiver overload—such as the Zarit scale—was conducted [16]. In this research, variables related to the educational intervention received by the patient and caregivers were not collected either, which could affect the interpretation of the observed results. In this sense, there is a need of to perform specific prospective and randomized clinical trials to evaluate the impact of care and educational interventions by the patient himself/herself as well as by relatives and professional caregivers. The results of the MOTIVATE-HF trial have recently been published, showing that structured motivational interviewing with HF patients and caregivers may have an impact on patient survival. These findings could not be analyzed in our study considering its retrospective design, as motivational interviewing was not included as a variable in the RICA registry [17].

5. Conclusions

Our study showed that the presence of a family caregiver in elderly patients with HF was associated with a lower readmission rate and a lower mortality rate at 120 days of follow-up. More prospective studies and clinical trials are needed to evaluate the impact of different types of caregivers on the outcome of patients with HF.

Supplementary Materials: The following supporting information can be downloaded at: https://www.mdpi.com/article/10.3390/jcm11123516/s1. Table S1: Baseline characteristics and outcomes of patients with HF with and without caregivers; Figure S1: Analysis of survival at one year in patients with heart failure with and without caregivers.

Author Contributions: Conceptualization, M.M.-B., N.L.-V., J.R.-G., M.C.M.-G., G.R.-L., E.M.-L., R.Q.-L., S.C.-G., A.G.-F., E.A., J.C.-C. and M.M.-P.-B.; methodology, M.M.-B., N.L.-V., J.R.-G., M.C.M.-G., G.R.-L., E.M.-L., R.Q.-L., S.C.-G., A.G.-F., E.A., J.C.-C. and M.M.-P.-B.; software, M.M.-B. and M.M.-P.-B.; validation, M.M.-B., N.L.-V. and M.M.-P.-B.; formal analysis, M.M.-B., N.L.-V. and M.M.-P.-B.; investigation, M.M.-B., N.L.-V., J.R.-G., M.C.M.-G., G.R.-L., E.M.-L., R.Q.-L., S.C.-G., A.G.-F., E.A., J.C.-C. and M.M.-P.-B.; resources, M.M.-B. and M.M.-P.-B.; data curation, M.M.-B., N.L.-V. and M.M.-P.-B.; writing—original draft preparation, M.M.-B., E.A., N.L.-V. and M.M.-P.-B.; writing—review and editing, M.M.-B., E.A., N.L.-V. and M.M.-P.-B.; visualization, M.M.-B., N.L.-V. and M.M.-P.-B.; supervision, M.M.-B. and M.M.-P.-B.; project administration, M.M.-P.-B. All authors have read and agreed to the published version of the manuscript.

Funding: This research received no external funding.

Institutional Review Board Statement: Approved by the Ethics Committee of the Hospital Universitario Reina Sofía de Córdoba and subsequently approved by each of the committees of the participating hospitals, code 18/349-E, with the last update approved by the CEIC on 9 August 2018.

Informed Consent Statement: Informed consent was obtained from all subjects involved in the study.

Data Availability Statement: Data is contained within the article.

Conflicts of Interest: The authors declare no conflict of interest.

References

1. Fernández-Casso, M.L.; Hernando-Arizaleta, L.; Palomar-Rodriguez, J.A.; Soria-Arcos, F.; Pascual-Figal, D.A. Trends and Characteristics of Hospitalization for Heart Failure in a Population Setting From 2003 to 2013. *Rev. Esp. Cardiol.* **2017**, *70*, 720–726. [CrossRef] [PubMed]
2. Calero-Molina, E.; Hidalgo, E.; Rosenfeld, L.; Verdú-Rotellar, J.M.; Verdú-Soriano, J.; Garay, A.; Alcoberro, L.; Jimenez-Marrero, S.; Garcimartin, P.; Yun, S.; et al. The relationship between self-care, long-term mortality, and heart failure hospitalization: Insights from a real-world cohort study. *Eur. J. Cardiovasc. Nurs.* **2022**, *21*, 116. [CrossRef] [PubMed]
3. Kitko, L.; McIlvennan, C.K.; Bidwell, J.T.; Dionne-Odom, J.N.; Dunlay, S.M.; Lewis, L.M.; Meadows, G.; Sattler, E.L.P.; Schulz, R.; Strömberg, A. American Heart Association Council on Cardiovascular and Stroke Nursing; Council on Quality of Care and Outcomes Research; Council on Clinical Cardiology; and Council on Lifestyle and Cardiometabolic Health. Family Caregiving for Individuals with Heart Failure: A Scientific Statement from the American Heart Association. *Circulation* **2020**, *141*, e864–e878. [CrossRef] [PubMed]
4. Riegel, B.; Moser, D.K.; Anker, S.D.; Appel, L.J.; Dunbar, S.B.; Grady, K.L.; on behalf of the American Heart Association Council on Cardiovascular Nursing; American Heart Association Council on Cardiovascular Nursing; American Heart Association Council on Clinical Cardiology; American Heart Association Council on Nutrition, Physical Activity, and Metabolism; et al. State of the science: Promoting self-care in persons with heart failure: A scientific statement from the American Heart Association. *Circulation* **2009**, *120*, 1141–1163. [CrossRef] [PubMed]
5. Riegel, B.; Moser, D.K.; Buck, H.G.; Dickson, V.V.; Dunbar, S.B.; Lee, C.S.; on behalf of the American Heart Association Council on Cardiovascular and Stroke Nursing; Council on Peripheral Vascular Disease; Council on Quality of Care and Outcomes Research. Self-care for the prevention and management of cardiovascular disease and stroke: A scientific statement for healthcare professionals from the American Heart Association. *J. Am. Heart Assoc.* **2017**, *6*, e006797. [CrossRef] [PubMed]
6. Albert, N.M. A systematic review of transitional-care strategies to reduce rehospitalization in patients with heart failure. *Heart Lung* **2016**, *45*, 100–113. [CrossRef] [PubMed]
7. Chung, M.L. Caregiving in Heart Failure. *J. Cardiovasc. Nurs.* **2020**, *35*, 229–230. [CrossRef] [PubMed]
8. Trullàs, J.C.; Formiga, F.; Montero, M.; Conde, A.; Casado, J.; Carrasco, F.J.; Díez, J.; Ceresuela, L.M.; Grupo RICA. Paradoja de la obesidad en la insuficiencia cardiaca. Resultados del Registro RICA [Paradox of obesity in heart failure: Results from the Spanish RICA Registry]. *Med. Clin.* **2011**, *137*, 671–677. [CrossRef] [PubMed]

9. Rogero-García, J.; García-Sainz, C. Caregiver Leave-Taking in Spain: Rate, Motivations, and Barriers. *J. Aging Soc. Policy* **2016**, *28*, 98–112. [CrossRef] [PubMed]
10. Chivite, D.; Formiga, F.; Corbella, X.; Conde-Martel, A.; Aramburu, Ó.; Carrera, M.; Dávila, M.F.; Pérez-Silvestre, J.; Manzano, L.; Montero-Pérez-Barquero, M.; et al. Basal functional status predicts one-year mortality after a heart failure hospitalization in elderly patients—The RICA prospective study. *Int. J. Cardiol.* **2018**, *254*, 182–188. [CrossRef] [PubMed]
11. Vest, A.R.; Chan, M.; Deswal, A.; Givertz, M.M.; Lekavich, C.; Lennie, T.; Litwin, S.E.; Parsly, L.; Rodgers, J.E.; Rich, M.W.; et al. Nutrition, Obesity, and Cachexia in Patients with Heart Failure: A Consensus Statement from the Heart Failure Society of America Scientific Statements Committee. *J. Card. Fail.* **2019**, *25*, 380–400. [CrossRef] [PubMed]
12. Kamath, D.Y.; Bhuvana, K.B.; Dhiraj, R.S.; Xavier, D.; Varghese, K.; Salazar, L.J.; Granger, C.B.; Pais, P.; Granger, B.B. Patient and caregiver reported facilitators of self-care among patients with chronic heart failure: Report from a formative qualitative study. *Wellcome Open Res.* **2020**, *5*, 10. [CrossRef] [PubMed]
13. Méndez-Bailón, M.; Jiménez-García, R.; Hernández-Barrera, V.; Comín-Colet, J.; Esteban-Hernández, J.; de Miguel-Díez, J.; de Miguel-Yanes, J.M.; Muñoz-Rivas, N.; Lorenzo-Villalba, N.; López-de-Andrés, A. Significant and constant increase in hospitalization due to heart failure in Spain over 15 year period. *Eur. J. Intern. Med.* **2019**, *64*, 48–56. [CrossRef] [PubMed]
14. Elkhateeb, O.; Salem, K. Patient and caregiver education levels and readmission and mortality rates of congestive heart failure patients. *East Mediterr. Health J.* **2018**, *24*, 345–350. [CrossRef] [PubMed]
15. Ktaa, S.; Polovina, M.; Rosano, G.; Abdin, A.; Anguita, M.; Lainscak, M.; Lund, L.H.; McDonagh, T.; Metra, M.; Mindham, R.; et al. European Society of Cardiology quality indicators for the care and outcomes of adults with heart failure. Developed by the Working Group for Heart Failure Quality Indicators in collaboration with the Heart Failure Association of the European Society of Cardiology. *Eur. J. Heart Fail.* **2022**, *24*, 132–142.
16. Ghasemi, M.; Arab, M.; Mangolian Shahrbabaki, P. Relationship Between Caregiver Burden and Family Functioning in Family Caregivers of Older Adults with Heart Failure. *J. Gerontol. Nurs.* **2020**, *46*, 25–33. [CrossRef] [PubMed]
17. Iovino, P.; Rebora, P.; Occhino, G.; Zeffiro, V.; Caggianelli, G.; Ausili, D.; Alvaro, R.; Riegel, B.; Vellone, E. Does motivational interviewing reduce health services use and mortality in heart failure patients? A secondary analysis of the MOTIVATE-HF trial. *Eur. J. Cardiovasc. Nurs.* **2021**, *20*, zvab060.093. [CrossRef]

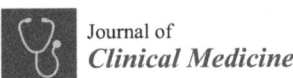

Article

Comparison of 3-Year Outcomes between Early and Delayed Invasive Strategies in Older and Younger Adults with Non-ST-Segment Elevation Myocardial Infarction Undergoing New-Generation Drug-Eluting Stent Implantation

Yong Hoon Kim [1,*,†], Ae-Young Her [1,†], Seung-Woon Rha [2,*], Cheol Ung Choi [2], Byoung Geol Choi [3], Ji Bak Kim [2], Soohyung Park [2], Dong Oh Kang [2], Ji Young Park [4], Sang-Ho Park [5] and Myung Ho Jeong [6]

1. Division of Cardiology, Department of Internal Medicine, Kangwon National University School of Medicine, Chuncheon 24289, Korea
2. Cardiovascular Center, Korea University Guro Hospital, Seoul 08308, Korea
3. Cardiovascular Research Institute, Korea University College of Medicine, Seoul 02841, Korea
4. Division of Cardiology, Department of Internal Medicine, Cardiovascular Center, Nowon Eulji Medical Center, Eulji University, Seoul 01830, Korea
5. Cardiology Department, Soonchunhyang University Cheonan Hospital, Cheonan 31151, Korea
6. Department of Cardiology, Cardiovascular Center, Chonnam National University Hospital, Gwangju 61469, Korea
* Correspondence: yhkim02@kangwon.ac.kr (Y.H.K.); swrha617@yahoo.co.kr (S.-W.R.)
† Yong Hoon Kim and Ae-Young Her contributed equally to this work as the first authors.

Abstract: We evaluated the 3-year clinical outcomes of early invasive (EI) and delayed invasive (DI) strategies in older and younger adults with non-ST-segment elevation myocardial infarction (NSTEMI) undergoing successful new-generation drug-eluting stent (DES) implantation to reflect current real-world practice. Overall, 4513 patients with NSTEMI were recruited from the Korea Acute Myocardial Infarction Registry-National Institute of Health and divided into two groups according to age: group A (age ≥ 65 years, n = 2253) and group B (age < 65 years, n = 2260). These two groups were further divided into two subgroups: group EI (A1 and B1) and DI (A2 and B2). The primary clinical outcome was the occurrence of major adverse cardiac and cerebrovascular events (MACCEs), defined as all-cause death, recurrent MI (re-MI), any repeat coronary revascularization, or stroke. The secondary clinical outcome was definite or probable stent thrombosis (ST). In both groups A and B, after multivariable-adjusted and propensity score-adjusted analyses, MACCE (group A, p = 0.137 and p = 0.255, respectively; group B, p = 0.171 and p = 0.135, respectively), all-cause death, cardiac death (CD), non-CD, re-MI, any repeat revascularization, stroke, and ST rates were similar between the EI and DI groups. When including only those with complex lesions, the primary and secondary clinical outcomes were not significantly different between the EI and DI groups. In the era of new-generation DESs, major clinical outcomes were not significantly different between the EI and DI strategies in both older and younger adults with NSTEMI.

Keywords: drug-eluting stent; elderly; non-ST-segment elevation myocardial infarction; percutaneous coronary intervention

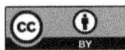

1. Introduction

In patients presenting with non-ST-segment elevation (NSTE) myocardial infarction (MI), the results of the Timing of Intervention in Acute Coronary Syndrome (TIMACS) trial [1] demonstrated that the outcomes of individuals who underwent routine early invasive (EI) strategy (coronary angiography [CAG] within 24 h of admission) did not differ greatly from those of individuals who underwent delayed invasive (DI) strategy in preventing the primary outcome, but it could reduce the rate of the composite secondary outcome of death, myocardial infarction, or refractory ischemia and was superior to DI in high-risk patients ($p = 0.003$) during a 6-month follow-up period. In a meta-analysis, the routine invasive strategy significantly reduced 5-year rates of cardiovascular death or MI compared to the selective invasive strategy ($p = 0.002$) [2]. Recently, in the Very Early Versus Deferred Invasive Evaluation Using Computerized Tomography study (VERDICT) [3] with a mean follow-up of 4.3 years, a very early strategy (median time from diagnosis to revascularization = 4.7 h) improved the primary outcome compared with the standard invasive treatment (hazard ratio [HR], 0.81; 95% confidence interval [CI], 0.67–1.01) in the high-risk subgroup, but it did not improve overall long-term clinical outcomes compared with an invasive strategy conducted within 2–3 days in patients with NSTE-acute coronary syndrome (ACS). Hence, pooled analyses of randomized trials [1] or meta-analyses [2,4,5] showed early benefit of the routine intervention, but long-term results are inconsistent, and the optimal timing of percutaneous coronary intervention (PCI) in NSTEMI has yet to be determined. According to the most recent European guidelines [6], the EI strategy is recommended in patients with at least one high-risk criterion, and the recommended diagnostic and interventional strategies for older and younger patients are the same (class I and level of evidence B). The American College of Cardiology/American Heart Association guidelines [7] recommend an EI strategy for initially stabilized high-risk patients with NSTE-ACS and a DI strategy as reasonable for high/intermediate-risk patients (class IIa and level of evidence B). Although information concerning the preferred treatment option between the EI and DI strategies in older and younger patients with NSTEMI could be important for the interventional cardiologist, the available data on this subject are limited. Furthermore, previous studies on the comparative outcomes between the EI and DI strategies were not limited to patients who received new-generation drug-eluting stents (DESs), thereby limiting their findings in reflecting the current real-world practices. In this study, we compared the 3-year major clinical outcomes in older and younger adults with NSTEMI who underwent new-generation DES implantation.

2. Methods

2.1. Study Population

A total of 13,104 patients with acute MI between November 2011 and December 2015 were recruited from the Korea Acute MI Registry-National Institute of Health (KAMIR-NIH) [8]. KAMIR-NIH is a nationwide prospective multicenter registry integrated from 20 high-volume centers in the Republic of Korea. Detailed information on this registry can be found on the website (http://www.kamir.or.kr, accessed on 1 November 2011). All patients aged ≥18 years at the time of hospital admission were included. The following patients were excluded from the study: (1) patients who did not undergo PCI ($n = 1369$, 10.4%); (2) those who underwent unsuccessful PCI (failed PCI ($n = 61$, 0.5%) and suboptimal PCI ($n = 94$, 0.7%)); (3) those who underwent balloon angioplasty ($n = 739$, 5.6%); (4) those who were treated with bare-metal stents or first-generation DESs ($n = 563$, 4.3%); (5) those who underwent coronary artery bypass grafting ($n = 38$, 0.3%); (6) those with ST-segment elevation myocardial infarction (STEMI, $n = 5342$, 40.8%), cardiogenic shock, or in-hospital death ($n = 228$, 1.7%); and (7) those who were unavailable for follow-up ($n = 157$, 1.2%). Overall, 4513 patients with NSTEMI who underwent successful new-generation DES implantation were included (Figure 1). The types of new-generation DESs used are listed in Table 1. These patients were divided into two groups according to their age: group A (age ≥ 65 years, $n = 2253$, 49.9%) and group B (age < 65 years, $n = 2260$, 50.1%). Subsequently, these two groups of patients were further divided into two subgroups: group EI (group A1 ($n = 1612$, 71.5%) or B1 ($n = 1688$, 74.7%)) and DI (group A2 ($n = 641$, 28.5%) and B2 ($n = 572$, 25.3%)) (Figure 1). Trained research coordinators at each center collected patient data using a web-based report form on the Internet-based Clinical Research and Trial management system, supported by a grant (2016-ER6304-02) from the Korean Centers for Disease Control and Prevention since November 2011 (Internet-based Clinical Research and Trial management system study No. C110016). The study was conducted in accordance with the ethical guidelines of the 2004 Declaration of Helsinki. The study was approved by the ethics committee of each participating center and the Chonnam National University Hospital Institutional Review Board ethics committee (CNUH-2011-172). All patients included in the study provided written informed consent prior to enrollment. They also completed a 3-year clinical follow-up via face-to-face interviews, phone calls, or chart reviews. All clinical events were evaluated by an independent event adjudication committee. The event adjudication process has previously been described by KAMIR investigators [8].

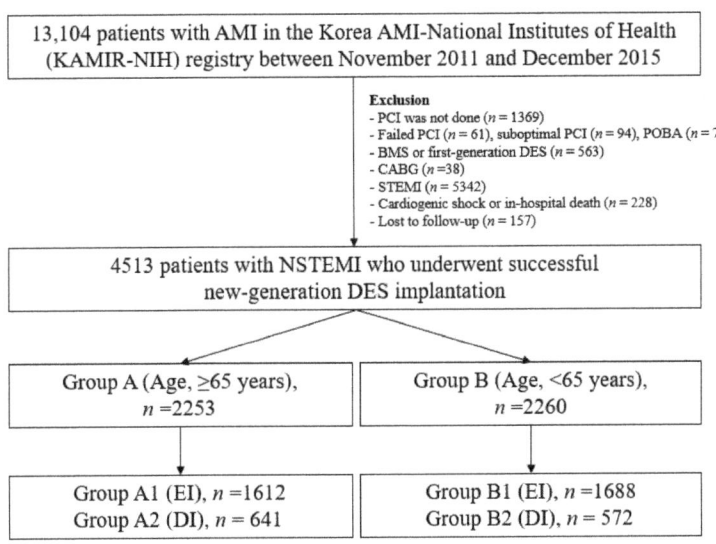

Figure 1. Flowchart. PCI, percutaneous coronary intervention; POBA, plain old balloon angioplasty; BMS, bare-metal stent; DES, drug-eluting stent; CABG, coronary artery bypass graft; STEMI, ST-segment-elevation myocardial infarction; NSTEMI, non-STEMI; EI, early invasive; DI, delayed invasive.

Table 1. Baseline characteristics and discharge medications.

Variables	Group A (Age, ≥65 Years, n = 2253)			Group B (Age, <65 Years, n = 2260)		
	Group A1 Early Invasive (n = 1612)	Group A2 Delayed Invasive (n = 641)	p Value	Group B1 Early Invasive (n = 1688)	Group B2 Delayed Invasive (n = 572)	p Value
Male, n (%)	927 (57.5)	371 (57.9)	0.872	1476 (87.4)	513 (89.7)	0.153
Age, years	74.3 ± 5.8	75.0 ± 5.9	0.007	54.4 ± 7.3	54.5 ± 7.2	0.760
LVEF, %	53.2 ± 10.6	51.6 ± 12.3	0.005	55.9 ± 9.4	55.1 ± 10.9	0.149
BMI, kg/m^2	23.2 ± 3.1	23.5 ± 3.3	0.048	25.0 ± 3.2	24.8 ± 3.1	0.120
SBP, mmHg	133.5 ± 26.4	135.4 ± 25.8	<0.001	137.0 ± 25.8	139.2 ± 25.8	0.087
DBP, mmHg	80.4 ± 15.7	81.3 ± 14.8	0.038	83.9 ± 15.8	83.8 ± 15.1	0.874
Symptom-to-door time, h	8.0 (3.0–28.6)	8.8 (2.7–45.3)	0.054	5.8 (2.0–19.3)	4.5 (1.6–23.9)	0.181
Door-to-balloon time, h	6.0 (2.9–16.1)	46.4 (31.1–71.6)	<0.001	6.9 (3.0–16.1)	43.2 (29.8–58.6)	<0.001
Killip class 3	181 (11.2)	98 (15.3)	0.011	65 (3.9)	34 (5.9)	0.044
Hypertension, n (%)	1050 (65.1)	427 (66.6)	0.505	662 (39.2)	243 (42.5)	0.183
Diabetes mellitus, n (%)	567 (35.2)	227 (35.4)	0.914	408 (24.2)	154 (26.9)	0.198
Dyslipidemia, n (%)	154 (9.6)	83 (12.9)	0.022	225 (13.3)	92 (16.1)	0.109
Previous MI, n (%)	136 (8.4)	48 (7.5)	0.496	73 (4.3)	388 (6.6)	0.033
Previous PCI, n (%)	112 (6.9)	33 (5.1)	0.128	66 (3.9)	34 (5.9)	0.046
Previous CABG, n (%)	6 (0.4)	3 (0.5)	0.720	2 (0.1)	1 (0.2)	0.749
Previous HF, n (%)	27 (1.7)	15 (2.3)	0.302	9 (0.5)	6 (1.0)	0.230
Previous stroke, n (%)	124 (7.7)	57 (8.9)	0.346	60 (3.6)	23 (4.0)	0.608
Current smokers, n (%)	324 (20.1)	102 (15.9)	0.023	921 (54.6)	309 (54.0)	0.846
Peak CK-MB, mg/dL	20.9 (6.4–78.6)	13.9 (5.0–42.6)	<0.001	29.0 (7.2–99.0)	15.6 (4.6–56.7)	<0.001
Peak Troponin-I, ng/mL	10.6 (2.1–22.1)	4.7 (1.1–18.9)	<0.001	14.3 (2.8–23.1)	5.4 (1.0–21.1)	<0.001
Blood glucose, mg/dL	158.6 ± 72.7	162.1 ± 80.2	0.338	153.6 ± 73.4	158.9 ± 79.6	0.157

Table 1. Cont.

Variables	Group A (Age, ≥65 Years, n = 2253)			Group B (Age, <65 Years, n = 2260)		
	Group A1 Early Invasive (n = 1612)	Group A2 Delayed Invasive (n = 641)	p Value	Group B1 Early Invasive (n = 1688)	Group B2 Delayed Invasive (n = 572)	p Value
Hs-CRP (mg/dL)	1.53 ± 3.24	1.78 ± 7.72	0.440	1.07 ± 2.50	1.11 ± 2.10	0.687
Serum creatinine (mg/L)	1.12 ± 1.15	1.26 ± 1.34	0.023	1.04 ± 1.27	1.21 ± 1.73	0.034
eGFR < 60 mL/min/1.73 m^2, n (%)	570 (35.4)	269 (42.0)	0.003	193 (11.4)	86 (15.0)	0.027
Total cholesterol, mg/dL	171.9 ± 43.3	171.7 ± 44.1	0.900	188.5 ± 43.1	185.3 ± 41.9	0.117
Triglyceride, mg/L	111.7 ± 71.8	112.8 ± 82.7	0.771	152.7 ± 96.3	156.2 ± 94.3	0.523
HDL cholesterol, mg/L	43.1 ± 11.4	44.5 ± 82.7	0.013	42.1 ± 10.8	42.2 ± 10.6	0.913
LDL cholesterol, mg/L	108.7 ± 34.7	106.0 ± 35.3	0.101	120.2 ± 36.8	116.9 ± 35.3	0.053
GRACE risk score	151.2 ± 34.5	154.4 ± 36.7	0.058	105.8 ± 28.4	106.5 ± 32.3	0.676
>140, n (%)	979 (60.7)	390 (60.8)	0.961	171 (10.1)	81 (14.2)	0.011
Atrial fibrillation, n (%)	93 (5.8)	44 (6.9)	0.329	26 (1.5)	13 (2.3)	0.265
ST-depression, n (%)	392 (24.3)	157 (24.5)	0.930	334 (19.8)	103 (18.0)	0.352
T-wave inversion, n (%)	370 (23.0)	155 (24.2)	0.534	291 (17.2)	119 (20.8)	0.060
Discharge medications, n (%)						
Aspirin, n (%)	1600 (99.3)	635 (99.1)	0.645	1678 (99.4)	568 (99.3)	0.778
Clopidogrel, n (%)	1251 (77.6)	540 (84.2)	<0.001	1065 (63.1)	406 (71.0)	0.001
Ticagrelor, n (%)	283 (17.6)	77 (12.0)	0.001	361 (21.4)	109 (19.1)	0.257
Prasugrel, n (%)	78 (4.8)	24 (3.7)	0.106	262 (15.5)	57 (10.0)	0.001
BBs, n (%)	1354 (84.0)	542 (84.6)	0.742	1491 (88.3)	485 (84.8)	0.029
ACEIs or ARBs, n (%)	1361 (84.4)	506 (78.9)	0.002	1423 (84.3)	462 (80.8)	0.051
Statin, n (%)	1534 (95.2)	601 (93.8)	0.178	1631 (96.6)	541 (94.6)	0.033
Anticoagulant, n (%)	50 (3.1)	25 (3.9)	0.362	11 (0.7)	10 (1.7)	0.024
Infarct-related artery						
Left main, n (%)	50 (3.1)	25 (3.9)	0.362	33 (2.0)	23 (4.0)	0.008
LAD, n (%)	684 (42.4)	286 (44.6)	0.346	723 (42.8)	238 (41.6)	0.625
LCx, n (%)	400 (24.8)	141 (22.0)	0.172	459 (27.2)	150 (26.2)	0.663
RCA, n (%)	478 (29.7)	189 (29.5)	0.959	473 (28.0)	161 (28.1)	0.957
Multivessel disease, n (%)	971 (60.2)	423 (66.0)	0.011	811 (48.0)	300 (52.4)	0.073
ACC/AHA type B2/C lesions	1373 (85.2)	544 (84.9)	0.854	1413 (83.7)	467 (81.6)	0.271
Pre-PCI TIMI flow grade 0/1	633 (39.3)	199 (31.0)	<0.001	760 (45.0)	177 (30.9)	<0.001
GP IIb/IIIa inhibitor	133 (8.3)	43 (6.7)	0.258	174 (10.3)	41 (7.2)	0.026
Transradial approach	781 (48.4)	309 (48.2)	0.926	959 (56.8)	292 (51.0)	0.017
IVUS/OCT, n (%)	346 (21.5)	174 (27.1)	0.004	421 (24.9)	202 (35.3)	<0.001
FFR, n (%)	27 (1.7)	23 (3.6)	0.010	33 (2.0)	24 (4.2)	0.005
Drug-eluting stents [a]						
ZES, n (%)	374 (23.2)	155 (24.2)	0.621	419 (24.8)	142 (24.8)	0.999
EES, n (%)	860 (53.3)	332 (51.8)	0.504	878 (52.0)	294 (51.4)	0.809
BES, n (%)	326 (20.2)	144 (22.5)	0.237	340 (20.1)	125 (21.9)	0.402
Others, n (%)	52 (3.2)	10 (1.6)	0.032	51 (3.0)	11 (1.9)	0.184
Stent diameter (mm)	3.04 ± 0.40	3.03 ± 0.41	0.531	3.12 ± 0.43	3.10 ± 0.44	0.196
Stent length (mm)	30.2 ± 14.4	31.1 ± 14.9	0.205	28.6 ± 13.2	29.8 ± 14.5	0.074
Number of stents	1.22 ± 0.46	1.26 ± 0.50	0.044	1.17 ± 0.42	1.22 ± 0.47	0.030

Values are means ± standard deviation or median (interquartile range) or numbers and percentages. The p values for continuous data were obtained from the unpaired t-test. The p values for categorical data from chi-square or Fisher's exact test. LVEF, left ventricular ejection fraction; BMI, body mass index; SBP, systolic blood pressure; DBP, diastolic blood pressure; MI, myocardial infarction; PCI, percutaneous coronary intervention; CABG, coronary artery bypass graft; HF, heart failure; CK-MB, creatine kinase myocardial band; Hs-CRP, high sensitivity C-reactive protein; eGFR, estimated glomerular filtration rate; HDL, high-density lipoprotein; LDL, low-density lipoprotein; GRACE, Global Registry of Acute Coronary Events; BBs, ß-blockers; ACEIs, angiotensin-converting enzyme inhibitors; ARBs, angiotensin receptor blockers; LAD, left anterior descending artery; LCx, left circumflex artery; RCA, right coronary artery; ACC/AHA, American College of Cardiology/American Heart Association; TIMI, thrombolysis in myocardial infarction; GP, glycoprotein; IVUS, intravascular ultrasound; OCT, optical coherence tomography; FFR, fractional flow reserve; ZES, zotarolimus-eluting stent; EES, everolimus-eluting stent; BES, biolimus-eluting stent. [a] Drug-eluting stents were composed of ZES (Resolute Integrity stent; Medtronic, Inc., Minneapolis, MN), EES (Xience Prime stent, Abbott Vascular, Santa Clara, CA; or Promus Element stent, Boston Scientific, Natick, MA), and BES (BioMatrix Flex stent, Biosensors International, Morges, Switzerland; or Nobori stent, Terumo Corporation, Tokyo, Japan).

2.2. Percutaneous Coronary Intervention and Medical Treatment

A transfemoral or transradial approach was performed in accordance with the general guidelines [9]. Aspirin (200–300 mg) and clopidogrel (300–600 mg), ticagrelor (180 mg), or prasugrel (60 mg) were prescribed to the patients as loading doses before PCI. After PCI, all patients were prescribed aspirin (100 mg/day) along with clopidogrel (75 mg/day), ticagrelor (90 mg twice a day), or prasugrel (5–10 mg/day) for at least 1 year. The access site, revascularization strategy, and selection of the DES were left to the discretion of the individual surgeons.

2.3. Study Definitions and Clinical Outcomes

NSTEMI was defined as the absence of persistent ST-segment elevation with increased levels of cardiac biomarkers and appropriate clinical context [6,7]. A successful PCI was defined as residual stenosis of <30% and thrombolysis in MI (TIMI) flow grade 3 in the infarct-related artery. EI strategy was defined as CAG performed within 24 h of admission [1]. Glomerular function for estimated glomerular filtration rate (eGFR) was calculated using the Chronic Kidney Disease Epidemiology Collaboration equation [10]. The GRACE risk score [11] was calculated for all patients. Complex lesions were defined as PCI for unprotected left main coronary disease, multivessel PCI, multiple stent implantation ($\geq$3 stents per patient), and cases with a total length of deployed stent >38 mm [12,13]. The primary clinical outcome was the occurrence of major adverse cardiac and cerebrovascular events (MACCE), which was defined by all-cause death, recurrent MI (re-MI), and any repeat coronary revascularization, including target lesion revascularization, target vessel revascularization (TVR), non-TVR, and stroke. According to the American Heart Association/American Stroke Association guidelines, an acute cerebrovascular event resulting in death or neurological deficit for >24 h or the presence of acute infarction demonstrated by imaging studies was defined as stroke [14]. All-cause death was considered a cardiac death (CD) unless an undisputed non-cardiac cause was present [15]. The secondary clinical outcome was definite or probable stent thrombosis (ST) during a 3-year follow-up period. ST was defined according to the definition provided by the Academic Research Consortium [16]. The definitions of re-MI, TLR, TVR, and non-TVR have been published previously [17].

2.4. Statistical Analyses

For continuous variables, differences between the groups were evaluated using unpaired *t*-tests. Data are expressed as the mean ± standard deviation or median (interquartile range). For discrete variables, differences between the groups were expressed as counts and percentages and were analyzed using the chi-squared or Fisher's exact tests. Univariate analysis was performed for all variables in the EI and DI groups with the *p*-value set at <0.05. Subsequently, we performed a multicollinearity test [18] between the included variables to confirm non-collinearity between them (Supplementary Table S1). Variance inflation factor (VIF) values were calculated to measure the degree of multicollinearity among the variables. A VIF of >5 indicated a high correlation [19]. When the tolerance value was <0.1 [20] or the condition index was >10 [19], the presence of multicollinearity was considered. Variables included in the multivariable Cox regression analysis were male sex, left ventricular ejection fraction (LVEF), body mass index, systolic blood pressure, diastolic blood pressure, symptom-to-door time, Killip class 3, hypertension, diabetes mellitus, dyslipidemia, previous PCI, previous heart failure, previous stroke, current smoker, peak creatine kinase myocardial band (CK-MB), peak troponin-I, serum creatinine, eGFR <60 mL/min/1.73 m^2, high-density lipoprotein cholesterol, low-density lipoprotein cholesterol, GRACE risk score >140, and clopidogrel, ticagrelor, prasugrel, angiotensin-converting enzyme inhibitor or angiotensin receptor blocker, and statin use. Moreover, to adjust for potential confounders, a propensity score (PS)-adjusted analysis was performed using a logistic regression model. We tested all potentially relevant variables, such as baseline clinical, angiographic, and procedural factors (Table 1). The c-statistic for the PS-matched (PSM) analysis in this study was 0.684. Patients in the EI group were matched to those in the DI group (1:1) using the nearest available pair-matching method according to PS. The subjects were matched with a caliper width of 0.01. This procedure yielded 2318 well-matched pairs (Supplementary Table S2). Various clinical outcomes were estimated using a Kaplan–Meier curve analysis, and group differences were compared using the log-rank test. Statistical significance was defined as a two-tailed *p*-value of <0.05. All statistical analyses were performed using SPSS software v. 20 (IBM; Armonk, NY, USA).

3. Results

3.1. Baseline Characteristics

Table 1 and Supplementary Tables S2 and S3 show the baseline, laboratory, angiographic, and procedural characteristics of the study population. In both groups, A and B, the mean values of peak CK-MB and troponin-I and the number of patients with pre-PCI TIMI flow grade 0/1 were higher in the EI group (group A1 or B1) than in the DI group (group A2 or B2). In contrast, patients who had Killip class 3 had reduced renal function (eGFR, <60 mL/min/1.73 m^2) and received clopidogrel as discharge medication; the mean serum creatinine level was 1.26 ± 1.34 vs. 1.12 ± 1.15 mg/L in group A2 vs. group A1 (p = 0.023), and 1.21 ± 1.73 vs. 1.04 ± 1.27 mg/L in group B2 vs. group B1 (p = 0.034); the use of intravascular ultrasound/optical coherent tomography/fractional flow rate was higher in the DI group than in the EI group. In group A, the mean value of LVEF, number of current smokers, and prescription rates of ticagrelor, ACEIs, or ARBs as discharge medications were higher in the EI group (group A1) than in the DI group (group A2). However, the mean age of enrolled patients; mean values of BMI, SBP, and DBP; number of patients with dyslipidemia and multivessel disease; and mean number of deployed stents were higher in the DI group (group A2) than in the EI group (group A1). In group B, the prescription rates of prasugrel, beta-blockers, and statin; use of glycoprotein IIb/IIIa inhibitors; and transradial approach rate were higher in the EI group (group B1) than in the DI group (group B2). In contrast, the number of patients with previous MI and PCI and higher GRACE risk scores (>140) were higher in the DI group (group B2) than in the EI group (group B1) (Table 1).

3.2. Clinical Outcomes

The 3-year major clinical outcomes are summarized in Table 2 and Figure 2. After multivariable-adjusted analysis, in group A, the MACCE (Figure 2A, adjusted HR (aHR), 1.198; 95% CI, 0.944–1.521; p = 0.137), all-cause death (Figure 2B, aHR, 1.150; p = 0.434), CD (Figure 2C, aHR, 1.100; p = 0.692), non-CD (Figure 2D, aHR, 1.207; p = 0.485), re-MI (Figure 2E, aHR, 1.061; p = 0.809), any repeat revascularization (Figure 2F, aHR, 1.247; p = 0.186), stroke (Figure 2G, aHR, 1.255; p = 0.394), and ST (definite or probable, Figure 2H, aHR, 2.969; 95% CI, 0.978–9.017; p = 0.055) rates were not significantly different between groups A1 and A2. In group B, the MACCE (aHR, 1.236; 95% CI, 0.913–1.673; p = 0.171), all-cause death (aHR, 1.065; p = 0.869), CD (aHR, 1.359; p = 0.527), non-CD (aHR, 1.447; p = 0.570), re-MI (aHR, 1.259; p = 0.478), any repeat revascularization (aHR, 1.289; p = 0.145), stroke (aHR, 1.523; p = 0.299), and ST (definite or probable, aHR, 4.152; 95% CI, 0.501–32.82; p = 0.101) rates were not significantly different between groups B1 and B2. In the total study population, MACCE (aHR, 1.199; 95% CI, 0.995–1.445; p = 0.056), all-cause death (aHR, 1.078; p = 0.636), CD (aHR, 1.060; p = 0.780), non-CD (aHR, 1.281; p = 0.313), re-MI (aHR, 1.034; p = 0.864), any repeat revascularization (aHR, 1.258; p = 0.056), stroke (aHR, 1.351; p = 0.175), and ST (definite or probable, aHR, 1.091; 95% CI, 0.449–2.651; p = 0.847) rates were not significantly different between the EI (group A1+B1) and DI (group A2+B2) groups (Table 2). These results were confirmed after PS-adjusted analysis. After PS-adjusted analysis in both groups A and B, the primary and secondary clinical outcomes were not significantly different between groups A1 and A2 or groups B1 and B2 (Table 2). To provide more meaningful insights with a cut-off age of 75 or 80 years, the major clinical outcomes were reanalyzed according to the two cut-off ages of the study population (Supplementary Tables S4 and S5). It was observed that regardless of the cut-off age, the primary and secondary clinical outcomes were not significantly different between groups A1 and A2 or groups B1 and B2.

Table 2. Comparison of clinical outcomes at 2 years.

Outcomes	Group A (Age, ≥65 Years, n = 2253)								
	Group A1 Early Invasive (n = 1612)	Group A2 Delayed Invasive (n = 641)	Log-Rank	Unadjusted HR (95% CI)	p	Multivariable-Adjusted [a] HR (95% CI)	p	Propensity score-Adjusted HR (95% CI)	p
MACCE	265 (16.4)	97 (15.1)	0.434	1.097 (0.869–1.384)	0.435	1.198 (0.944–1.521)	0.137	1.176 (0.889–1.500)	0.255
All-cause death	118 (7.5)	47 (7.5)	0.997	0.999 (0.713–1.401)	0.997	1.150 (0.810–1.633)	0.434	1.269 (0.850–1.894)	0.244
Cardiac death	63 (4.0)	27 (4.3)	0.749	0.929 (0.592–1.458)	0.749	1.100 (0.687–1.761)	0.692	1.127 (0.694–1.913)	0.659
Non-cardiac death	55 (3.5)	20 (3.2)	0.729	1.095 (0.656–1.826)	0.729	1.207 (0.712–2.043)	0.485	1.487 (0.803–2.753)	0.207
Recurrent MI	60 (3.9)	24 (3.9)	0.980	0.994 (0.619–1.595)	0.980	1.061 (0.654–1.722)	0.809	1.035 (0.584–1.653)	0.907
Any repeat revascularization	146 (9.4)	50 (8.1)	0.325	1.175 (0.852–1.620)	0.326	1.247 (0.899–1.730)	0.186	1.236 (0.843–1.710)	0.277
Stroke	44 (2.8)	22 (3.6)	0.380	0.796 (0.477–1.327)	0.381	1.255 (0.745–2.114)	0.394	1.067 (0.570–2.000)	0.839
ST (definite or probable)	8 (0.5)	6 (1.0)	0.231	0.529 (0.184–1.525)	0.239	2.969 (0.978–9.017)	0.055	1.490 (0.421–5.281)	0.537
Outcomes	Group B (Age, <65 Years, n = 2260)								
	Group B1 Early Invasive (n = 1688)	Group B2 Delayed Invasive (n = 572)	Log-Rank	Unadjusted HR (95% CI)	p	Multivariable-Adjusted [a] HR (95% CI)	p	Propensity score-Adjusted HR (95% CI)	p
MACCE	185 (11.0)	56 (9.8)	0.457	1.120 (0.831–1.510)	0.458	1.236 (0.913–1.673)	0.171	1.317 (0.918–1.890)	0.135
All-cause death	24 (1.5)	14 (2.5)	0.098	0.577 (0.299–1.116)	0.102	1.065 (0.506–2.239)	0.869	1.583 (0.614–4.085)	0.342
Cardiac death	13 (0.8)	10 (1.8)	0.044	0.438 (0.192–0.999)	0.050	1.359 (0.525–3.517)	0.527	1.024 (0.212–2.984)	0.925
Non-cardiac death	11 (0.7)	4 (0.7)	0.892	0.924 (0.294–2.901)	0.892	1.447 (0.405–5.172)	0.570	1.505 (0.517–6.102)	0.342
Recurrent MI	42 (2.4)	13 (2.3)	0.784	1.091 (0.586–2.032)	0.784	1.259 (0.666–2.382)	0.478	1.147 (0.746–2.411)	0.717
Any repeat revascularization	155 (9.2)	43 (7.6)	0.246	1.221 (0.871–1.711)	0.247	1.289 (0.917–1.813)	0.145	1.347 (0.921–2.018)	0.149
Stroke	17 (1.0)	10 (1.8)	0.151	0.569 (0.260–1.242)	0.157	1.523 (0.688–3.369)	0.299	1.446 (0.551–3.109)	0.454
ST (definite or probable)	10 (0.6)	1 (0.2)	0.218	3.376 (0.432–26.37)	0.246	4.152 (0.501–32.82)	0.101	2.984 (0.310–23.68)	0.344
Outcomes	Early Invasive Group A1 + B1 (n = 3300)	Delayed Invasive Group A2 + B2 (n = 1213)	Log-Rank	Unadjusted HR (95% CI)	p	Multivariable-Adjusted [a] HR (95% CI)	p	Propensity Score-Adjusted HR (95% CI)	p
MACCE	450 (13.6)	153 (12.6)	0.380	1.086 (0.904–1.304)	0.380	1.199 (0.995–1.445)	0.056	1.225 (0.998–1.528)	0.071
All-cause death	142 (4.3)	61 (5.1)	0.295	0.852 (0.631–1.150)	0.295	1.078 (0.790–1.470)	0.636	1.130 (0.798–1.630)	0.512
Cardiac death	76 (2.3)	37 (3.1)	0.154	0.752 (0.508–1.144)	0.155	1.060 (0.704–1.595)	0.780	1.058 (0.655–1.521)	0.807
Non-cardiac death	66 (2.0)	24 (2.0)	0.980	1.006 (0.631–1.605)	0.980	1.281 (0.792–2.074)	0.313	1.451 (0.821–2.566)	0.200
Recurrent MI	102 (3.2)	37 (3.1)	0.960	1.010 (0.693–1.471)	0.960	1.034 (0.706–1.516)	0.864	1.029 (0.654–1.498)	0.902
Any repeat revascularization	301 (9.3)	93 (7.9)	0.132	1.195 (0.947–1.508)	0.133	1.258 (0.994–1.591)	0.056	1.235 (0.975–1.575)	0.075
Stroke	61 (1.9)	32 (2.7)	0.095	0.696 (0.454–1.067)	0.097	1.351 (0.875–2.087)	0.175	1.037 (0.635–1.812)	0.792
ST (definite or probable)	18 (0.6)	7 (0.6)	0.893	0.942 (0.393–2.255)	0.893	1.091 (0.449–2.651)	0.847	1.001 (0.351–2.553)	0.999

MACCE, major adverse cardiac and cerebrovascular events; ST, stent thrombosis; HR, hazard ratio; CI, confidence interval; LVEF, left ventricular ejection fraction; BMI, body mass index; SBP, systolic blood pressure; DBP, diastolic blood pressure; DM, diabetes mellitus; PCI, percutaneous coronary intervention; HF, heart failure; CK-MB, creatine kinase myocardial band; eGFR, estimated glomerular filtration rate; HDL, high-density lipoprotein; LDL, low-density lipoprotein; GRACE, Global Registry of Acute Coronary Events; ACEIs, angiotensin-converting enzyme inhibitors; ARBs, angiotensin receptor blockers. [a] Adjusted by male sex, LVEF, BMI, SBP, DBP, symptom-to-door time, Killip class 3, hypertension, DM, dyslipidemia, previous PCI, previous HF, previous stroke, current smoker, peak CK-MB, peak troponin-I, serum creatinine, eGFR < 60 mL/min/1.73 m^2, HDL-cholesterol, LDL-cholesterol, GRACE risk score >140, clopidogrel, ticagrelor, prasugrel, ACEI or ARB, and statin.

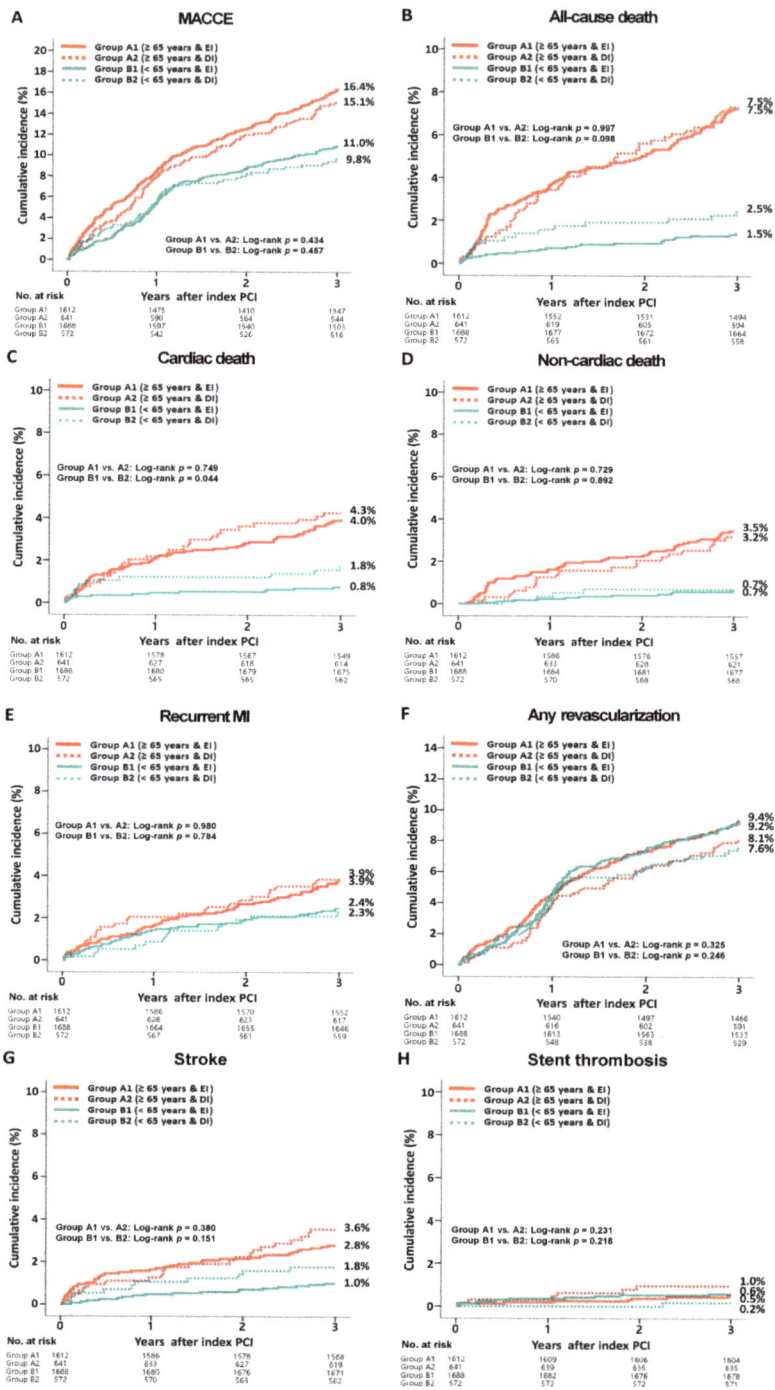

Figure 2. Kaplan-Meier curved analysis for MACCE (**A**), all-cause death (**B**), cardiac death (**C**), non-cardiac death (**D**), recurrent MI (**E**), any repeat revascularization (**F**), stroke (**G**), and stent thrombosis (**H**). MACCE, major adverse cardiac and cerebrovascular events; MI, myocardial infarction; PCI, percutaneous coronary intervention; EI, early invasive; DI, delayed invasive.

For further assessment of major clinical outcomes between the EI and DI groups of groups A and B, we compared these major clinical outcomes by limiting the study population to patients with complex lesions (Table 3). The number of patients with complex lesions in each group was >40% (group A1, 49.6%; group A2, 55.5%; group B1, 40.9%; group B2, 46.5%) (Figure 3). The MACCE rates were similar between the EI and DI groups (group A1 vs. group A2; aHR, 1.149; 95% CI, 0.843–1.564; p = 0.379; group B1 vs. group B2; aHR, 1.136; 95% CI, 0.754–1.713; p = 0.542) (Table 3). The ST (definite or probable) rates were also similar between the EI and DI groups (group A1 vs. group A2; aHR, 3.777; 95% CI, 0.673–116.94; p = 0.139; group B1 vs. group B2; aHR, 1.140; 95% CI, 0.030–43.82; p = 0.944, Table 3). Additionally, all-cause death, CD, non-CD, re-MI, any repeat revascularization, and stroke rates were not significantly different between the EI and DI groups after adjustment (Table 3). Figure 4 shows the subgroup analysis for MACCE in groups A and B. The results of the subgroup analysis using the Cox logistic regression model revealed that all subgroups, except for those showing significant p-for-interaction, demonstrated comparable MACCE rates in this study.

Table 3. Comparison of clinical outcomes in patient with complex coronary lesions.

Outcomes	Group A (Age, ≥65 Years, n = 2253)						
	Group A1 Early Invasive (n = 799)	Group A2 Delayed Invasive (n = 356)	Log-Rank	Unadjusted HR (95% CI)	p	Multivariable-Adjusted [a] HR (95% CI)	p
MACCE	141 (17.6)	61 (17.1)	0.829	1.034 (0.765–1.396)	0.829	1.149 (0.843–1.564)	0.379
All-cause death	64 (8.2)	27 (7.7)	0.814	1.056 (0.673–1.655)	0.814	1.254 (0.784–2.006)	0.345
Cardiac death	31 (4.0)	16 (4.5)	0.632	0.863 (0.472–1.578)	0.632	1.021 (0.539–1.934)	0.949
Non-cardiac death	33 (4.2)	11 (3.2)	0.404	1.336 (0.675–2.643)	0.406	1.616 (0.794–3.286)	0.185
Recurrent MI	31 (4.0)	14 (4.1)	0.966	0.986 (0.525–1.854)	0.966	1.097 (0.574–2.097)	0.780
Any repeat revascularization	76 (9.9)	35 (10.3)	0.893	0.973 (0.652–1.452)	0.893	1.041 (0.691–1.568)	0.849
Stroke	25 (3.2)	14 (4.1)	0.490	0.795 (0.413–1.529)	0.491	1.338 (0.688–2.601)	0.391
ST (definite or probable)	4 (0.5)	3 (0.9)	0.488	0.592 (0.133–2.646)	0.493	3.777 (0.673–16.94)	0.139
Outcomes	Group B (Age, <65 Years, n = 977)						
	Group B1 Early Invasive (n = 691)	Group B2 Delayed Invasive (n = 286)	Log-Rank	Unadjusted HR (95% CI)	p	Multivariable-Adjusted [a] HR (95% CI)	p
MACCE	89 (12.9)	33 (12.4)	0.892	1.028 (0.689–1.533)	0.892	1.136 (0.754–1.713)	0.542
All-cause death	12 (1.7)	10 (3.8)	0.062	0.458 (0.198–1.061)	0.068	1.005 (0.384–2.629)	0.991
Cardiac death	7 (1.0)	6 (2.3)	0.136	0.446 (0.150–1.327)	0.147	0.968 (0.285–3.288)	0.958
Non-cardiac death	5 (0.7)	4 (1.5)	0.258	0.476 (0.128–1.774)	0.269	1.026 (0.174–6.046)	0.978
Recurrent MI	14 (2.0)	5 (1.9)	0.892	1.073 (0.687–2.980)	0.892	1.347 (0.471–3.856)	0.579
Any repeat revascularization	74 (10.8)	25 (9.6)	0.614	1.124 (0.714–1.768)	0.614	1.136 (0.716–1.802)	0.589
Stroke	6 (0.9)	8 (3.1)	0.013	0.293 (0.098–0.815)	0.019	2.923 (0.949–9.002)	0.062
ST (definite or probable)	1 (0.1)	1 (0.4)	0.480	3.383 (0.024–6.117)	0.497	1.140 (0.030–43.82)	0.944

MACCE, major adverse cardiac and cerebrovascular events; ST, stent thrombosis; HR, hazard ratio; CI, confidence interval; LVEF, left ventricular ejection fraction; BMI, body mass index; SBP, systolic blood pressure; DBP, diastolic blood pressure; DM, diabetes mellitus; PCI, percutaneous coronary intervention; HF, heart failure; CK-MB, creatine kinase myocardial band; eGFR, estimated glomerular filtration rate; HDL, high-density lipoprotein; LDL, low-density lipoprotein; GRACE, Global Registry of Acute Coronary Events; ACEIs, angiotensin-converting enzyme inhibitors; ARBs, angiotensin receptor blockers. [a] Adjusted by male sex, LVEF, BMI, SBP, DBP, symptom-to-door time, Killip class 3, hypertension, DM, dyslipidemia, previous PCI, previous HF, previous stroke, current smoker, peak CK-MB, peak troponin-I, serum creatinine, eGFR < 60 mL/min/1.73 m^2, HDL-cholesterol, LDL-cholesterol, GRACE risk score > 140, clopidogrel, ticagrelor, prasugrel, ACEI or ARB, statin.

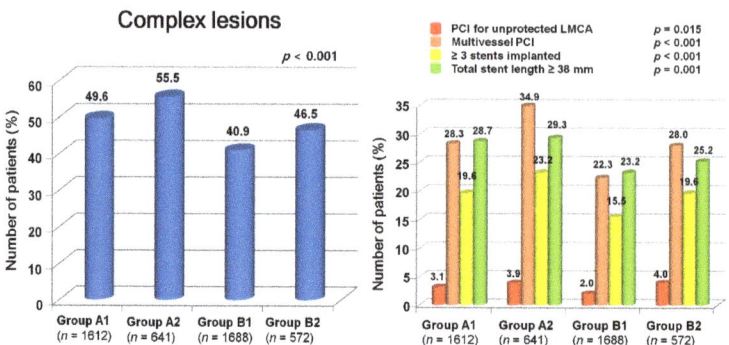

Figure 3. Distribution of complex lesions in the 4 groups. Group A1, ≥65 years and early invasive; Group A2, ≥65 years and delayed invasive; Group B1, <65 years and early invasive; Group B2, <65 years and delayed invasive, PCI percutaneous coronary intervention, LMCA left main coronary artery.

A ≥65 years

Subgroup	Early invasive	Delayed invasive	HR (95% CI)	p value	p-for interaction
All patients	265/1612	97/641	1.09 (0.86–1.38)	0.435	
Sex					0.188
Male	160/927	56/371	1.16 (0.85–1.57)	0.329	
Female	105/685	41/270	1.00 (0.70–1.44)	0.961	
LVEF, %					0.461
<50	106/514	54/241	0.91 (0.66–1.27)	0.606	
≥50	159/1098	43/400	1.38 (0.98–1.93)	0.062	
Hypertension					0.006
Yes	192/1050	67/427	1.18 (0.89–1.56)	0.231	
No	73/562	30/214	0.92 (0.60–1.41)	0.714	
Diabetes mellitus					0.160
Yes	102/567	45/227	0.90 (0.63–1.28)	0.569	
No	163/1045	52/414	1.26 (0.92–1.72)	0.141	
eGFR (mL/min/1.73m²)					0.048
<60	125/570	51/269	1.18 (0.85–1.63)	0.319	
≥60	140/1042	46/372	1.09 (0.78–1.52)	0.589	
GRACE risk score					0.013
≤140	181/979	70/390	1.25 (0.81–1.94)	0.301	
>140	84/633	27/251	1.03 (0.78–1.36)	0.800	
Mutivessel disease					0.139
Yes	141/799	61/356	1.03 (0.76–1.39)	0.829	
No	124/813	36/285	1.22 (0.84–1.78)	0.276	

B <65 years

Subgroup	Early invasive	Delayed invasive	HR (95% CI)	p value	p-for interaction
All patients	185/1688	56/572	1.12 (0.83–1.51)	0.458	
Sex					0.740
Male	160/1476	50/513	1.11 (0.81–1.52)	0.510	
Female	25/212	6/59	1.15 (0.47–2.82)	0.747	
LVEF, %					0.772
<50	51/356	15/131	1.26 (0.71–2.24)	0.479	
≥50	134/1332	41/441	1.07 (0.76–1.53)	0.670	
Hypertension					0.001
Yes	92/662	22/243	1.57 (0.98–2.50)	0.057	
No	93/1026	34/329	0.86 (0.58–1.28)	0.465	
Diabetes mellitus					<0.001
Yes	65/408	28/408	0.85 (0.55–1.33)	0.496	
No	120/1280	28/1280	1.41 (0.93–2.13)	0.098	
eGFR (mL/min/1.73m²)					0.098
<60	37/193	17/86	0.96 (0.54–1.70)	0.894	
≥60	148/1495	39/486	1.24 (0.87–1.76)	0.231	
GRACE risk score					0.084
≤140	160/1517	15/491	1.26 (0.90–1.78)	0.175	
>140	25/171	41/81	0.78 (0.41–1.48)	0.458	
Complex lesions					0.027
Yes	89/691	33/266	1.02 (0.68–1.53)	0.892	
No	96/997	23/306	1.29 (0.85–2.04)	0.267	

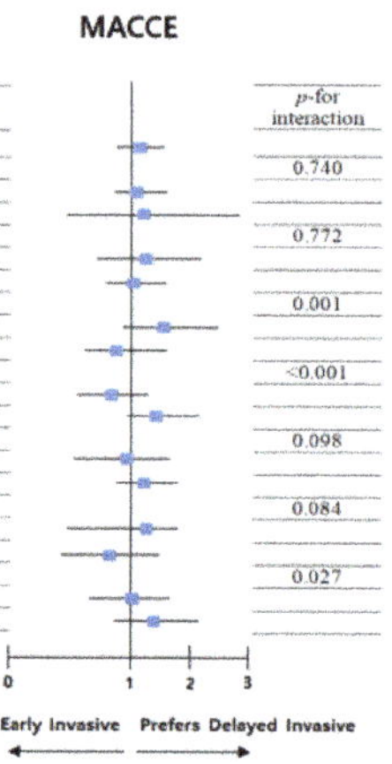

Figure 4. Subgroup analysis for MACCE in older (**A**) and younger (**B**) adults. MACCE, major adverse cardiac events; HR, hazard ratio; CI, confidence interval; LVEF, left ventricular ejection fraction; eGFR, estimated glomerular filtration rate; GRACE, Global Registry of Acute Coronary Events.

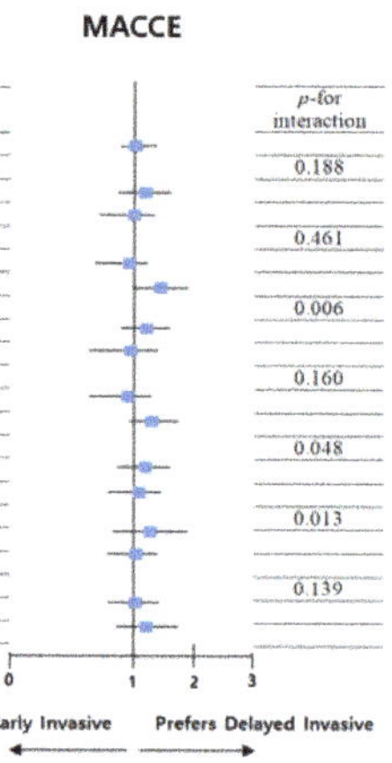

4. Discussion

The main findings of this prospective observational study were as follows: (1) in both older and younger groups, after multivariable-adjusted and PS-adjusted analyses, MACCE, all-cause death, CD, non-CD, re-MI, any repeat revascularization, stroke, and ST (definite or probable) rates were similar between the EI and DI groups; (2) even after limiting the study population to patients who had complex lesions in both older and younger groups, the primary and secondary clinical outcomes were not significantly different between the EI and DI groups.

The merits of the EI strategy include early identification of significant lesions, early revascularization, and facilitation of earlier discharge from a facility [21]. In contrast, the DI strategy may provide adequate time for optimal medical treatment to decrease the thrombus burden and improve plaque stability [21]. In general, older individuals presenting with ACS tend to have clinical complexity, frailty, and high-risk coronary lesions [22]. Moreover, the clinical presentation of NSTE-ACS in older adults is atypical [10], and the electrocardiographic changes are less frequent in older patients than in younger patients [23]. Because of evidence-based therapy, there was a significant decrease in mortality and morbidities associated with ACS [24]. However, the improvements in ACS treatment strategy have not equally improved outcomes for older adults [7]. Additionally, there is a paucity of evidence to guide the selection of the EI or DI strategy in elderly patients with NSTE-ACS [25]. Although previous reports [26,27] demonstrated significant beneficial effects of the EI strategy compared with conservative treatment in elderly patients with NSTE-ACS, these studies were not performed in the era of new-generation DESs and did not compare clinical outcomes between the EI and DI strategies. We know that the 3-year follow-up period in this study was insufficient to estimate long-term clinical outcomes. To overcome insufficient information concerning comparative clinical outcomes between the EI and DI strategies in older and younger adults with NSTEMI undergoing successful new-generation DES implantation, we attempted to investigate the 3-year clinical outcomes, which were not a long time. The definition of older adults is controversial. In general, a person aged ≥ 60 or 65 years is considered an older adult [28]. The average age at which individuals experience a first heart attack is 65.8 years for men and 70.4 years for women [29]. Additionally, based on the Consensus Development Conference on Diabetes and Older Adults (age ≥ 65 years) convened by the American Diabetes Association in February 2012 [30] and another report [31], which showed that multimorbidity and polypharmacy are highly prevalent among adults aged ≥ 65 years, we set the cut-off age at ≥ 65 years for older adults in our study.

In the case of neointimal hyperplasia and repeated revascularization, a DES, in which a pharmaceutically active agent is coated onto a bare-metal stent (BMS) along with a drug-carrying polymer, is used to lower the risks posed by BMSs [7]. Although DESs are carefully designed to reduce ST, the risk of late ST and restenosis is seen with DES use in clinical trials [7,32]. The introduction of the 1G-DES (Cypher and Taxus) revolutionized the field of interventional cardiology, but second-generation DESs (2G-DES; Xience, Promus) are the gold standard of stent technology because they not only resolved the problems associated with 1G-DES (such as inflammation and restenosis) but also decreased the mortality rate [33].

The current guidelines suggest that older patients with NSTE-ACS should be considered for invasive management with CAG and PCI [6,7]. However, the key study underpinning the current guidelines [6,7] was the TIMACS trial [1]. Although this study [1] showed valuable results for understanding the beneficial effect of EI CAG in patients with ACS, this study was conducted between April 2003 and June 2008; approximately 45% of the cases used BMSs, and the type of DES was not confined to the new-generation DES. Additionally, <60% of the patients underwent PCI. In our study, in both older and younger groups, the major clinical outcomes were not significantly different between the EI and DI groups after adjustments (multivariable or PS-adjusted) during a 3-year follow-up period. Regarding the limitations of the TIMACS trial [1], our study results could be more impactful with respect to reflecting the current real-world practices. As shown in Table 3, we performed additional analysis to clearly estimate long-term clinical outcomes between the EI and DI groups. Even after considering patients with complex lesions [16,17], the 3-year major clinical outcomes were not significantly different between the two groups (Table 3). Subgroup analyses for MACCE in groups A and B (Figure 4) showed that all subgroups except for those showing significant p-for-interaction had comparable MACCE rates.

The proportion of men decreased with age in group A ($\geq$65 years) compared with group B (<65 years) in our study. Additionally, comorbidities including hypertension, diabetes mellitus, previous MI, previous HF, previous stroke, and renal insufficiency (eGFR <60 mL/min/1.73 m^2) were more prevalent in group A than in group B (Table 1). Therefore, the patient characteristics in this study are consistent with previously published data [29,34]. This increasing prevalence of cardiovascular disease with aging has been attributed to several age-related changes, including vascular wall elasticity, coagulation, the hemostatic system, and endothelial dysfunction [35–37]. Hence, age-related decline in organ function could increase cardiovascular diseases [37].

An age subgroup analysis [31] from the Treat Angina with Aggrastat and Determine Cost of Therapy with an Invasive or Conservative Strategy—Thrombolysis in Myocardial Infarction 18 (TACTICS-TIMI 18) trial [38] showed that the EI strategy yielded a greater absolute (4.1% vs. 1%) and relative (42% vs. 20.4%) risk reduction in mortality or MI at 30 days in the $\geq$65 years of age subgroup compared with younger patients. However, this benefit coexisted with a 3-fold higher risk of major bleeding with the EI strategy in patients $\geq$75 years of age (16.6% vs. 6.5%; $p = 0.009$). Thus, compared with younger patients, older patients gain greater absolute and relative benefits from the EI strategy but with increased bleeding risk [10]. However, similar to the TIMACS trial [1], the types of deployed stents were not confined to new-generation DESs in these studies [31,38].

The current guideline [6] suggests that the management of older patients should be based on ischemic and bleeding risks, estimated life expectancy, comorbidities, the need for non-cardiac surgery, quality of life, frailty, cognitive and functional impairment, patient values and preferences, and estimated risks and benefits of revascularization. We agree with this suggestion. Interestingly, in the era of new-generation DESs, the major clinical outcomes were not significantly different between the EI and DI strategies in both older and younger adults with NSTEMI during a 3-year follow-up period in our study. In the present study, although the population size may have been insufficient to provide meaningful results, 20 tertiary high-volume university hospitals participated in the registry. Therefore, we believe that our results could provide helpful information to interventional cardiologists in terms of the long-term effects of the EI and DI strategies in older and younger adults with NSTEMI undergoing successful new-generation DES implantation. Based on our results, we can conclude that elderly patients with several comorbidities and a relatively mild NSTEMI would receive a more "planned" (hence delayed) treatment. It is reassuring to note that this does not lead to inferior clinical outcomes. However, we could not completely explain the comparable clinical outcomes between the various study groups. It may be an important shortcoming of the non-randomized registry study.

In our study, although the number of patients with multivessel disease (average > 55%) and type B2/C lesions (average > 80%) were higher, the LVEF was normal (average > 62%). The number of patients with multivessel disease and type B2/C lesions in our study may have increased after applying the exclusion criteria, as shown in Figure 1. Moreover, the baseline characteristics of our study are similar to those in recent publications based on the KAMIR-NIH [39,40].

This study had some limitations. First, although this study was based on a prospective observational registry, it is not a randomized controlled study, and there may have been selection bias. Second, bleeding is a serious complication that occurs after PCI in older adults [26,27]; however, anti-platelet therapy after 1 year index PCI was different among physicians; therefore, we could not include bleeding as an outcome parameter in our study during the 3-year follow-up period—this is a major shortcoming of our study. Third, because we set the cut-off age for older adults at ≥65 years, our results may change according to different cut-off ages. Fourth, despite the multivariable and PS-adjusted analyses, variables that were not included in the data registry may have affected the study outcome. Fifth, the 3-year follow-up period was insufficient to evaluate long-term adverse events. Sixth, although the number of coronary bifurcation lesions, type and incidence of procedural complications (no-reflow, coronary dissections, etc.), characteristics of calcified coronary lesions, and use of rotational atherectomy may have impacted the outcome and important variables for long-term prognosis, these variables were not mandatory in the KAMIR-NIH data. Hence, we could not provide this information in our study. Finally, there were substantial differences between the EI and DI cohorts. For example, the fact that peak troponin was higher and TIMI flow 0/1 was more often present in the EI groups indicates a selection bias for more severe NSTEMI cases being treated earlier (which is to be expected in the registry setting). Yet, the DI group had more comorbidities. The PS-adjusted analysis attempts to compensate for this but is still not ideal. To really prove that the EI strategy does not improve outcomes compared with the DI strategy, a randomized trial is required.

5. Conclusions

In conclusion, in both older and younger adults with NSTEMI, the EI and DI strategies showed comparable clinical outcomes after successful new-generation DES implantation during a 3-year follow-up period. However, to clarify the differences in clinical outcomes between these two reperfusion strategies in those patients, further randomized, large-scale, and long-term follow-up studies are needed.

Supplementary Materials: The following supporting information can be downloaded at: https://www.mdpi.com/article/10.3390/jcm11164780/s1. Table S1: Results of collinearity test for MACCE, Table S2: Comparison of baseline characteristics before and after PSM, Table S3: Baseline characteristics of the total study population. Table S4: Clinical outcomes between the age ≥ 75 years and <75 years groups at 2 years. Table S5: Clinical outcomes between the age ≥ 80 years and <80 years groups at 2 years.

Author Contributions: Conceptualization, Y.H.K., A.-Y.H., S.-W.R., C.U.C., B.G.C., J.B.K., S.P., D.O.K., J.Y.P., S.-H.P. and M.H.J.; Data curation, Y.H.K., A.-Y.H., B.G.C., S.P. and D.O.K.; Formal analysis, Y.H.K., A.-Y.H., B.G.C., S.P. and D.O.K.; Funding acquisition, M.H.J.; Investigation, Y.H.K., A.-Y.H., S.-W.R., C.U.C., B.G.C., J.B.K., S.P., D.O.K., J.Y.P., S.-H.P. and M.H.J.; Methodology, Y.H.K., A.-Y.H., S.-W.R., C.U.C., B.G.C., J.B.K., S.P., D.O.K., J.Y.P., S.-H.P. and M.H.J.; Project administration, Y.H.K., A.-Y.H., S.-W.R., C.U.C., J.B.K., J.Y.P., S.-H.P. and M.H.J.; Resources, S.-W.R., C.U.C., B.G.C., J.B.K., S.P., D.O.K. and M.H.J.; Software, Y.H.K., A.-Y.H., J.B.K., S.P. and D.O.K.; Supervision, Y.H.K., S.-W.R. and M.H.J.; Validation, Y.H.K., A.-Y.H., S.-W.R., C.U.C., B.G.C., J.B.K., S.P., D.O.K. and M.H.J.; Visualization, Y.H.K., A.-Y.H., S.-W.R., C.U.C., B.G.C., J.B.K., S.P., D.O.K. and M.H.J.; Writing—original draft, Y.H.K. and A.-Y.H.; Writing—review and editing, Y.H.K., A.-Y.H., S.-W.R., C.U.C., B.G.C., J.B.K., S.P., D.O.K., J.Y.P., S.-H.P. and M.H.J. All authors have read and agreed to the published version of the manuscript.

Funding: This research was supported by a fund (2016-ER6304-02) by Research of Korea Centers for Disease Control and Prevention.

Institutional Review Board Statement: The study was conducted according to the guidelines of the Declaration of Helsinki and approved by the Chonnam National University Hospital Institutional Review Board (IRB) ethics committee (protocol code CNUH-2011-172 and 1 March 2011).

Informed Consent Statement: Informed written consent was obtained from all subjects involved in this study.

Data Availability Statement: Data are contained within the article or supplementary material.

Acknowledgments: Investigators of KAMIR-NIH (Korea Acute Myocardial Infarction Registry-National Institutes of Health) Myung Ho Jeong, Chonnam National University Hospital, Gwangju, Korea, Young Jo Kim, Yeungnam University Medical Center, Daegu, Korea, Chong Jin Kim, Kyunghee University Hospital at Gangdong, Seoul, Korea, Myeong Chan Cho, Chungbuk National University

Hospital, Cheongju, Korea, Hyo-Soo Kim, Seoul National University Hospital, Seoul, Korea, Hyeon-Cheol Gwon, Samsung Medical Center, Seoul, Korea, Ki Bae Seung, Seoul St. Mary's Hospital, Seoul, Korea, Dong Joo Oh, Korea University Guro Hospital, Seoul, Korea, Shung Chull Chae, Kyungpook National University Hospital, Daegu, Korea, Kwang Soo Cha, Pusan National University Hospital, Busan, Korea, Junghan Yoon, Wonju Severance Christian Hospital, Wonju, Korea, Jei-Keon Chae, Chonbuk National University Hospital, Jeonju, Korea, Seung Jae Joo, Jeju National University Hospital, Jeju, Korea, Dong-Ju Choi, Seoul National University Bundang Hospital, Bundang, Korea, Seung-Ho Hur, Keimyung University Dongsan Medical Center, Daegu, Korea, In Whan Seong, Chungnam National University Hospital, Daejeon, Korea, Doo Il Kim, Inje University Haeundae Paik Hospital, Busan, Korea, Seok Kyu Oh, Wonkwang University Hospital, Iksan, Korea, Tae Hoon Ahn, Gachon University Gil Medical Center, Incheon, Korea, Jin-Yong Hwang, Gyeongsang National University Hospital, Jinju, Korea.

Conflicts of Interest: The authors declare they do not have anything to disclose regarding conflict of interest with respect to this manuscript.

References

1. Mehta, S.R.; Granger, C.B.; Boden, W.E.; Steg, P.G.; Bassand, J.P.; Faxon, D.P.; Afzal, R.; Chrolavicius, S.; Jolly, S.S.; Widimsky, P.; et al. Early versus delayed invasive intervention in acute coronary syndromes. *N. Engl. J. Med.* **2009**, *360*, 2165–2175. [CrossRef]
2. Fox, K.A.; Clayton, T.C.; Damman, P.; Pocock, S.J.; de Winter, R.J.; Tijssen, J.G.; Lagerqvist, B.; Wallentin, L. Long-term outcome of a routine versus selective invasive strategy in patients with non-ST-segment elevation acute coronary syndrome a meta-analysis of individual patient data. *J. Am. Coll. Cariol.* **2010**, *55*, 2435–2445. [CrossRef] [PubMed]
3. Kofoed, K.F.; Kelbæk, H.; Hansen, P.R.; Torp-Pedersen, C.; Høfsten, D.; Kløvgaard, L.; Holmvang, L.; Helqvist, S.; Jørgensen, E.; Galatius, S.; et al. Early Versus Standard Care Invasive Examination and Treatment of Patients With Non-ST-Segment Elevation Acute Coronary Syndrome. *Circulation* **2018**, *138*, 2741–2750. [CrossRef] [PubMed]
4. Jobs, A.; Mehta, S.R.; Montalescot, G.; Vicaut, E.; Van't Hof, A.W.J.; Badings, E.A.; Neumann, F.J.; Kastrati, A.; Sciahbasi, A.; Reuter, P.G.; et al. Optimal timing of an invasive strategy in patients with non-ST-elevation acute coronary syndrome: A meta-analysis of randomised trials. *Lancet* **2017**, *390*, 737–746. [CrossRef]
5. Bonello, L.; Laine, M.; Puymirat, E.; Lemesle, G.; Thuny, F.; Paganelli, F.; Michelet, P.; Roch, A.; Kerbaul, F.; Boyer, L. Timing of Coronary Invasive Strategy in Non-ST-Segment Elevation Acute Coronary Syndromes and Clinical Outcomes: An Updated Meta-Analysis. *JACC Cardiovasc. Interv.* **2016**, *9*, 2267–2276. [CrossRef]
6. Collet, J.P.; Thiele, H.; Barbato, E.; Barthélémy, O.; Bauersachs, J.; Bhatt, D.L.; Dendale, P.; Dorobantu, M.; Edvardsen, T.; Folliguet, T.; et al. 2020 ESC Guidelines for the management of acute coronary syndromes in patients presenting without persistent ST-segment elevation. *Eur. Heart J.* **2021**, *42*, 1289–1367. [CrossRef]
7. Amsterdam, E.A.; Wenger, N.K.; Brindis, R.G.; Casey, D.E., Jr.; Ganiats, T.G.; Holmes, D.R., Jr.; Jaffe, A.S.; Jneid, H.; Kelly, R.F.; Kontos, M.C.; et al. 2014 AHA/ACC Guideline for the Management of Patients with Non-ST-Elevation Acute Coronary Syndromes: A report of the American College of Cardiology/American Heart Association Task Force on Practice Guidelines. *J. Am. Coll. Cardiol.* **2014**, *64*, e139–e228. [CrossRef]
8. Kim, J.H.; Chae, S.C.; Oh, D.J.; Kim, H.S.; Kim, Y.J.; Ahn, Y.; Cho, M.C.; Kim, C.J.; Yoon, J.H.; Park, H.Y.; et al. Multicenter Cohort Study of Acute Myocardial Infarction in Korea-Interim Analysis of the Korea Acute Myocardial Infarction Registry-National Institutes of Health Registry. *Circ. J.* **2016**, *80*, 1427–1436. [CrossRef]
9. Grech, E.D. ABC of interventional cardiology: Percutaneous coronary intervention. II: The procedure. *BMJ* **2003**, *326*, 1137–1140. [CrossRef]
10. Levey, A.S.; Stevens, L.A.; Schmid, C.H.; Zhang, Y.L.; Castro, A.F., 3rd; Feldman, H.I.; Kusek, J.W.; Eggers, P.; Van Lente, F.; Greene, T.; et al. A new equation to estimate glomerular filtration rate. *Ann. Intern. Med.* **2009**, *150*, 604–612. [CrossRef]
11. Pieper, K.S.; Gore, J.M.; FitzGerald, G.; Granger, C.B.; Goldberg, R.J.; Steg, G.; Eagle, K.A.; Anderson, F.A.; Budaj, A.; Fox, K.A. Validity of a risk-prediction tool for hospital mortality: The Global Registry of Acute Coronary Events. *Am. Heart J.* **2009**, *157*, 1097–1105. [CrossRef] [PubMed]
12. Choi, K.H.; Song, Y.B.; Lee, J.M.; Lee, S.Y.; Park, T.K.; Yang, J.H.; Choi, J.H.; Choi, S.H.; Gwon, H.C.; Hahn, J.Y. Impact of Intravascular Ultrasound-Guided Percutaneous Coronary Intervention on Long-Term Clinical Outcomes in Patients Undergoing Complex Procedures. *JACC Cardiovasc. Interv.* **2019**, *12*, 607–620. [CrossRef] [PubMed]
13. Valgimigli, M.; Bueno, H.; Byrne, R.A.; Collet, J.P.; Costa, F.; Jeppsson, A.; Jüni, P.; Kastrati, A.; Kolh, P.; Mauri, L.; et al. 2017 ESC focused update on dual antiplatelet therapy in coronary artery disease developed in collaboration with EACTS: The Task Force for dual antiplatelet therapy in coronary artery disease of the European Society of Cardiology (ESC) and of the European Association for Cardio-Thoracic Surgery (EACTS). *Eur. Heart J.* **2018**, *39*, 213–260. [PubMed]
14. Sacco, R.L.; Kasner, S.E.; Broderick, J.P.; Caplan, L.R.; Connors, J.J.; Culebras, A.; Elkind, M.S.; George, M.G.; Hamdan, A.D.; Higashida, R.T.; et al. An updated definition of stroke for the 21st century: A statement for healthcare professionals from the American Heart Association/American Stroke Association. *Stroke* **2013**, *44*, 2064–2089. [CrossRef] [PubMed]

15. Lee, J.M.; Rhee, T.M.; Hahn, J.Y.; Kim, H.K.; Park, J.; Hwang, D.; Choi, K.H.; Kim, J.; Park, T.K.; Yang, J.H.; et al. Multivessel Percutaneous Coronary Intervention in Patients With ST-Segment Elevation Myocardial Infarction With Cardiogenic Shock. *J. Am. Coll. Cardiol.* **2018**, *71*, 844–856. [CrossRef]
16. Cutlip, D.E.; Windecker, S.; Mehran, R.; Boam, A.; Cohen, D.J.; van Es, G.A.; Steg, P.G.; Morel, M.A.; Mauri, L.; Vranckx, P.; et al. Clinical end points in coronary stent trials: A case for standardized definitions. *Circulation* **2007**, *115*, 2344–2351. [CrossRef]
17. Kim, Y.H.; Her, A.Y.; Jeong, M.H.; Kim, B.K.; Lee, S.Y.; Hong, S.J.; Shin, D.H.; Kim, J.S.; Ko, Y.G.; Choi, D.; et al. Impact of renin-angiotensin system inhibitors on long-term clinical outcomes in patients with acute myocardial infarction treated with successful percutaneous coronary intervention with drug-eluting stents: Comparison between STEMI and NSTEMI. *Atherosclerosis* **2019**, *280*, 166–173. [CrossRef]
18. Vatcheva, K.P.; Lee, M.; McCormick, J.B.; Rahbar, M.H. Multicollinearity in Regression Analyses Conducted in Epidemiologic Studies. *Epidemiology* **2016**, *6*, 227. [CrossRef]
19. Kim, J.H. Multicollinearity and misleading statistical results. *Korean J. Anesthesiol.* **2019**, *72*, 558–569. [CrossRef]
20. Kalantari, S.; Khalili, D.; Asgari, S.; Fahimfar, N.; Hadaegh, F.; Tohidi, M.; Azizi, F. Predictors of early adulthood hypertension during adolescence: A population-based cohort study. *BMC Public Health* **2017**, *17*, 915. [CrossRef]
21. Mahendiran, T.; Nanchen, D.; Meier, D.; Gencer, B.; Klingenberg, R.; Räber, L.; Carballo, D.; Matter, C.M.; Lüscher, T.F.; Windecker, S.; et al. Optimal Timing of Invasive Coronary Angiography following NSTEMI. *J. Interv. Cardiol.* **2020**, *2020*, 8513257. [CrossRef] [PubMed]
22. Kitagawa, T.; Yamamoto, H.; Urabe, Y.; Tsushima, H.; Utsunomiya, H.; Tatsugami, F.; Awai, K.; Kihara, Y. Age- and sex-related differences in coronary plaque high-risk features in patients with acute coronary syndrome assessed by computed tomography angiography. *Int. J. Cardiol.* **2014**, *174*, 744–747. [CrossRef] [PubMed]
23. Rosengren, A.; Wallentin, L.; Simoons, M.; Gitt, A.K.; Behar, S.; Battler, A.; Hasdai, D. Age, clinical presentation, and outcome of acute coronary syndromes in the Euroheart acute coronary syndrome survey. *Eur. Heart J.* **2006**, *27*, 789–795. [CrossRef] [PubMed]
24. Fox, K.A.; Steg, P.G.; Eagle, K.A.; Goodman, S.G.; Anderson, F.A., Jr.; Granger, C.B.; Flather, M.D.; Budaj, A.; Quill, A.; Gore, J.M. Decline in rates of death and heart failure in acute coronary syndromes, 1999–2006. *JAMA* **2007**, *297*, 1892–1900. [CrossRef] [PubMed]
25. González Ferrero, T.; Álvarez Álvarez, B.; Cordero, A.; Martinón Martínez, J.; Cacho Antonio, C.; Sestayo-Fernández, M.; Bouzas-Cruz, N.; Antúnez Muiños, P.; Casas, C.A.J.; Otero García, Ó.; et al. Early angiography in elderly patients with non-ST-segment elevation acute coronary syndrome: The cardio CHUS-HUSJ registry. *Int. J. Cardiol.* **2022**, *351*, 8–14. [CrossRef] [PubMed]
26. Bauer, T.; Koeth, O.; Jünger, C.; Heer, T.; Wienbergen, H.; Gitt, A.; Zahn, R.; Senges, J.; Zeymer, U. Effect of an invasive strategy on in-hospital outcome in elderly patients with non-ST-elevation myocardial infarction. *Eur. Heart J.* **2007**, *28*, 2873–2878. [CrossRef]
27. Bach, R.G.; Cannon, C.P.; Weintraub, W.S.; DiBattiste, P.M.; Demopoulos, L.A.; Anderson, H.V.; DeLucca, P.T.; Mahoney, E.M.; Murphy, S.A.; Braunwald, E. The effect of routine, early invasive management on outcome for elderly patients with non-ST-segment elevation acute coronary syndromes. *Ann. Intern. Med.* **2004**, *141*, 186–195. [CrossRef]
28. Kim, Y.H.; Her, A.Y.; Jeong, M.H.; Kim, B.K.; Hong, S.J.; Park, S.H.; Kim, B.G.; Kim, S.; Ahn, C.M.; Kim, J.S.; et al. Outcomes between prediabetes and type 2 diabetes mellitus in older adults with acute myocardial infarction in the era of newer-generation drug-eluting stents: A retrospective observational study. *BMC Geriatr.* **2021**, *21*, 653. [CrossRef]
29. Alexander, K.P.; Newby, L.K.; Cannon, C.P.; Armstrong, P.W.; Gibler, W.B.; Rich, M.W.; Van de Werf, F.; White, H.D.; Weaver, W.D.; Naylor, M.D.; et al. Acute coronary care in the elderly, part I: Non-ST-segment-elevation acute coronary syndromes: A scientific statement for healthcare professionals from the American Heart Association Council on Clinical Cardiology: In collaboration with the Society of Geriatric Cardiology. *Circulation* **2007**, *115*, 2549–2569.
30. Kirkman, M.S.; Briscoe, V.J.; Clark, N.; Florez, H.; Haas, L.B.; Halter, J.B.; Huang, E.S.; Korytkowski, M.T.; Munshi, M.N.; Odegard, P.S.; et al. Diabetes in older adults. *Diabetes Care* **2012**, *35*, 2650–2664. [CrossRef]
31. Barnett, K.; Mercer, S.W.; Norbury, M.; Watt, G.; Wyke, S.; Guthrie, B. Epidemiology of multimorbidity and implications for health care, research, and medical education: A cross-sectional study. *Lancet* **2012**, *380*, 37–43. [CrossRef]
32. Roffi, M.; Patrono, C.; Collet, J.P.; Mueller, C.; Valgimigli, M.; Andreotti, F.; Bax, J.J.; Borger, M.A.; Brotons, C.; Chew, D.P.; et al. 2015 ESC Guidelines for the management of acute coronary syndromes in patients presenting without persistent ST-segment elevation: Task Force for the Management of Acute Coronary Syndromes in Patients Presenting without Persistent ST-Segment Elevation of the European Society of Cardiology (ESC). *Eur. Heart J.* **2016**, *37*, 267–315. [PubMed]
33. Kim, Y.H.; Her, A.Y.; Jeong, M.H.; Kim, B.K.; Hong, S.J.; Kim, S.; Ahn, C.M.; Kim, J.S.; Ko, Y.G.; Choi, D.; et al. Effects of stent generation on clinical outcomes after acute myocardial infarction compared between prediabetes and diabetes patients. *Sci. Rep.* **2021**, *11*, 9364. [CrossRef]
34. Tegn, N.; Abdelnoor, M.; Aaberge, L.; Endresen, K.; Smith, P.; Aakhus, S.; Gjertsen, E.; Dahl-Hofseth, O.; Ranhoff, A.H.; Gullestad, L.; et al. Invasive versus conservative strategy in patients aged 80 years or older with non-ST-elevation myocardial infarction or unstable angina pectoris (After Eighty study): An open-label randomised controlled trial. *Lancet* **2016**, *387*, 1057–1065. [CrossRef]
35. Abbate, R.; Prisco, D.; Rostagno, C.; Boddi, M.; Gensini, G.F. Age-related changes in the hemostatic system. *Int. J. Clin. Lab. Res.* **1993**, *23*, 1–3. [CrossRef] [PubMed]
36. Brandes, R.P.; Fleming, I.; Busse, R. Endothelial aging. *Cardiovasc. Res.* **2005**, *66*, 286–294. [CrossRef] [PubMed]
37. Usta, C.; Bedel, A. Update on pharmacological treatment of acute coronary syndrome without persistent ST segment elevation myocardial infarction in the elderly. *J. Geriatr. Cariol.* **2017**, *14*, 457–464.

38. Cannon, C.P.; Weintraub, W.S.; Demopoulos, L.A.; Vicari, R.; Frey, M.J.; Lakkis, N.; Neumann, F.J.; Robertson, D.H.; DeLucca, P.T.; DiBattiste, P.M.; et al. Comparison of early invasive and conservative strategies in patients with unstable coronary syndromes treated with the glycoprotein IIb/IIIa inhibitor tirofiban. *N. Engl. J. Med.* **2001**, *344*, 1879–1887. [CrossRef]
39. Cho, K.H.; Han, X.; Ahn, J.H.; Hyun, D.Y.; Kim, M.C.; Sim, D.S.; Hong, Y.J.; Kim, J.H.; Ahn, Y.; Hwang, J.Y.; et al. KAMIR-NIH Investigators. Long-Term Outcomes of Patients With Late Presentation of ST-Segment Elevation Myocardial Infarction. *J. Am. Coll. Cardiol.* **2021**, *77*, 1859–1870. [CrossRef]
40. Kim, Y.; Bae, S.; Johnson, T.W.; Son, N.H.; Sim, D.S.; Hong, Y.J.; Kim, S.W.; Cho, D.K.; Kim, J.S.; Kim, B.K.; et al. Role of Intravascular Ultrasound-Guided Percutaneous Coronary Intervention in Optimizing Outcomes in Acute Myocardial Infarction. *J. Am. Heart Assoc.* **2022**, *11*, e023481. [CrossRef]

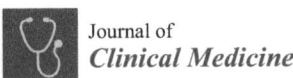

Article

Management and Outcomes in the Elderly with Non-ST-Elevation Acute Coronary Syndromes Admitted to Spoke Hospitals with No Catheterization Laboratory Facility

Francesca Mantovani [1,*], Gianluca Campo [2], Elisa Guerri [1], Francesco Manca [1], Massimo Calzolari [1], Giovanni Tortorella [3], Sergio Musto D'Amore [1], Gianluca Pignatelli [1], Vincenzo Guiducci [1] and Alessandro Navazio [1]

[1] Cardiology Unit, Azienda USL-IRCCS di Reggio Emilia, Viale Risorgimento 80, 42123 Reggio Emilia, Italy
[2] Cardiology Unit, Cardiovascular Institute, Translational Medicine Department, University of Ferrara, 44121 Ferrara, Italy
[3] Cardiology Unit, AUSL di Parma, Ospedale Vaio-Fidenza, 43036 Vaio, Italy
* Correspondence: francy_manto@hotmail.com

Abstract: Background: Contemporary guidelines advocate for early invasive strategy with coronary angiography in patients with non-ST-elevation acute coronary syndromes (NSTE-ACS). Still, the impact of an invasive strategy in older patients remains controversial and may be challenging in spoke hospitals with no catheterization laboratory (cath-lab) facility. Purpose: The purpose of this study was to analyse the characteristics and outcomes of patients ≥80 years old with NSTE-ACS admitted to spoke hospitals. Methods: Observational–retrospective study of all consecutive NSTE-ACS patients admitted to two spoke hospitals of our cardiology network, where a service strategy (same-day transfer between a spoke hospital and a hub centre with a cath-lab facility in order to perform coronary angiography) was available. Patients were followed up for 1 year after the admission date. Results: From 2013 to 2017, 639 patients were admitted for NSTE-ACS; of these, 181 (28%) were ≥80 years old (median 84, IQR 82–89) and represented the study cohort. When the invasive strategy was chosen (in 105 patients, or 58%), 98 patients (93%) were initially managed with a service strategy, whereas the remainder of the patients were transferred from the spoke hospital to the hub centre where they completed their hospital stay. Of the patients managed with the service strategy, a shift of strategy after the invasive procedure was necessary for 10 (10%). These patients remained in the hub centre, while the rest of the patients were sent back to the spoke hospitals, with no adverse events observed during the back transfer. The median time to access the cath-lab was 50 h (IQR 25–87), with 73 patients (70%) reaching the invasive procedure <72 h from hospital admission. A conservative strategy was associated with: older age, known CAD, clinical presentation with symptoms of LV dysfunction, lower EF, renal failure, higher GRACE score, presence of PAD and atrial fibrillation (all $p < 0.03$). At the 1-year follow-up, the overall survival was significantly higher in patients treated with an invasive strategy compared to patients managed conservatively (94% ± 2 vs. 54% ± 6, $p < 0.001$; HR: 10.4 [4.7–27.5] $p < 0.001$), even after adjustment for age, serum creatinine, known previous CAD and EF (adjusted HR: 2.0 [1.0–4.0]; $p < 0.001$). Conclusions: An invasive strategy may confer a survival benefit in the elderly with NSTE-ACS. The same-day transfer between a spoke hospital and a hub centre with a cath-lab facility (service strategy) is safe and may grant access to the cath-lab in a timely fashion, even for the elderly.

Keywords: elderly; service strategy; coronary artery angiography; acute coronary syndrome; spoke hospital; same-day transfer

Citation: Mantovani, F.; Campo, G.; Guerri, E.; Manca, F.; Calzolari, M.; Tortorella, G.; D'Amore, S.M.; Pignatelli, G.; Guiducci, V.; Navazio, A. Management and Outcomes in the Elderly with Non-ST-Elevation Acute Coronary Syndromes Admitted to Spoke Hospitals with No Catheterization Laboratory Facility. *J. Clin. Med.* 2022, 11, 6179. https://doi.org/10.3390/jcm11206179

Academic Editors: Claudio Montalto, Nuccia Morici and Aung Myat

Received: 21 July 2022
Accepted: 18 October 2022
Published: 20 October 2022

Publisher's Note: MDPI stays neutral with regard to jurisdictional claims in published maps and institutional affiliations.

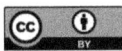

Copyright: © 2022 by the authors. Licensee MDPI, Basel, Switzerland. This article is an open access article distributed under the terms and conditions of the Creative Commons Attribution (CC BY) license (https://creativecommons.org/licenses/by/4.0/).

1. Background

Recent evidence has shown the advantages of an early invasive strategy (coronary angiography ± percutaneous coronary intervention (PCI)) for patients with intermediate–

high-risk non-ST-segment elevation acute coronary syndrome (NSTEACS) admitted to a hospital; such strategy is now recommended in the international guidelines [1]. However, these recommendations are based on large randomized trials with a mean age of participants of ~65 years and, since few patients in their 80s were enrolled, the survival benefit cannot be presupposed to translate to these patients [2]. In routine clinical practice, frail patients with several comorbidities are more likely to be treated non-invasively, whereas the fittest patients are more likely to undergo invasive management. Therefore, the rate of invasive coronary angiography declines with age; only 38% of patients with NSTEMI who are older than 80 years receive a coronary angiogram, compared with 78% of those aged 60 years or younger [3]. Moreover, practice gaps in patients' management have been noticed between hospitals with or without a catheterization laboratory (cath-lab) facility (hub centres vs. spoke centres) [4–8]. The service strategy is explained as the same-day transfer between the referring non-invasive spoke hospital and the hub centre with cath-lab facility; it has been shown to be a safe option and to minimise these inconsistencies [9–14]. The aim of this study was to retrospectively analyse the implementation of the service strategy and the 1-year outcomes of the elderly admitted in spoke hospitals of an Italian cardiology network.

2. Methods

2.1. Study Population and Data Collection

We retrospectively enrolled all consecutive patients aged ≥80 years [15], admitted to two spoke hospitals of our cardiology network in Reggio (Guastalla and Castelnovo nè Monti) and diagnosed with NSTEACS from January 2013 to December 2017.

NSTEACS patients were detected in data retrieved from hospital administrative systems using discharge diagnoses codes for non-ST-segment elevation myocardial infarction (NSTEMI) and unstable angina (UA) (International Classification of Diseases, Ninth Revision, Classification Modification, or ICD-9, codes: 410.7, 411.1, 411.81 and 411.89). The study population was divided into two groups according to the management chosen: invasive vs. conservative.

Hospital notes were examined for more information, whenever they were judged to be needed. All-cause death was the endpoint of the study. Follow-up information for death was acquired from the national death index, where the status of all citizens is securely and constantly updated and is 100% complete. Indeed, in Italy, it is mandatory by law that all deceased patients are instantly recorded in this national data bank. Since the present retrospective analysis did not alter the contemporary clinical practice in the reported institutions, the regulatory authorities did not require any supplementary written informed consent for data gathering. The ordinary written consent for coronary angiography and data privacy was acquired from all patients.

2.2. The Cardiology Network

Reggio Emilia is an area of the Italian Emilia-Romagna region with nearly 532,000 inhabitants. Hospitals are organized according to their facilities as follows: (a) one hub hospital with intensive cardiac care unit (ICCU) and catheterisation laboratory (cath-lab) with 24/7 service for primary PCI (Reggio Emilia); (b) two spoke hospitals with ICCU (Guastalla and Castelnovo nè Monti), whose data are object of the present study; (c) three spoke hospitals with internal medicine departments and cardiology consultation services without ICCU (Correggio, Scandiano, Montecchio) Figure 1.

Patients with NSTEACS, triaged by the emergency medical system or self-presenting, were generally admitted to the nearest hospital with ICCU, regardless of the presence of a catheterization laboratory. Only patients with NSTEACS and haemodynamic-instability criteria were sent straight to the hub centre. In the spoke hospitals, the NSTEACS patients' appropriateness for coronary angiography ± PCI was at the discretion of the clinician, after a stratification of ischaemic and bleeding risk with the GRACE score, and consideration of comorbidities and clinical status. If coronary angiography was suggested, the hub centre would be contacted to plan the procedure. According to the clinical case, patients could be managed with service strategy (see below definition), or with a strategy of transfer from the spoke hospital to the hub centre, where patients underwent coronary angiography ± PCI and concluded their hospital stay with no return to the spoke centre.

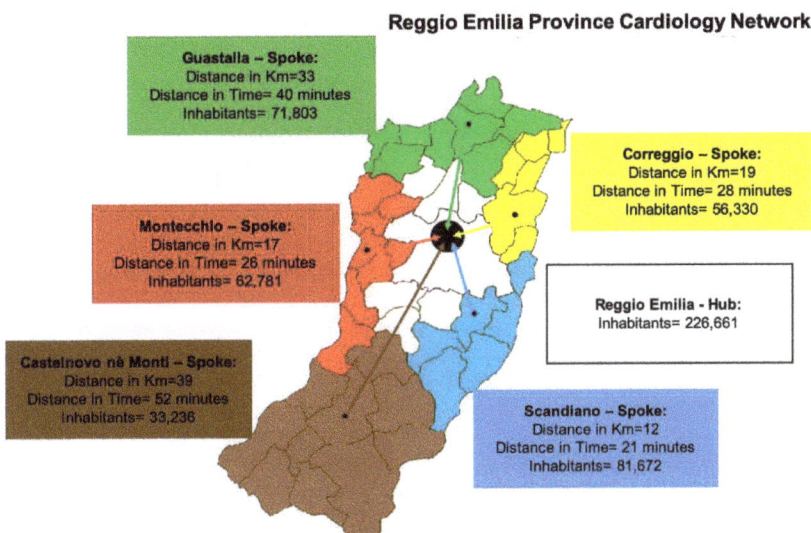

Figure 1. The cardiology network in Reggio Emilia. Six hospitals serve the Province of Reggio Emilia. Hospitals are organized according to their facilities: one invasive hub hospital with catheterisation laboratory (cath-lab) with 24/7 service (Reggio Emilia) and five non-invasive spoke hospitals (Guastalla and Castelnovo nè Monti, whose data are the object of the present study and Correggio, Scandiano, Montecchio). The distance between the spokes and the hub centres are expressed in km and time.

2.3. Service Strategy: Description

The service strategy has been formerly illustrated in detail in [11,13,14].

To briefly illustrate this strategy, the NSTEACS patients hospitalised in spoke hospitals were transferred to the cath-lab of the hub centre the day of coronary angiography. Once there, the interventional cardiologist revised the medical record and re-evaluated the suitability for the procedure. Then, coronary angiographies ± PCI were performed. All invasive procedures were performed according to the standard interventional technique. Medical therapy (including heparin, P2Y12 receptor inhibitors, aspirin, glycoprotein IIb/IIIa inhibitors and bivalirudin) was ordered according to contemporary guidelines [1].

After the coronary angiography, patients were monitored in the cath-lab recovery room for nearly 4–5 h. After this time (and within the same day), patients were sent back to the referring spoke centre, attended by basic-life-support-certified staff.

Severe angiographic complications, hemodynamic instability or logistical motivations were considered as reasons preventing the return to the referral centre.

2.4. Endpoint

The principal objective of the present study was to describe: (a) characteristics; (b) management and strategy chosen; (c) time between hospital admission to spoke centres and cath-lab access; and (d) outcomes in terms of all-cause death of patients ≥80 years old with NSTE-ACS admitted to spoke hospitals.

3. Statistical Analysis

Continuous variables were expressed as mean ± standard deviation (SD) or mean and interquartile range (IQR) and were compared by the unpaired t-test. Categorical variables were expressed as counts and percentages and the comparison was performed by the chi-square test.

Kaplan–Meier curves were constructed to show survival according to strategy chosen (invasive or conservative). Univariate and multivariable Cox proportional hazards models were used to assess the association between strategy and the risk of death; the risk was presented as hazard ratio (HR) and 95% confidence interval (CI).

The level of statistical significance was set at 5% ($p < 0.05$) and all statistical analyses were carried out using SPSS (version 15 for Windows).

4. Results

4.1. Demographic and Clinical Characteristics of the Study Population

Table 1 shows the main baseline characteristics of the study population.

Table 1. Demographic and clinical characteristics of the study population.

Table	Invasive Strategy, $n = 105$ (58%)	Conservative Strategy $n = 76$ (42%)	Total $n = 181$	p Value
Age, years	84 ± 3	88 ± 5	86 ± 4	<0.001
Male sex, n (%)	51 (49%)	43 (57%)	94 (52%)	0.28
Weight, kg	72 ± 12	63 ± 13	70 ± 12	0.005
BMI	26 ± 4	24 ± 4	26 ± 4	0.02
Smoke habit, n (%)	4 (4%)	2 (3%)	6 (3%)	0.1
Dyslipidaemia, n (%)	68 (65%)	23 (30%)	91 (50%)	<0.001
Diabetes, n (%)	25 (24%)	19 (25%)	44 (23%)	0.48
Hypertension, n (%)	79 (75%)	54 (71%)	133 (73%)	0.44
Known CAD, n (%)	38 (36%)	44 (56%)	82 (45%)	0.009
Clinical presentation: -Unstable angina, n (%) -NSTEMI, n (%)	25 (24%) 80 (76%)	11 (14%) 65 (86%)	36 (20%) 145 (80%)	0.12
Clinical presentation: -symptoms of LV dysfunction, n (%)	9 (9%)	37 (49%)	46 (25%)	<0.001
Serum creatinine, mg/dL	1.1 ± 0.5	1.5 ± 0.8	1.2 ± 0.6	<0.001
Chronic renal failure requiring dialysis	1 (1%)	3 (4%)	4 (2%)	<0.001
EF, %	50 ± 11	44 ± 13	47 ± 12	0.002
GRACE score	170 ± 26	186 ± 33	176 ± 29	0.001
Severe COPD, n (%)	8 (8%)	11 (14%)	19 (11%)	0.13
PAD, n (%)	22 (21%)	37 (49%)	59 (32%)	<0.001
Atrial fibrillation/flutter, n (%)	12 (11%)	18 (47%)	30 (17%)	0.004
Length of hospital stay, days	6.0 ± 3.5	6.5 ± 3.7	6.5 ± 3.6	0.37

Table legend: BMI (body mass index); CAD (coronary artery disease); NSTEMI (non-ST elevation myocardial infarction); LV (left ventricle); EF (ejection fraction); COPD (chronic obstructive pulmonary disease); PAD (peripheral-artery disease).

From January 2013 to December 2017, 639 consecutive patients were admitted to spoke centres with a diagnosis of NSTEACS. Of these, 181 (28%) were ≥80 years old and represented the study cohort. The median age of the study population was 84 (IQR 82–89) years old. The most frequent clinical presentation was non-ST elevation myocardial infarction in 145 patients (80%); the remainder of the patients presented with unstable angina. Forty-six patients (25%) showed clinical signs of left-ventricular dysfunction and one hundred fifty-one patients (83%) were in sinus rhythm at admission. The proportion of cardiovascular risk factors in the study population comprised: smoke habit in 39%, dyslipidaemia in 50%, diabetes in 23%, arterial hypertension in 73% and known previous CAD in 45%. Major comorbidities in the study population showed the presence of severe chronic kidney disease requiring dialyses in 2%, severe chronic obstructive pulmonary disease (COPD) in 11% and peripheral-artery disease (PAD) in 32%.

Left-ventricle ejection fraction (LVEF) was 47 ± 12%. Serum creatinine was 1.2 ± 0.6 mg/dL. The calculated GRACE score was 176 ± 29.

The study cohort was divided into two groups according to management: invasive strategy in 105 (58%) while the remainder were managed with the conservative strategy. Figure 2.

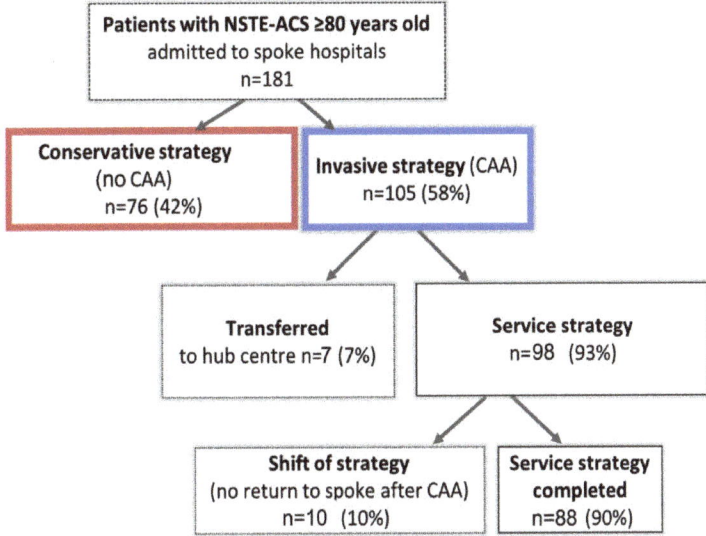

Figure 2. Study population according to the chosen management of NSTE-ACS (non-ST-elevation acute coronary syndrome); CAA (coronary artery angiography).

4.2. Management Strategy and Time between Spoke Admission and Access to the Cath-Lab

When the invasive strategy was chosen, 98 patients (93%) were initially managed with a service strategy, whereas the rest of the patients (7%) were transferred from the spoke hospital to the hub centre and completed their hospital stay without returning to the spoke centre for clinical or organizational reasons. Of the patients initially managed with the service strategy, a shift of strategy was necessary after the invasive procedure for 10 (10%) and the patients remained in the hub centre until discharged home with no return to the spoke hospital, mainly for clinical reasons; the rest of patients were sent back to the spoke hospitals, with no adverse events observed during the transfer. Figure 2. The median time for access to the cath-lab was 50 h (IQR 25–87), with 73 patients (70%) reaching the invasive procedure <72 h from hospital admission and 23 patients (22%) reaching the invasive procedure in <24 h. The mean hospital-stay length was 6 ± 3 days (median value 5 days; IR 4–8).

4.3. Conservative vs. Invasive Strategy

In the elderly, the conservative strategy was chosen in 76 patients (42%). Conservative strategy was found to be associated with older age, smallest body mass index, higher prevalence of known CAD, clinical presentation with symptoms of LV dysfunction, lower

EF, worse renal failure, higher GRACE score, higher prevalence of PAD and atrial fibrillation (all $p < 0.03$). The choice of strategy did not affect the length of hospital stay ($p = 0.37$).

At 1-year follow-up, the overall survival was significantly higher in patients treated with the invasive strategy compared to patients managed conservatively (94% ± 2 vs. 54% ± 6, $p < 0.001$; HR: 10.4 [4.7–27.5] $p < 0.001$), even after adjustment for age, serum creatinine, known previous CAD and EF (adjusted HR: 2.0 [1.0–4.0]; $p < 0.001$). Figure 3.

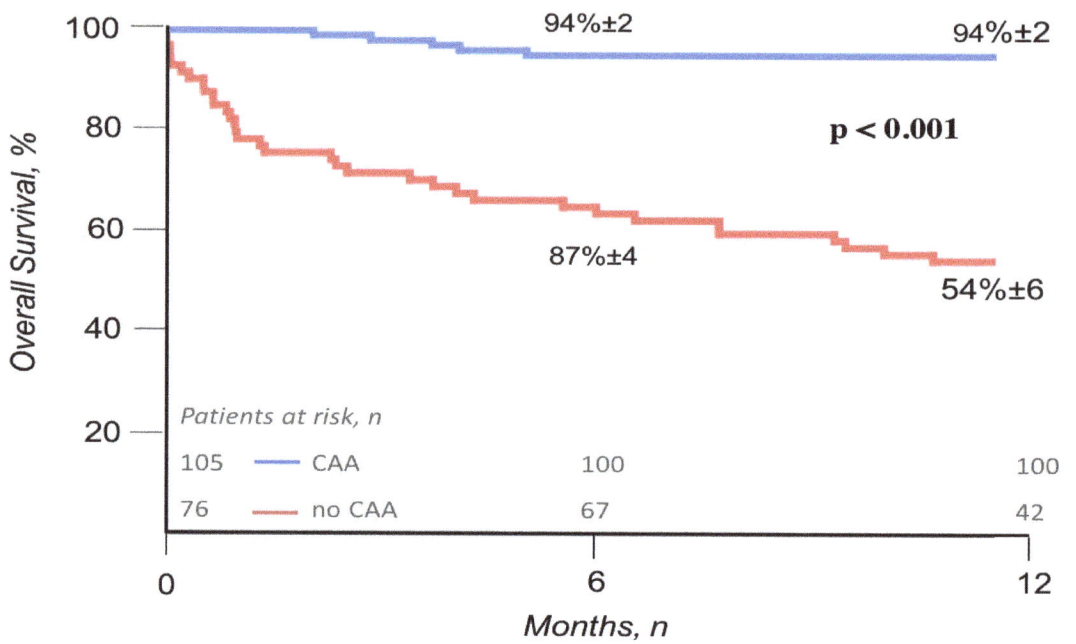

Figure 3. Overall 1-year survival after NSTEACS in patients treated with invasive strategy (blue line) and conservative strategy (red line). Figure legend: CAA (coronary artery angiography).

4.4. Discussion

Our observational–retrospective study showed that, in our provincial cardiology network, the treatment of elderly people admitted to spoke hospitals with NSTEACS was characterised as follows: (a) they were managed invasively in more than half of cases; (b) the invasive strategy conferred a 1-year survival benefit compared to the conservative strategy; (c) the service strategy represented an effective and safe strategy to ensure access to the cath-lab in a timely fashion (<72 h) in the vast majority of elderly patients (70%).

The elderly (aged 80 or older) characterize a growing proportion of the patients presenting with NSTEMI, but these patients are much less likely to receive invasive management.

Data from the National Inpatient Sample database in the USA indicated that 78% of patients with NSTEMI aged 60 years or younger underwent coronary angiography, compared with 38% of patients aged 81 years or older [3]. In the SENIOR-NSTEMI study, 49% of eligible patients from five tertiary centres in UK underwent invasive management during their index admission [16].

In our study, 58% of patients older than 80 years underwent coronary angiography.

These differences in treatment strategy between elderly and younger patients likely reflect insufficient data to guide clinical practice. In fact, recommendations are based on large randomized trials with a mean age of participants of ~65 years and, since few patients in their 80s were enrolled, the survival benefit cannot be assumed to translate to these patients [2]. Treatment decisions are habitually made in the elderly within the clinical context of a delicate evaluation of risks and benefits according to comorbidities and estimated life expectancy. Particularly, clinicians fear bleeding risk and the risk of acute kidney injury in decision making regarding the decision around invasive management in the elderly. In a sub-study of the Randomized ANTARCTIC Trial, clinically relevant bleeding events were observed in 20% of elderly patients undergoing percutaneous coronary angiography for an ACS and were strongly associated with further stroke occurrence [17]. Rather than the antiplatelet therapy, comorbidities and an age > 85 years predicted bleeding outcomes in this elderly population [17]. Moreover, the elderly are at incremented risk of acute kidney injury due to several aging-related factors, such as nephrosclerosis, inflammation and vascular changes [18,19]. Between older adults undergoing cardiac catheterization for acute myocardial infarction in the SILVER-AMI study, nearly one in five experienced acute kidney injury [20]. Development of acute kidney injury after coronary angiography is associated with worse outcomes [21], including increased length of stay, excess costs, progression to end-stage renal disease and mortality, with predictors that largely mirrored those described in previous studies of younger patients [20].

In our study, patients managed with the conservative strategy were associated with: older age; smallest body mass index; higher prevalence of known CAD; known complex coronary lesions in most cases being previously judged to not be treatable by percutaneous coronary intervention; clinical presentation with symptoms of LV dysfunction; lower EF; worse renal failure; higher GRACE score; higher prevalence of PAD (possibly complicating in the choice of arterial accesses) and atrial fibrillation (raising concerns about bleeding risk on triple-anticoagulant therapy); and having worse prognosis at 1-year follow-up.

Despite international guidelines continuing to recommend that older patients be considered for invasive management and revascularization (class IIa recommendation) [1,22,23], these recommendations are based on small randomised trials (Italian Elderly ACS [24] (invasive group n = 154 and non-invasive group n = 159) and the After Eighty trial [15] (invasive group n = 229 and non-invasive group n = 228)) and small post hoc subgroup analyses of randomised trials (TACTICS-TIMI 18 [25] and FIR [26]) that have evaluated invasive management versus non-invasive management for NSTEMI in patients aged 75–80 years or older. Moreover, a meta-analysis pooling of these data did not find evidence that invasive management reduced mortality at long-term follow-up [27]. In the SENIOR-NSTEMI study, the adjusted cumulative 5-year mortality was 36% in the invasive management group vs. 55% in the non-invasive management group (adjusted hazard ratio 0.68, 95% CI 0.55–0.84). Therefore, the survival advantage of invasive compared with non-invasive management appeared to extend to patients with NSTEMI who are aged 80 years or older [16]. The ongoing SENIOR-RITA trial aims to randomly assign 1668 patients with NSTEMI aged 75 years or older to receive invasive or non-invasive management. The primary outcome is a composite of cardiovascular death and non-fatal myocardial infarction, and the planned follow-up is 5 years; the study is estimated to be completed in 2024 [28].

In absence of convincing evidence from randomised trials, a few studies from registries [29–31] have indicated a benefit from invasive therapy, but the findings might have been amplified by immortal time bias [32] and the inclusion of very frail patients who were certain to be managed non-invasively [33]. Studies of temporal trends from registry data in the US and Europe suggest that, over the past two decades, the progressive switch from a non-invasive to a more invasive approach in older patients with NSTEMI has been accompanied by declining mortality [3,34,35].

Moreover, the admission to a tertiary (hub) centre with a cath-lab facility or to a spoke centre without a cath-lab facility might make a difference in treatment choice, especially for the elderly.

Several studies have described a distinct scenario in spoke centres with no cath-lab facilities compared to tertiary centres [6–8,36]. In the Italian BLITZ 2 registry, just 36% of patients admitted to spoke hospitals were managed with an invasive strategy [36]. The restricted number of available beds in hub centres with a cath-lab has been indicated as potential cause of this discrepancy between centres. In addition, in NSTEACS patients, the correct timing for coronary angiography plays a central role [22,23]. Guidelines suggested an invasive strategy during the same hospital stay and, if possible, within 72 h from admission [1,23]; this timeframe has recently been further lowered to <24 h [22].

While the number of patients with NSTE-ACS needing early coronary angiography is expected to grow, the number of available beds in hub hospitals may not increase accordingly.

Consequently, a possible solution to these discrepancies is to establish fast-track lines for patients in need of coronary angiography ± PCI treatments. Therefore, a healthcare model based on service strategy (patients' same-day transfer back to the spoke-referring hospital after invasive procedure) has been judged to solve the bed-shortage at hub centres. After coronary angiography and ad hoc PCI, previous studies showed that patients with NSTEACS might be safely re-transferred to the spoke hospital after a few hours of observation [11,13,14,37]. Our previous study on ~1000 patients with NSTEACS managed with a service strategy confirmed that the adoption of this strategy in our province network is safe and allowed access to coronary angiography in a timely fashion [38]. Traditionally, in our regional network, the percentage of patients with NSTEACS referred for coronary angiography from spoke to hub centres was relatively high (73%, 95% CI 71.5–74.5%) and a service strategy was significantly associated with early access to the cath-lab and with a consequent reduction in the hospital stay length [37]. The present study confirms the available evidence even in the subgroup of patients aged older than 80 years.

5. Limits of the Study

Limitations should be taken into account in the interpretation of the present data.

The main limitations of our study relate to its observational–retrospective nature and its small sample size. In addition, we did not have information on whether there was a differential receipt of evidence-based cardiac care in the non-invasive management group, including prescription of medications.

Moreover, we acknowledge that the elderly patients managed with the conservative strategy may have several confounding factors which might be associated with the worst outcomes (cancer, severe frailty, high bleeding risk, etc.) compared to patients managed with the invasive strategy. These factors have not been fully adjusted with multivariate analysis.

However, thus far, there are no data in the literature on management and outcomes on elderly NSTEACS patients admitted to spoke hospitals. Therefore, we believe our study may be of interest despite its limitations.

6. Conclusions

This study provides supporting evidence for an invasive approach for treatment of elderly people with NSTEACS.

However, this group of patients is still undertreated, especially when admitted to spoke centres with no cath-lab facilities. A well-organised network with a service strategy for early access to coronary angiography is safe and could guarantee access to cath-labs, even for patients older than 80 years with NSTEACS who have been admitted to the spoke hospitals.

Author Contributions: Conceptualization, F.M. (Francesca Mantovani), E.G. and V.G.; Data curation, F.M. (Francesca Mantovani), E.G., M.C., G.T., S.M.D., G.P. and V.G.; Formal analysis, F.M. (Francesca Mantovani); Methodology, F.M. (Francesca Mantovani), G.C. and V.G.; Supervision, A.N.; Validation, G.C. and V.G.; Writing—original draft, F.M. (Francesca Mantovani), G.C., F.M. (Francesco Manca), M.C. and V.G.; Writing—review & editing, F.M. (Francesca Mantovani), G.C., E.G., F.M. (Francesco Manca), M.C., G.T., S.M.D., G.P., V.G and A.N. All authors have read and agreed to the published version of the manuscript.

Funding: This research received no external funding.

Institutional Review Board Statement: The study was conducted in accordance with the Declaration of Helsinki, and approved by the Institutional Review Board of Azienda USL-IRCCS di Reggio-Emilia, protocol number 2022/71621 date 1 June 2022.

Informed Consent Statement: Not applicable.

Data Availability Statement: Not applicable.

Acknowledgments: We express our thanks to data managers Rosa Maria De Mola and Linda Valli for their substantial and competent work in contributing to this study.

Conflicts of Interest: The authors declare that there are no conflict of interest.

References

1. Roffi, M.; Patrono, C.; Collet, J.P.; Mueller, C.; Valgimigli, M.; Andreotti, F.; Bax, J.J.; Borger, M.A.; Brotons, C.; Chew, D.P.; et al. 2015 ESC Guidelines for the management of acute coronary syndromes in patients presenting without persistent ST-segment elevation: Task Force for the Management of Acute Coronary Syndromes in Patients Presenting without Persistent ST-Segment Elevation of the European Society of Cardiology (ESC). *Eur. Heart J.* **2016**, *37*, 267–315. [CrossRef]
2. Sinclair, H.; Kunadian, V. Coronary revascularisation in older patients with non-ST elevation acute coronary syndromes. *Heart* **2016**, *102*, 416–424. [CrossRef]
3. Rashid, M.; Fischman, D.L.; Gulati, M.; Tamman, K.; Potts, J.; Kwok, C.S.; Ensor, J.; Shoaib, A.; Mansour, H.; Zaman, A.; et al. Temporal trends and inequalities in coronary angiography utilization in the management of non-ST-Elevation acute coronary syndromes in the U.S. *Sci. Rep.* **2019**, *9*, 240. [CrossRef]
4. Toleva, O.; Westerhout, C.M.; Senaratne, M.P.J.; Bode, C.; Lindroos, M.; Sulimov, V.A.; Montalescot, G.; Newby, L.K.; Giugliano, R.P.; Van de Werf, F.; et al. Practice patterns and clinical outcomes among non-ST-segment elevation acute coronary syndrome (NSTE-ACS) patients presenting to primary and tertiary hospitals: Insights from the EARLY glycoprotein IIb/IIIa inhibition in NSTE-ACS (EARLY-ACS) trial. *Catheter. Cardiovasc. Interv.* **2014**, *84*, 934–942. [CrossRef]
5. Mehta, R.H.; Chen, A.Y.; Ohman, E.M.; Gibler, W.B.; Peterson, E.D.; Roe, M.T.; Investigators, C.N.Q.I.I. Influence of transfer-in rates on quality of care and outcomes at receiving hospitals in patients with non-ST-segment elevation myocardial infarction. *Am. Heart J* **2010**, *160*, 405–411. [CrossRef]
6. Fox, K.A.; Goodman, S.G.; Anderson, F.A., Jr.; Granger, C.B.; Moscucci, M.; Flather, M.D.; Spencer, F.; Budaj, A.; Dabbous, O.H.; Gore, J.M.; et al. From guidelines to clinical practice: The impact of hospital and geographical characteristics on temporal trends in the management of acute coronary syndromes. The Global Registry of Acute Coronary Events (GRACE). *Eur. Heart J.* **2003**, *24*, 1414–1424. [CrossRef]
7. Di Chiara, A.; Chiarella, F.; Savonitto, S.; Lucci, D.; Bolognese, L.; De Servi, S.; Greco, C.; Boccanelli, A.; Zonzin, P.; Coccolini, S.; et al. Epidemiology of acute myocardial infarction in the Italian CCU network: The BLITZ study. *Eur. Heart J.* **2003**, *24*, 1616–1629. [CrossRef]
8. Vavalle, J.P.; Lopes, R.D.; Chen, A.Y.; Newby, L.K.; Wang, T.Y.; Shah, B.R.; Ho, P.M.; Wiviott, S.D.; Peterson, E.D.; Roe, M.T.; et al. Hospital length of stay in patients with non-ST-segment elevation myocardial infarction. *Am. J. Med.* **2012**, *125*, 1085–1094. [CrossRef]
9. Abdelaal, E.; Rao, S.V.; Gilchrist, I.C.; Bernat, I.; Shroff, A.; Caputo, R.; Costerousse, O.; Pancholy, S.B.; Bertrand, O.F. Same-Day Discharge Compared with Overnight Hospitalization after Uncomplicated Percutaneous Coronary Intervention a Systematic Review and Meta-Analysis. *JACC Cardiovasc. Interv.* **2013**, *6*, 99–112. [CrossRef]
10. Agarwal, S.; Thakkar, B.; Skelding, K.A.; Blankenship, J.C. Trends and Outcomes after Same-Day Discharge after Percutaneous Coronary Interventions. *Circ. Cardiovasc. Qual. Outcomes* **2017**, *10*, e003936. [CrossRef]
11. Andersen, J.G.; Kløw, N.-E.; Johansen, O. Safe and feasible immediate retransfer of patients to the referring hospital after acute coronary angiography and percutaneous coronary angioplasty for patients with acute coronary syndrome. *Eur. Heart J. Acute Cardiovasc. Care* **2013**, *2*, 256–261. [CrossRef]
12. Brayton, K.M.; Patel, V.G.; Stave, C.; de Lemos, J.A.; Kumbhani, D.J. Same-day discharge after percutaneous coronary intervention: A meta-analysis. *J. Am. Coll. Cardiol.* **2013**, *62*, 275–285. [CrossRef] [PubMed]
13. Do, D.H.; Dalery, K.; Gervais, A.; Harvey, J.; Lepage, S.; Maltais, A.; Nguyen, M. Same-day transfer of patients with unstable angina and non-ST segment elevation myocardial infarction back to their referring hospital after angioplasty. *Can. J. Cardiol.* **2006**, *22*, 405–409. [CrossRef]
14. Vendrametto, F.; Oberhollenzer, R.; Pitscheider, W. Percutaneous coronary intervention and immediate re-transfer to the referring hospital for patients with acute coronary syndrome. A single-center experience. *G. Ital. Di Cardiol.* **2006**, *7*, 281–286.
15. Tegn, N.; Abdelnoor, M.; Aaberge, L.; Endresen, K.; Smith, P.; Aakhus, S.; Gjertsen, E.; Dahl-Hofseth, O.; Ranhoff, A.H.; Gullestad, L.; et al. Invasive versus conservative strategy in patients aged 80 years or older with non-ST-elevation myocardial infarction or unstable angina pectoris (After Eighty study): An open-label randomised controlled trial. *Lancet* **2016**, *387*, 1057–1065. [CrossRef]
16. Kaura, A.; Sterne, J.A.C.; Trickey, A.; Abbott, S.; Mulla, A.; Glampson, B.; Panoulas, V.; Davies, J.; Woods, K.; Omigie, J.; et al. Invasive versus non-invasive management of older patients with non-ST elevation myocardial infarction (SENIOR-NSTEMI): A cohort study based on routine clinical data. *Lancet* **2020**, *396*, 623–634. [CrossRef]
17. Lattuca, B.; Cayla, G.; Silvain, J.; Cuisset, T.; Leclercq, F.; Manzo-Silberman, S.; Saint-Etienne, C.; Delarche, N.; El Mahmoud, R.; Carrie, D.; et al. Bleeding in the Elderly: Risk Factors and Impact on Clinical Outcomes after an Acute Coronary Syndrome, a Sub-study of the Randomized ANTARCTIC Trial. *Am. J. Cardiovasc. Drugs* **2021**, *21*, 681–691. [CrossRef]

18. Coca, S.G. Acute kidney injury in elderly persons. *Am. J. Kidney Dis.* **2010**, *56*, 122–131. [CrossRef]
19. Anderson, S.; Eldadah, B.; Halter, J.B.; Hazzard, W.R.; Himmelfarb, J.; Horne, F.M.; Kimmel, P.L.; Molitoris, B.A.; Murthy, M.; O'Hare, A.M.; et al. Acute kidney injury in older adults. *J. Am. Soc. Nephrol.* **2011**, *22*, 28–38. [CrossRef]
20. Dodson, J.A.; Hajduk, A.; Curtis, J.; Geda, M.; Krumholz, H.M.; Song, X.; Tsang, S.; Blaum, C.; Miller, P.; Parikh, C.R.; et al. Acute Kidney Injury Among Older Patients Undergoing Coronary Angiography for Acute Myocardial Infarction: The SILVER-AMI Study. *Am. J. Med.* **2019**, *132*, e817–e826. [CrossRef]
21. Tsai, T.T.; Patel, U.D.; Chang, T.I.; Kennedy, K.F.; Masoudi, F.A.; Matheny, M.E.; Kosiborod, M.; Amin, A.P.; Messenger, J.C.; Rumsfeld, J.S.; et al. Contemporary incidence, predictors, and outcomes of acute kidney injury in patients undergoing percutaneous coronary interventions: Insights from the NCDR Cath-PCI registry. *JACC Cardiovasc. Interv.* **2014**, *7*, 1–9. [CrossRef] [PubMed]
22. Collet, J.P.; Thiele, H.; Barbato, E.; Barthelemy, O.; Bauersachs, J.; Bhatt, D.L.; Dendale, P.; Dorobantu, M.; Edvardsen, T.; Folliguet, T.; et al. 2020 ESC Guidelines for the management of acute coronary syndromes in patients presenting without persistent ST-segment elevation. *Eur. Heart J.* **2021**, *42*, 1289–1367. [CrossRef]
23. Amsterdam, E.A.; Wenger, N.K.; Brindis, R.G.; Casey, D.E., Jr.; Ganiats, T.G.; Holmes, D.R., Jr.; Jaffe, A.S.; Jneid, H.; Kelly, R.F.; Kontos, M.C.; et al. 2014 AHA/ACC Guideline for the Management of Patients with Non-ST-Elevation Acute Coronary Syndromes: A report of the American College of Cardiology/American Heart Association Task Force on Practice Guidelines. *J. Am. Coll. Cardiol.* **2014**, *64*, e139–e228. [CrossRef] [PubMed]
24. Savonitto, S.; Cavallini, C.; Petronio, A.S.; Murena, E.; Antonicelli, R.; Sacco, A.; Steffenino, G.; Bonechi, F.; Mossuti, E.; Manari, A.; et al. Early aggressive versus initially conservative treatment in elderly patients with non-ST-segment elevation acute coronary syndrome: A randomized controlled trial. *JACC Cardiovasc. Interv.* **2012**, *5*, 906–916. [CrossRef] [PubMed]
25. Bach, R.G.; Cannon, C.P.; Weintraub, W.S.; DiBattiste, P.M.; Demopoulos, L.A.; Anderson, H.V.; DeLucca, P.T.; Mahoney, E.M.; Murphy, S.A.; Braunwald, E. The effect of routine, early invasive management on outcome for elderly patients with non-ST-segment elevation acute coronary syndromes. *Ann. Intern. Med.* **2004**, *141*, 186–195. [CrossRef] [PubMed]
26. Damman, P.; Clayton, T.; Wallentin, L.; Lagerqvist, B.; Fox, K.A.; Hirsch, A.; Windhausen, F.; Swahn, E.; Pocock, S.J.; Tijssen, J.G.; et al. Effects of age on long-term outcomes after a routine invasive or selective invasive strategy in patients presenting with non-ST segment elevation acute coronary syndromes: A collaborative analysis of individual data from the FRISC II-ICTUS-RITA-3 (FIR) trials. *Heart* **2012**, *98*, 207–213. [CrossRef]
27. Gnanenthiran, S.R.; Kritharides, L.; D'Souza, M.; Lowe, H.C.; Brieger, D.B. Revascularisation compared with initial medical therapy for non-ST-elevation acute coronary syndromes in the elderly: A meta-analysis. *Heart* **2017**, *103*, 1962–1969. [CrossRef] [PubMed]
28. ClinicalTrial.org The British Heart Foundation SENIOR-RITA. Trial (SENIOR-RITA). Available online: https://clinicaltrials.gov/ct2/show/NCT03052036 (accessed on 8 June 2022).
29. Gierlotka, M.; Gasior, M.; Tajstra, M.; Hawranek, M.; Osadnik, T.; Wilczek, K.; Kalarus, Z.; Lekston, A.; Zembala, M.; Polonski, L. Outcomes of invasive treatment in very elderly Polish patients with non-ST-segment-elevation myocardial infarction from 2003–2009 (from the PL-ACS registry). *Cardiol. J.* **2013**, *20*, 34–43. [CrossRef] [PubMed]
30. Bauer, T.; Koeth, O.; Junger, C.; Heer, T.; Wienbergen, H.; Gitt, A.; Zahn, R.; Senges, J.; Zeymer, U.; Acute Coronary Syndromes Registry, I. Effect of an invasive strategy on in-hospital outcome in elderly patients with non-ST-elevation myocardial infarction. *Eur. Heart J.* **2007**, *28*, 2873–2878. [CrossRef]
31. Devlin, G.; Gore, J.M.; Elliott, J.; Wijesinghe, N.; Eagle, K.A.; Avezum, A.; Huang, W.; Brieger, D.; Investigators, G. Management and 6-month outcomes in elderly and very elderly patients with high-risk non-ST-elevation acute coronary syndromes: The Global Registry of Acute Coronary Events. *Eur. Heart J.* **2008**, *29*, 1275–1282. [CrossRef] [PubMed]
32. Suissa, S. Immortal time bias in pharmaco-epidemiology. *Am. J. Epidemiol.* **2008**, *167*, 492–499. [CrossRef]
33. Giobbie-Hurder, A.; Gelber, R.D.; Regan, M.M. Challenges of guarantee-time bias. *J. Clin. Oncol.* **2013**, *31*, 2963–2969. [CrossRef]
34. Elbadawi, A.; Elgendy, I.Y.; Ha, L.D.; Mahmoud, K.; Lenka, J.; Olorunfemi, O.; Reyes, A.; Ogunbayo, G.O.; Saad, M.; Abbott, J.D. National Trends and Outcomes of Percutaneous Coronary Intervention in Patients >/=70 Years of Age with Acute Coronary Syndrome (from the National Inpatient Sample Database). *Am. J. Cardiol.* **2019**, *123*, 25–32. [CrossRef] [PubMed]
35. Schoenenberger, A.W.; Radovanovic, D.; Windecker, S.; Iglesias, J.F.; Pedrazzini, G.; Stuck, A.E.; Erne, P.; Investigators, A.P. Temporal trends in the treatment and outcomes of elderly patients with acute coronary syndrome. *Eur. Heart J.* **2016**, *37*, 1304–1311. [CrossRef] [PubMed]
36. Di Chiara, A.; Fresco, C.; Savonitto, S.; Greco, C.; Lucci, D.; Gonzini, L.; Mafrici, A.; Ottani, F.; Bolognese, L.; De Servi, S.; et al. Epidemiology of non-ST elevation acute coronary syndromes in the Italian cardiology network: The BLITZ-2 study. *Eur. Heart J.* **2006**, *27*, 393–405. [CrossRef] [PubMed]
37. Campo, G.; Menozzi, M.; Guastaroba, P.; Vignali, L.; Belotti, L.M.; Casella, G.; Berti, E.; Solinas, E.; Guiducci, V.; Biscaglia, S.; et al. Same-day transfer for the invasive strategy of patients with non-ST-segment elevation acute coronary syndrome admitted to spoke hospitals: Data from the Emilia-Romagna Regional Network. *Eur. Heart J. Acute Cardiovasc. Care* **2016**, *5*, 428–434. [CrossRef] [PubMed]
38. Mantovani, F.; Guiducci, V.; Colaiori, I.; Pignatelli, G.; Manca, F.; Guerri, E.; Calzolari, M.; Catellani, E.; Reverzani, A.; Navazio, A. Service strategy for the early referral to catheterization laboratory of patients admitted with non-ST-elevation acute coronary syndromes in spoke hospitals: 5-year results of the Reggio Emilia province network. *G Ital. Cardiol.* **2020**, *21*, 807–815. [CrossRef]

MDPI
St. Alban-Anlage 66
4052 Basel
Switzerland
www.mdpi.com

Journal of Clinical Medicine Editorial Office
E-mail: jcm@mdpi.com
www.mdpi.com/journal/jcm

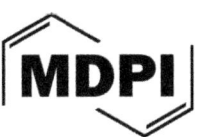

Disclaimer/Publisher's Note: The statements, opinions and data contained in all publications are solely those of the individual author(s) and contributor(s) and not of MDPI and/or the editor(s). MDPI and/or the editor(s) disclaim responsibility for any injury to people or property resulting from any ideas, methods, instructions or products referred to in the content.

www.ingramcontent.com/pod-product-compliance
Lightning Source LLC
LaVergne TN
LVHW070612100526
838202LV00012B/625